Mindfulness in Behavioral Health

Series Editor
Nirbhay N. Singh
Medical College of Georgia
Georgia Regents University
Augusta, Georgia, USA

More information about this series at http://www.springer.com/series/8678

Akihiko Masuda · William T. O'Donohue
Editors

Handbook of Zen, Mindfulness, and Behavioral Health

Springer

Editors
Akihiko Masuda
Department of Psychology
University of Hawaii at Manoa
Honolulu, HI
USA

William T. O'Donohue
Department of Psychology
University of Nevada
Reno, NV
USA

ISSN 2195-9579 ISSN 2195-9587 (electronic)
Mindfulness in Behavioral Health
ISBN 978-3-319-54593-6 ISBN 978-3-319-54595-0 (eBook)
DOI 10.1007/978-3-319-54595-0

Library of Congress Control Number: 2017933065

Printed on acid-free paper

This Springer imprint is published by Springer Nature
The registered company is Springer International Publishing AG
The registered company address is: Gewerbestrasse 11, 6330 Cham, Switzerland

This book is dedicated to our wives, Migdalia and Jane

Contents

Editors and Contributors

About the Editors

Akihiko Masuda Ph.D. is an assistant professor of clinical psychology at University of Hawaii at Manoa. He was on the Georgia State University faculty between 2007 and 2016 (assistant professor 2007–2013; associate professor with tenure 2013–2016). Dr. Masuda was born and raised in Nagano, Japan, and moved to the USA for his psychology career. His primary areas of interest include acceptance- and mindfulness-based behavioral therapies, diversity, and Zen Buddhism. He is the author of more than 80 peer-reviewed papers and chapters. He is the editor of the book, *Mindfulness and Acceptance in Multicultural Competency* (New Harbinger, 2014).

William T. O'Donohue Ph.D. is a professor of clinical psychology at the University of Nevada, Reno. He has published research on evidence-based practice in behavioral health, focusing on cognitive behavior therapy. Dr. O'Donohue has published more than 80 books and 300 journal articles and chapters. He served as a principle investigator on a number of grants that have focused on the transfer of technology to practice, including a grant investigating transferring integrated care to a variety of medical settings in Hawaii.

Contributors

Josh Bartok Greater Boston Zen Center, Boundless Way Zen, Cambridge, USA

Shoryu Bradley Gyobutsuji Zen Monastery, Kingston, USA

Kenneth Po-Lun Fung University of Toronto, Toronto, Canada

Gordon M. Greene Spring Green Dojo, Spring Green, WI, USADepartment of Family Medicine, University of Wisconsin School of Medicine and Public Health, Madison, WI, USAMeriter Hospital, Madison, WI, USA, Spring Green, WI, USA

Holly Hazlett-Stevens University of Nevada, Reno, USA

Sungjin Im University of Nevada, Reno, USA

Kiyozumi Seijun Ishii Komazawa University, Tokyo, Japan

Shudo Ishii Komazawa University, Tokyo, Japan

Kenneth P. Kushner Department of Family Medicine and Community Health, University of Wisconsin, Madison, Wi, USA

Peiwei Li Springfield College, Springfield, USA

Marsha Linehan University of Washington, Seattle, USA

Akihiko Masuda University of Hawaii, Honolulu, HI, USA

Daiko Matsuyama Taizoin Zen Buddhist Temple, Kyoto, Japan

Takashi Ogawa Komazawa University, Tokyo, Japan

Hidetaka Shuryu Okajima Aichigakuin University, Aichi, Japan

Shohaku Okumura Sanshin Zen Community, Bloomington, USA

William T. O'Donohue University of Nevada, Reno, NV, USA

Daniel Rodriguez Ramirez University of California Santa Cruz, Santa Cruz, USA

Lizabeth Roemer University of Massachusetts Boston, Boston, USA

Kayla Sargent University of Hawaii, Honolulu, HI, USA

Mike K. Sayama Chozen-ji, International Zen Dojo, Honolulu, HI, USA

Jeffrey Schneider San Francisco Zen Center, California, USA

Kenshu Sugawara Aichi Gakuin University, Aichi, Japan

Tairyu Tsunoda Komazawa University, Setagaya, Tokyo, Japan

Josephine Pui-Hing Wong Ryerson University, Toronto, Canada

Norma Wong Institute of Zen Studies, Honululu, HI, USA

Rosan Yoshida Missouri Zen Center, Webster Groves, MO, USA

Introduction: Zen, Mindfulness, and Behavioral Health

William T. O'Donohue, Akihiko Masuda and Kayla Sargent

Keywords
Zen · Buddhism · Behavioral health · Cognitive behavioral therapy (CBT) · Mindfulness

The rationale for this book is fourfold. First, in recent decades, there has been increased interest in the implication of mindfulness for improving a wide variety of problems in behavioral health (Brown et al. 2007; Hayes et al. 2004; Hofmann et al. 2010). We think this generally is an adaptive trend as there is significant research showing a wide variety of beneficial effects of mindfulness techniques both alone and as an adjunctive treatment with conventional cognitive behavioral techniques (Hazlett-Stevens, this volume). This is particularly important as these interventions seem to be helpful for problems that are epidemic in behavioral health, such as depression, anxiety, and chronic pain. Buddhism is the ultimate source for the construct of mindfulness (Kabat-Zinn 2003; Robins 2002; Van Gordon et al. 2015a, b); thus, part of the rationale of this book is that it might be useful to explore this root source in more detail with the focus on Zen Buddhism. This exploration might result in a deeper understanding of mindfulness as it can reveal its context and the system of interrelated beliefs that help define it.

Second, we pose the question of whether it is optimal to pluck a technique or construct such as mindfulness or acceptance from one interrelated body of beliefs and apply them within another. What, if anything, is lost when this is done? Is there any sort of bastardization of the mindfulness technique when it is stripped of its historical and conceptual context in Buddhism? We see this as a serious intellectual and applied dilemma (Li et al., this volume), and this book attempts to explore this issue.

Third, we argue that in the first part of the twenty-first century, there is a paucity of meaningful theory underlying our applied systems; further, we posit that finding and understanding meaning may be an important element not only in decreasing behavioral health problems but also in flourishing and improving our well-being

W.T. O'Donohue (✉)
University of Nevada, Reno, NV, USA
e-mail: wto@unr.edu

A. Masuda · K. Sargent
University of Hawaii at Manoa, Honolulu, USA
e-mail: amasuda4@hawaii.edu

K. Sargent
e-mail: kaylansargent@gmail.com

A. Masuda and W.T. O'Donohue (eds.), *Handbook of Zen, Mindfulness, and Behavioral Health*, Mindfulness in Behavioral Health, DOI 10.1007/978-3-319-54595-0_1

(Seligman 2011). Zen, a branch of Buddhism, might also be able to provide some content for creating meaning in positive psychology. Thus, in this text, there are chapters on a wide variety of subjects that look into broader life domains such as self, goals, desires, death, meaning, and relationships.

Fourth and finally, there has been some recent interest in Buddhism more broadly construed in an empirical wing of behavioral health, such as cognitive behavioral therapy (CBT; Gilbert 2010; Tirch et al. 2016). Buddhism and CBT share some foundational commonalities: Both assert that a key part of human suffering is due to problematic cognitive states. At the same time, it is fair to say that the specifics of the pathologies differ: Cognitive therapy is focused mostly on irrationality or a problematic attributional style, whereas Buddhism emphasizes desire, attachment to particular beliefs, and a lack of present moment awareness (i.e., mindfulness). It might also be fair to say that Buddhism is oriented toward deeper meta-cognitive processes that give rise to a myriad of individual automatic thoughts and irrational ideas rather than individual cognitions one by one.

Another key difference is that *rationality* itself is seen as part of the problem in some schools of Buddhism, such as Zen Buddhism (Ogawa, this volume), and in CBT, it clearly is seen as the desired end state—the solution. For example, Zen *koans* (公案; a paradoxical anecdote or riddle, used in Zen Buddhism practice) attempt to help students overcome and transcend rationality in order to attain the experience of enlightenment, one aim of Zen (see Matsuyama, this volume). In an important sense, Zen is simply not a discursive enterprise—even the content of a book can be seen as a distraction from the more important practice of just sitting or returning to the original wholeness. Psychotherapy, on the other hand, *is* a discursive enterprise.

Zen and Buddhism seem to advocate for an enlightened state, *satori*, in which a person experiences significant freedom and liberation from the problematic cognitive states that have plagued them historically (see Shudo Ishii; Masuda; Okumura; and Ogawa, this volume for Zen's account of enlightenment). On the other hand, CBT in general has not defined such an end state; in contrast, it seems to assert that life will continually be a challenge cognitively, advocating that our clients *can* get better, but there is always more to know, always more evidence to collect, and always a way to improve one's reasoning.

At a theoretical level, there are interesting similarities between the ideas of Buddhism and a deprivation analysis of behavior therapy (Timberlake 1995; Timberlake and Allison 1974). Buddhism, of course, suggests that happy feelings are fleeting and that desire will constantly rear its ugly head, causing the individual to be discontent. Deprivation theory suggests the same. The notion of a free operant suggests that there is an ideal condition in which a human can engage in their optimal level of access to their entire range of reinforcers (i.e., just enough chocolate, beach time, reading, skiing, time with each friend, and sleep): not too much and not too little. If there is either too much or too little, the event counts either as a punisher (if too much) or as a reinforcer (if too little). However, because this optimal, free operant rate is never actually experienced by any human; the result is similar to the Buddhist notion that humans are often in a state of desire and unhappiness and that excessive *or* inactive pursuit of desires can never bring happiness.

Buddhism is much more concerned with selfishness than CBT. It is fair to say that being selfless and having compassion toward others are not central concerns of CBT in Western cultures; rather, they are commonly set aside to be addressed by Western religious communities which often fail to interact with the scientific pursuit of evidence-based therapies. It is interesting to speculate whether or not these values would receive a hostile reaction by most cognitive behavior analysts.

Another difference is that Zen practice is generally seen as involving a large commitment, including disciplined practice usually over the span of a few decades (Dogen et al. 1995;

Uchiyama and Okumura 2014). CBT has a much simpler, less committed view: 16 one-hour sessions and reading a self-help book may be sufficient to rid oneself of problematic states or even to flourish (Seligman 2011).

Yet another difference is the individual's attitude toward the teacher. Although both share a basic view of the interaction between the student and the master as teaching and learning, in Zen Buddhism, the master is often an absolute authority to be respected and obeyed. In CBT, the therapist is seen as a teacher but one who is fallible, and a skeptical attitude toward all is promoted. This is certainly not a master–student relationship, wherein a clear social hierarchy exists.

Both Zen Buddhism and CBT focus on language; Zen Buddhism in particular focuses on the role of internal talk, discouraging dualistic views of how we understand words (e.g., Suzuki 1994, 1996). CBT shares in these concerns about language. A common interchange between a therapist and client may involve reframes like the following:

> Therapist: You are using the word 'catastrophe'—don't you think this is too strong—can you say instead you 'don't prefer' this?

However, it is also fair to say that perhaps to its detriment, CBT has not been sufficiently concerned with linguistics and a deeper understanding of problematic and non-problematic language. For example, CBT has been generally concerned with semantics (i.e., word meaning) instead of syntax (i.e., linguistic structure). O'Donohue and Ferguson (2016), for example, has suggested that the use of syntax (e.g., passive voice) in sex offenders when describing their abusive experiences may be significant. It would be interesting for both Zen and CBT to be explored from a more sophisticated linguistic perspective as Zen tends to have a larger sense of the ineffable—what transcends language—what cannot be said.

Another difference is in the style of communication. Zen sometimes engages in what might be taken as very indirect communication that involves mental gymnastics to understand. Alternatively, CBT engages in more direct communication. For example, Zen sometimes communicates using verses like the following:

> The bamboo shadows are sweeping the stairs
> But no dust is stirred
> The moonlight penetrates the depth of the pool
> But no trace is left in the water (Senzaki and Strout-McCandless 1953, p. 22).

Sometimes in Zen, language use is intentionally provocative and therefore quite different than CBT. For example, Zen sometimes uses direct contradictions to communicate; for example, there is talk of the "gateless gate" (Senzaki and Strout-McCandless 1953, p. 30). In one koan, a monk says, "The flag is moving." Another monk says, "The wind is moving." The former clings to the entity of the flag; the latter has a broader view but does not understand true emptiness. The Sixth Patriarch responds to them with, "The flag is not moving. The wind is not moving. The mind is moving." (pg. 38). Zen also communicates through poignant stories; CBT generally does not. For example:

> Nan-in, a master during the Mejia era, received a university professor who came to inquire about Zen.
> Nan-in served tea. He poured his visitor's cup full and then kept on pouring.
> The professor watched the overflow until he could no longer restrain himself. "It is overfull. No more will go in."
> "Like this cup," Nan-in replied, "You are full of your own opinions and speculations. How can I show you Zen unless you first empty your cup?" (pgs. 30–31)

Zen sees mediation as a key process; CBT does not. Cognitive behavior therapists, with the exception of the more recent mindfulness-based practitioners, seldom recommend meditation, and Zen masters do not encourage students to engage in rational scrutiny of their beliefs or learn skills to more effectively engage reinforcers.

Zen Buddhism, even when practiced in the USA, has deep connections with Japanese culture (Masuda, this volume), whereas CBT has deeper connections to American culture. Typically, when one studies Zen, one learns some Japanese phrases, may be guided toward Japanese martial arts, may be exposed to Japanese aesthetics, may study Japanese history, may eat

Japanese food, and may engage in other traditions like taking one's shoes off before entering a room.

Another difference is that Zen is more asocial—one practices meditation along side others and under a master, but it is a much more private, personal, and internal undertaking—mediation is a turning inward. Certainly, Zen suggests that one treats others with kindness, compassion, and honesty, but Zen is a looking inward such that aloneness and one's inner experience are paramount. In contrast, CBT places significantly more emphasis on a person's social context. Couples therapy and communication training are of explicit concern, social support is taken as an important variable, social skills are taught (e.g., to children with autism), and even one's cultural social context is seen as key.

Another difference is that Zen Buddhism utilizes terms that are fairly central and upon first glance appear to be inconsistent with the general metaphysical commitments of CBT. *Dharma*, for example, has no equivalent in CBT theory, which takes no position on an afterlife as it typically is beyond its scope of concerns, similar to how a chemist takes no such position either. Many other terms have no obvious overlap with conventional CBT: *karma*, *hara*, *koans*, etc. However, a metaphysical commonality is that neither is a theology; that is, neither postulates a god. Although these both share another part of a metaphysical stance in that both believe the universe is lawful, CBTs suggest that science is needed to determine these laws whereas Zen suggests that Buddha has discovered the most relevant laws already. Buddhism has in it a stronger critique of dualism, suggesting that all is one. CBT practitioners, on the other hand, are more content with a wide range of dichotomies and distinctions.

CBT does not contain an internal, intrinsically tied ethic. Buddhism does: right speech, right livelihood, etc. CBT has adopted ethical codes as part of its organizational structure, and it is fair to say that an epistemology may be internal to it.

One legitimate concern is that in some important ways, clinical science and Zen come from two very different traditions. Clinical science is less concerned with individual claims but much more concerned with epistemology, the process by which evidence and warrants are produced for claims. Zen, in stark contrast, appears to be much more concerned with content of claims, which are often associated with historical exegesis (i.e., what Buddha and other masters have said) and personal subjective experience, thus much less concerned with the scientific method.

How ought these contrasting traditions be viewed? First, we believe that there is nothing in Zen Buddhism that is directly contradictory to simultaneously also embracing science. The claims contained in Zen Buddhism can be put to scientific test. There is a distinction made in the philosophy of science between the context of discovery and the context of justification (Reichenbach 1938). In the context of discovery, interesting claims are formulated; in the context of justification, these claims are put to the test. Zen, we argue, has a potentially important role in the context of discovery; it may provide interesting content for further scientific investigation.

Second, Houts (2009) has provided an interesting contrast between two ways of making sense of the world using what he calls the tradition of Athens and the tradition of Jerusalem. He suggested that main differences in the two traditions can be captured in the table below:

Basic conceptual differences between thought categories of Athens and Jerusalem

Athenian Pole	Jerusalem Pole
Detachment/Objectivity/ Universal	Involvement/Subjectivity/ Particular
Chronos	Kairos
Being	Becoming
Logic/Reason	Decision/Emotion/Will
Necessary/Inevitable	Contingent

Houts (2009) further stated:

> At the other end of the universal-versus-particular-pole lies the individual instance. In focusing on this way of thinking, the individual person and what goes on in the emotionally laden and

embodied musings of the heart are the focus of concern and the model for how to think. The Hebraic and early Christian texts of the bible are filled with examples of stories about individuals. Teaching is conducted by concrete example rather than abstract principle (even though this too occurs especially as the texts themselves came to be influence by Hellenistic and Roman thought). God speaks to Abraham and to Job in all of their particularity, and from these particular stories about individuals, religious institutions later constructed principles, rules, and more abstracted generalities of theology and ethics. In the sayings of Jesus, one often finds teaching in the form of parables which are specific stories presented as pictures and intended to call the hearers to immediate action in the context of the presentation and the life situation of Jesus (Jeremias 1963). Some of the clearest exposition of this relative emphasis on the particular as contrasted with the universal can be found in Kierkegaard whose works have done much to clarify the differences between biblical and Greek thought. Kierkegaard often juxtaposes the emphasis on the individual as opposed to the abstract "mankind" and the preeminence of the subjective over the objective (Kierkegaard et al. 1962). In this way of thinking, thought moves from some defining, overwhelming, and revealing experience (the exodus from Egypt, the resurrection of Jesus) outward instead of moving from some postulates of reason and on to rational arguments. Truth is obtained not from detachment but from engagement and commitment to some particular tradition encountered in powerful experiences.... In this biblical way of life, the purpose of living is to be engaged rather than detached. The "real" world is to be found in commitment, engagement, and emotionally charged faithfulness to something not seen with the light of reason, but only encountered when reason, logic, and those ways of comportment fail and breakdown in self contradiction and limit (pp. 262–264).

Zen shares this epistemic orientation with Christianity and many of the same contrasts apply to it and science. Psychologists have been dubious and even hostile toward Christianity (Cummings et al. 2009), but much more open to Zen and Buddhism. However, this suggests that Zen may be associated with a different way of knowing—a more personal one—more akin to the way you know you love your daughter—knowledge that is independent from science but no less secure and possibly even more important to the individual. It would be unwise to reject Zen Buddhism simply because it represents a different way of knowing than that represented by the scientific method. Houts (2009) stated further:

> From the standpoint of the [protestant] tradition, an argument for God is like a bake sale for Bill Gates. This is succinct way of highlighting the stark difference between the biblical and the Greek traditions regarding the place of rationality and logic, where in the latter tradition logic is the supreme arbiter of what is rational and what is not. From the culture of Athens, we have inherited the traditions of critical reflection and the use of rational argument to settle points of disagreement. From the dialogues of Socrates to the *Principia Mathematica* of Russell and Whitehead (Whitehead and Russell 1910), rationality and its bedrock, logic, have been the central force of western philosophy as well as a chief ingredient in synthesizing theological expositions. In contrast to this rational emphasis on reasoned argument and the well-crafted treatise, the biblical traditions featured illustrative stories, recitation of great moments for decision and action, poetry, riddles, grand fantastic visions, and prophesy. At various times in the history of western culture, the conflict between these two very different modes of thought and expression has erupted in solitary thinkers and even in the culture at large (p. 268).

The reader will see in the chapters that follow that Zen, too, communicates the personal through stories, riddles, and personal commitment (see Ogawa; Matsuyama, this volume). It is also interesting to note that Martin Luther and the advent of the Protestant tradition illustrate the conflict between a dominant rationalist tradition from Athens and the eruption of a contrary tradition from Jerusalem. Luther is often quoted for having said, "Reason is the Devil's whore." Zen too can have a distrustful stance toward reason. Thus, it is also the case that clinical psychology must embrace this question if science is the only way knowledge is produced. If so, how is this reconciled with everyday, personal knowledge, the kind that confirms that you love your child, that genocide is wrong, or that you dislike red wine? This, too, is knowledge, but it is not the product of science.

These numerous differences are the reason why glib suggestions that Zen and CBT ought to be integrated are problematic. Combining the two is not like combining water and rum but in some ways much more like combining oil and water; there *are* incompatibilities. It seems much more reasonable to suggest something softer like a "Zen-informed CBT," but until these incompatibilities and inconsistencies are resolved, a stronger synthesis is not possible.

Varieties of Buddhism

In this book, we consider one variety of Buddhism—Zen Buddhism. There are others, and others have also captured the attention of psychologists in recent years such as the Tibetan Buddhism of the Dali Lama. There are many commonalities across Buddhist practices, such as the Four Noble Truths and the Eightfold path. Differences exist as well. It is beyond the scope of this book to attempt an accurate exegesis of each and to isolate all the points of contention. This is an exercise more relevant to scholars of Buddhism. Regardless, we want to offer a cautionary tale here that one should not assume in reading this text that there are no differences; as a non-denominational or interdisciplinary Buddhist, one should at least be aware of the major differences. For example, the Rinzai branch of Zen in Japan is more oriented toward martial arts practice and the problems of the samurai, whereas Tibetan Buddhism is relatively more pacifist, and this latter orientation would generally be more acceptable to the average CBT practitioner.

Considerations for Implementing Zen Within Behavioral Health

The underlying purpose of this text is to provide behavioral health professionals with a broader and deeper understanding of how Zen conceptualizes our field, to better understand what Zen has to say about the concept of behavioral health as we view it in the West. Further, it is important to us that the voices and perspectives sharing their knowledge and expertise on these topics have first-hand experience with Zen. Monks, academics, practitioners, students, researchers, and teachers alike have contributed to offer a comprehensive and diverse analysis of behavioral health from a Zen perspective.

As Masuda and Sargent in this volume point out, basic linguistic and epistemological differences between Western and Zen worldviews prevent traditional Zen practices from transmitting in their exact forms and interpretations globally. This is evidenced in history given changes and adaptations of Buddhism observed as it reached China from India, Japan from China, etc. That is, as Zen "outsiders" make sense of Zen within their own cultures, the ways in which Zen is implemented and practiced morph and cannot overlap completely with native forms. Zen-like practices have emerged with immense popularity across the globe, particularly within the field of behavioral health. And out of each transmission arises change of some sort, such that the identification of a "true" or "pure" Zen is no longer possible. Because of this, we have also argued that an array of behaviors can be conducted in the Buddha way.

The Limits of Mindfulness and Zen

The use of mindfulness is a good example of a Zen concept being transmitted and therefore changed as it is applied in a new context. As noted above, the field of behavioral health has become increasingly interested in mindfulness and Zen practices because of their salutary effects found on various psychological and health outcomes (see Hazlett-Stevens, Kushner, this volume). Given these favorable outcomes, mindfulness and Zen practices are used as a means to overcome internalizing issues (e.g., depression, anxiety, and pain) and to promote greater behavioral adaptation (Monteiro et al. 2015). Practitioners of diverse theoretical orientations now use forms of mindfulness as a way to improve therapeutic effectiveness and increase client functioning. Mindfulness-based cognitive therapy (MBCT) incorporates mindfulness practices (i.e., mindfulness meditation) into traditional CBT methods in order to help clients decenter, thereby disengaging with symptoms of depression that create dysfunction in their daily lives (e.g., self-criticism). It has also been used to prevent relapse in addicted populations (Ma and Teasdale 2004). Mindfulness-based stress reduction (MBSR) employs mindfulness meditation to alleviate suffering for people who are chronically ill, suffering with physical and psychosomatic symptoms. These therapeutic approaches have been effective in their stated goals (Grossman et al. 2004), and deeper exploration has pointed to probable cognitive mechanisms for the effectiveness of these approaches: A recent meta-analysis revealed that among the many studies evaluating MBCT and MBSR, changes in cognitive and emotional reactivity constituted the strongest mechanism underlying the behavioral changes that occur following MBCT and MBSR practices implemented in therapy (Gu et al. 2015), with other consistent mechanisms including changes in mindfulness, rumination, and worry.

In the non-secular domain, Zen Buddhism does not advocate the practice of mindfulness or meditation for the purpose of attaining these ends. Zen Buddhism also states that practicing Zen with the intention to gain these ends can be detrimental, especially doing so in the extreme (see Bartok and Roemer, this volume). In Zen literature, practicing Zen with the intention of gaining something is called *bonpu Zen* (Broughton 2009; Uchiyama et al. 2004). Dogen Zenji (道元禅師; 1200–1253), the founder of the Soto school of Zen in Japan, stated that one must practice Zen simply for the sake of it, instead (Dogen et al. 2011). In doing so, according to Dogen, the Buddha Way naturally unfolds (Okumura 2010).

In Zen, the Buddha Way is the ongoing pursuit of self-enlightenment (i.e., embodiment of true self or nature) or the perfection of self through the self with an earnest endeavor for the benefit of mankind and all sentient beings (Japan Buddhist Federation 1978). For this reason, many Zen Buddhist scholars and practitioners perceive that mindfulness and Zen practices in behavioral health appear narrow in scope (see Li and Ramirez; Masuda and Sargent, this volume). Whereas the pursuit of desire for the cessation of suffering (i.e., depression and anxiety) or the attainment of happiness certainly could bolster quality of life, Zen also advocates that one must direct efforts outward to external surroundings. In this sense, the self is blended into the whole. In the practice of mindfulness, this is the point where Zen Buddhism and Western behavioral health seem to diverge from one another. Throughout this book, various authors discuss the holistic perspective of Zen Buddhism and how mindfulness practices from this perspective differ from some of the commonly held styles of mindfulness practice in the field of behavioral health.

The Limits of Cognitive Behavior Therapy and Zen

Applied behavior analysis, which can be construed as either a part of CBT or a competitor (O'Donohue and Ferguson 2016), has been concerned that there may be what is called a "technical drift" in its development (Baer 1981). The core of this concern was that behavior analytic techniques would be used without proper understanding of their roots in learning theory or their relationships to the wider theory of radical behaviorism. Similar concerns can be raised about techniques of CBT. For example, can a technique related to the content of this book, mindfulness, be understood in terms of experimental cognitive psychology? If not, is this a problem for contemporary cognitive psychology, or mindfulness, or both? What happens to CBT if it becomes an eclectic grab bag of techniques that have dubious relationships to one another and unclear relationships to fundamental psychological principles found in learning and cognition?

The Limits of Acceptance- and Mindfulness-Based Cognitive Behavior Therapies and Zen

The influence of mindfulness and related approaches is likely to continue as a dominant force in the field of behavioral health, especially in the area of psychotherapy, for the next several years (Norcross et al. 2013). The expansion of mindfulness- and acceptance-based cognitive behavioral therapies (Hayes et al. 2004, 2011), such as acceptance and commitment therapy (ACT; Hayes et al. 1999, 2012), dialectical behavior therapy (Linehan 1993), mindfulness-based cognitive therapy (MBCT; Segal et al. 2002), and mindfulness-based stress reduction (MBSR; Kabat-Zinn 1990), has contributed substantially to this movement.

As noted above, the mindfulness movement seen in the field of behavioral health for the past 10 years is generally encouraging, as it sheds light on an alternative direction in the pursuit of happiness and flourishing. On the other hand, according to Zen Buddhism, when the standpoints of the therapist and client from which these mindfulness- and acceptance-based treatments are practiced are narrow and rigidly applied, they are likely to amplify sufferings unique to human beings.

Zen Buddhism emphasizes the importance of oneness and wholeness (e.g., experiencing the self as one blending into the environment and surroundings) that goes beyond linguistic categorizations and differentiations. It is this standpoint from which Zen Buddhism advocates for mindfulness, acceptance, and compassion—not from the standpoint of judgement (e.g., good vs. bad) or self as a separate being that one should cling to or isolate from others.

Take an ACT clinical case as an example. The practice of acceptance and commitment to values-consistent activities are the hallmarks of ACT practice (Hayes et al. 1999). As noted extensively in this book (see Fung et al., this volume), acceptance is a behavior of becoming open to whatever one is experiencing as it is without any efforts to change it, whereas the commitment to valued actions is the purposeful and intentional behavioral effort made to engage in the activities that are meaningful to the self. In sum, when the standpoint of these practices is too narrow, they end up serving as mood-altering and self-protection strategies that may paradoxically isolate the client from his or her whole personal experience as well as from his or her surroundings. ACT emerged partially in response to the pitfall derived from narrow and rigid standpoints regarding therapy and self inherent within some traditional CBT approaches. In fact, ACT and Zen Buddhism share many philosophical assumptions (e.g., act of person in a context as the fundamental unit of understanding). Highlighting the importance of clarifying one's standpoint, the originators of ACT caution clinicians not to practice it without thorough understanding of its conceptual and philosophical underpinnings (Hayes et al. 1999, 2012).

Looking Forward

Research on CBT, ACT, and mindfulness-based therapy practices tells us what can be accomplished in behavioral health when traditional practices are parsed out and implemented in isolation for utilitarian purposes. As you will learn in subsequent chapters, this utilitarian approach is, in fact, not Zen at all from a theoretical perspective. At the same time, utilitarian behaviors are a large part of life in all cultures, including those in which Zen originated. People have always and will continue to behave in ways that produce desired results: They will work toward careers that suit their interests, they will save money to afford vacations, they will harvest crops at specific times to create optimal return on investment and optimal flavor on the table, and in this sense, it is hard to claim that Zen and goal-directed behaviors cannot coexist. As such, psychologists, practitioners, and researchers will continue to study human behavior with the goal in mind to achieve some sort of influence over it in the service of better quality of life at individual and community levels.

Given that these goal-directed behaviors will persist in various contexts, we want to acknowledge the inherent discrepancies in what appear to be the underlying goals of Zen and behavioral health, but we also want to paint a picture of what a Zen-informed behavioral health might look like. As the chapters of this book explain in detail, Zen is not one thing. It is not *zazen*, it is not mindfulness, it is not concentration, it is not reading koans, and it is not the absence of pleasure or suffering. At its core, Zen is the culmination of all things that are both interconnected and independent, and we can understand the process of behavioral health similarly: Human beings and the ways in which we function in our environments are interconnected and independent. They can also be made predictable through scientific exploration, much like gardening or preparing food can. Gardening and cooking can both be utilitarian, yet they can also be processes that help us to experience the Buddha Way. Thus, the very best treatments will rely upon psychological theory, practice, and research that views people in this light. Rather than seeing a "mindfulness" practice in a therapeutic setting as a Zen practice per se, we can instead ask ourselves if our mindfulness practice, or our thought record, or our exposure technique is implemented with the client's functioning as a *whole person* in mind. Are we considering our client's *whole* context? Are we helping them to experience their lives in the here-and-now via our treatments, or have we implemented a given technique as a Band-Aid for a very specific symptom? For example, if we implement a treatment that helps an adolescent with bulimia nervosa reduce purging behaviors, but upon follow-up we observe that she began cutting her thighs, we may have been successful at symptom reduction, but we failed to address the client's functioning as a *whole* person and missed the underlying mechanism of her dysregulation because of our narrow focus on a single symptom. Using meditation or acceptance in this isolated manner does not constitute Zen-informed behavioral health—rather, a perspective of wholeness and an appreciation for the here-and-now in therapy and in research more closely bridges the gap between Zen and our field.

Philosophically Informed Behavioral Health and What Zen May Have to Offer

It may be important to develop a philosophically informed theory of behavioral health that includes key insights from Zen's perspective. Some ideas that Zen may offer to behavioral health include:

1. Although not uniquely (see Houts above), Zen illustrates another complementary epistemology of personal, experiential knowledge.
2. Zen offers other key insights that provide a broader and thus more useful structure of meaning, something suggested by some contemporary theorists, such as Seligman (2011), as important to flourishing and living a vital life.
3. Zen can provide an important meta-criticism to irrational ideas that lead to the some of the kinds of human suffering psychotherapists find that their patients encounter. This includes the craving to feel no pain or to "have it all." Zen suggests that life is always bitter sweet and that desire is the root of a lot of our pain. Should psychotherapists help their clients simplify their lives, accepting some of the pain of life as inevitable? This is in direct contrast to the view that the client comes to us with goals (e.g., desires), and it is the CBT therapist's role to help them gain these, much as an architect helps a client design and build a 14 bedroom house.
4. Zen might help CBT realize that both the body and the mind are important. Zen is literally an *embodied* view of the psychology of a person. CBT has traditionally been much more concerned with unembodied ideas.
5. Zen can provide an interesting analysis about living more simply. A popular view of the professional role of the psychotherapist has been that the psychotherapist serves as the architect and the client as the individual who defines the goal. But what if the client wants

too much? What if the client is what might be called from a Zen perspective a hungry ghost: a slave to ever perpetuating desires? Ought the psychotherapist take a meta-perspective and see the proliferation of want as the real problem? A popular Zen meme distributed on social media follows:

Do one thing at a time.
Do it slowly and deliberately.
Do it completely.
Do less.
Put space between things.
Develop rituals.
Designate time for certain things.
Devote time to sitting.
Smile and serve others.
Make cleansing and cooking become meditation.
Think about what is necessary.
Live simply.

6. Zen provides another structure by which to view thoughts, which are phenomena of obvious importance in cognitive behavior therapy. Zen, like CBT, suggests a distancing from thoughts, a view that thoughts are not inevitable but are products of a complex system of causes. Zen doesn't suggest that the way to influence thoughts is through rational disputation; rather, the process of meditation changes the person in such a way that thoughts change. Thus, potentially, there is another pathway to modify problematic thoughts, especially automatic thoughts.

Overview of Chapters

To address the four foci described at the beginning of this chapter, we have gathered experts from the field of Zen Buddhism, mindfulness-based interventions, and behavioral health in Japan and the USA. In terms of the structure, the present volume consists of four parts. Part I is the overview of Zen Buddhism in terms of history and sociocultural background as well as its relevance to Western behavioral health. The aim of Part I is to elucidate key historical and situational contexts of Zen Buddhism where the constructs of mindfulness, acceptance, and compassion were originally emerged. Following the present chapter, Shudo Ishii, Ph.D., an emeritus of Komazawa University, the oldest Soto-Zen Buddhism university, presents the history of Zen Buddhism in China and highlight its core perspective on enlightenment, practice, and everyday living (Chapter "Zen and Zen Buddhism: An Overview"). As discussed extensively elsewhere (Dumoulin 2005), the history of Zen Buddhism is traced back to Gautama Buddha (Shakamuni Buddha; 釈迦牟尼仏陀) of India in the sixth century B.C., the founder of the Buddhist religion. His teaching was then transmitted to China by Bodhidharma (菩提達磨) in the sixth century, and the practice of Bodhidharma became the foundation of Zen Buddhism. Even today, the core perspectives systematized in China remain central in Zen Buddhism.

Zen Buddhism was then transmitted to Japan in twelfth century, and there its teachings were blended into the native Japanese culture (Japan Buddhist Federation 1978; Suzuki 2010). As mentioned above, understanding Japanese culture is crucial for learning Zen Buddhism in the West in part because many sects of Zen Buddhism in the West trace their origins back to Zen Buddhism practices systematized in Japan. As such, Akihiko Masuda, Ph.D., of University of Hawaii, presents the intricate relation between Zen Buddhism and Japanese culture (see Chapter "Zen and Japanese Culture").

Part II of this volume then delineates the core features of Zen Buddhism, including its fundamental attitudes toward practice and everyday living, sitting zen mediation, paradoxical and illogical discourse, and its unique account of body and language. These chapters are written by internationally recognized Japanese Zen Buddhist scholars and practitioners. In Chapter "What is Zen?: The Path of Just Sitting," Rev. Shohaku Okumura Roshi, an internationally known Japanese Soto-Zen monk, presents the heart of Zen Buddhism by sharing his personal journey of the Buddha Way. More specifically, the heart of Zen Buddhism is described as the practice of what D.T. Suzuki called "pure subjectivity" (Suzuki 1996), and it is inherently personal and experiential (Uchiyama and Okumura 2014; Uchiyama et al. 2004). Okumura's chapter captures the extraordinariness of living consistent with the Buddha Way in seemingly ordinary aspects of everyday living.

Zazen (坐禅; sitting mediation) and *koan* (公案; a seemingly paradoxical anecdote or riddle) are the hallmarks of Zen Buddhism practice. Whereas many behavioral health practitioners may have heard of these practices, their core features and aims are often misunderstood. In Chapter "A Brief Note on Zazen," Rev. Tairyu Tsunoda Roshi of Komazawa University introduces the ideal attitude for practicing zazen. Many of us think that zazen is for strengthening our mind and body or attaining a sense of peace, kindness, and tranquility. However, Tsunoda Roshi argues for the importance of practicing zazen for the sake of zazen, without being caught up in the desire attached achieving these ends. Subsequently, in Chapter "The role and the present significance of Koans," Rev. Daiko Matsuyama, an internationally recognized Rinzai Zen monk, presents the process and aims of *koan*-based practice and uncovers the reason why a *koan*-based practice has been developed into its current form, which appears quite odd for Westerners.

Zen Buddhist practice characterized by *zazen* and *koan* is the historically and contextually situated act of a person as a whole, not merely the practice of mind or that of body. From this standpoint, Zen Buddhism presents its unique account of body, mind, and language (Wright 1992). In Chapter "Zen and Body," Kenshu Sugawara, Ph.D., of Aichi Gakuin University, another well-known Soto-Zen Buddhism university in Japan, highlights the Zen account of body where the body is construed as being more than a physical entity. Dr. Sugawara also elucidates the role of body for fully experiencing the Buddha Way in everyday living. Following the Zen account of body, Takashi Ogawa, Ph.D., of Komazawa University, presents the role of linguistic processes and discourse in Zen Buddhism practice (see Chapter "Zen and Language: Zen Mondo and Koan"). Zen's account of language, communication, and reasoning is one of the most widely discussed topics in the intersection of Zen Buddhism, philosophy, and psychological science (Gergen 1983; Kasulis 1981; Wright 1992). Ogawa argues that, unlike some misconceptions, Zen does not reject language or reasoning, and that it plays a crucial role in Zen Buddhist practice, although the linguistic practice of Zen is not like the one we are familiar to.

Part III of this book highlights the Zen Buddhism account of some of the key psychological constructs fundamental to understanding our sense of identity and well-being, such as self, desire, forgiveness, and everyday living (Gilbert and Irons 2005; Markus and Kitayama 1991; Menahem and Love 2013). As noted above, Buddhism is known for its unique treatment of human desire. Zen Buddhism argues that even some of the appropriate desires (e.g., desire for our own child's wellness) are detrimental especially when they are excessive. In Chapter "Zen and Desire," Seijun Ishii, Ph.D., of Komazawa University outlines a Zen account of desire from its perspective of human being as well as the link between practice and the attainment of enlightenment. Following the Zen account of desire, Hidetaka Okajima, Ph.D., of Aichi Gakuin University, presents a Zen Buddhist account of self and personality and its link to the concept of human desire and enlightenment (see Chapter "Zen, Self, and Personality"). In Zen Buddhism literature, the terms self and desire are often used interchangeably. Okajima argues that Zen practice is a way to integrate various personal experiences into the sense of self that is more than an individual self; further, the Buddha Way is this way of experiencing self.

As an ancient Chinese Zen master, Mazu Dahui (馬祖道一; 709–778) stated that the practice of Zen Buddhism should not be disjointed from everyday living (Poceski 2015); rather, the Buddha Way (e.g., the expression of true self and proper way to relate to desire) should be manifest in any given moment of our lives. Mike Sayama, Ph.D., a Rinzai Zen master, presents Zen's perspective about everyday living and demystifies Zen-consistent living by sharing his own everyday life (Chapter "Every Day Is a Fine Day").

In addition to the constructs of mindfulness and acceptance, other popular psychological terms in the field of behavioral health are compassion and forgiveness (Neff 2003). For example, many psychologists now believe that forgiveness is an essential aspect of psychological well-being (Menahem and Love 2013). Rev. Shoryu Bradley, the Dharma heir of Shohaku Okumura, presents a Zen account of forgiveness (Chapter "Zen and Forgiveness") and highlights how the sense of forgiveness in Zen Buddhism unfolds in everyday life as well as how it is linked to greater compassion toward humanity and all sentient beings. Finally, the last chapter of Part III by Rev. Rosan Daido, a Roshi, presents Zen principles as a value system that may serve as an ethical guide for scientists and consumers of scientific knowledge, the purpose of which is to protect humanity and our global ecosystem (Chapter "Zen and Science: Zen as an Ethical Guideline for Scientists' Conducts").

Part IV, the last section of this book, focuses on issues emerging within the intersection of Zen, mindfulness, and behavioral health. Zen and mindfulness practices are known for their salutary effects, and Part IV starts with Kenneth Kushner, Ph.D., of University of Wisconsin, Madison, also a Rinzai Zen master, who presents the current state of evidence of Zen on psychological and health outcomes (see Chapter "Zen and Behavioral Health: A Review of the Evidence"). Following Kushner Roshi, Peiwei Li, Ph.D., and her colleague of Springfield College introduce the history and current trends of cross-fertilization between Zen Buddhism and psychotherapies. They also raise concerns about the bastardization of mindfulness practice in the field of behavioral health with being too narrow in focus (see Chapter "Zen and Psychotherapy"). Subsequently, Akihiko Masuda, Ph.D., and Kayla Sargent of University of Hawaii present Zen Buddhist thought on the concept and practice of psychopathology, arguing that many of the differences between Zen and behavioral health in their account of psychopathology are epistemological, rather than empirical (Chapter "Zen's Thoughts on Psychopathology and Wellness"). They also argue that Zen's holistic and functional account present an alternative way of making sense of human psychopathology.

Zen Buddhism is holistic, transient, and inclusive in its epistemological standpoint, and it treats mindfulness from this standpoint. In Chapter "What Is Measured by Self-report Measures of Mindfulness?: Conceptual and Measurement Issues," Sungjin Im of University of Nevada, Reno reviews most commonly used self-report measures of mindfulness and their validities. He also elucidates conceptual and practical drift of mindfulness from its Eastern origin. Subsequently, Rev. Josh Bartok Roshi and Liz Roemer, Ph.D., of University of Massachusetts Boston, a co-founder of Acceptance-Based Behavior Therapy (Roemer and Orsillo 2005), present a Zen Buddhist account of acceptance and mindfulness (Chapter "Remembering and receiving: Mindfulness and acceptance in Zen"). More specifically, they show how the practice of mindfulness and acceptance is integrated into cognitive and behavioral practice, while remaining true to each tradition with the focus on the therapists' attitudes toward their work and their clients. Following Rev Bartok Roshi and Dr. Roemer, Marsha Linehan, Ph.D., the founder of Dialectical Behavior Therapy (DBT; Linehan 1993) and Kayla Sargent present subtle and yet extremely important overlaps between behavior therapy and Zen Buddhism (Chapter "Brief Thoughts on Zen and Behavior Therapy"). This is followed by Holly Hazlett-Stevens, Ph.D., of University of Nevada, Reno's chapter on similarities and differences between Zen Buddhism and CBT using a CBT framework (Chapter "Zen, Mindfulness, and Cognitive-Behavior Therapy") and by Kenneth Fung, M.D. and his colleague of University of Toronto's discussion of the association between Zen Buddhism and acceptance and commitment therapy (ACT) in Chapter "Acceptance and Commitment Therapy and Zen Buddhism."

Finally, the last three chapters of Part IV delineate the application/embodiment of Zen Buddhism teaching in various applied settings. In particular, Gordon Greene, Ph.D., of University of Wisconsin School of Medicine and Public Health as well as a Rinzai Zen master, shares his experience as a hospital chaplain (Chapter "Zen, Pain, Suffering and Death"), and Norma Wong Roshi presents the application of Zen principles for professionals and advocates who work for survivors of trauma and violence (Chapter "Application of Zen Practices and Principles for Professionals/Advocates Who Work for Survivors of Trauma and Violence"). Finally, Jeffrey Schneider, Roshi of San Francisco Zen Center, describes and reflects upon his work as a Zen priest with prison populations (Chapter "Zen Incarcerated: A Personal Essay").

Editors' Notes on Translated Chapters

Many chapters written by Japanese authors were originally composed in Japanese by these authors and then translated into English by one of the editors of this volume (A.M.) and his graduate assistant, Kayla Sargent. We, the editors of the volume, specify these translated chapters by presenting the names of translators under the chapter author at the first page of these chapters. We do so in part because we would like to take the full responsibility for the errors and mistakes of the English versions of these chapters.

It is important to inform the reader that the English versions of these chapters differ from the original Japanese versions in two major ways, although we made our best effort to present the contents of the original versions as closely as possible in the translated version. One domain of difference is the sentence and paragraph structure. Japanese communication style at times appears too indirect, subtle, and repetitive for Western audiences as they are accustomed to reading. As such, we have restructured some of the paragraphs to sound more direct and linear. Second, in the translated versions of chapters, we have added sentences and paragraphs further explaining some of the basic terms (e.g., *koan*, *zazen*) used in Zen Buddhism, key figures (e.g., Dogen Zenji), as well as its core teachings (e.g., enlightenment). Some of these additions were drawn from other sources that were not included in the original versions of chapter. Whereas these changes may enhance the readability for Western audiences, they may have obscured the unique features or nuances of Zen Buddhism teachings and the authors' intensions.

References

Baer, D. M. (1981). A flight of behavior analysis. *The Behavior Analyst, 4*(2), 85–91.

Broughton, J. L. (2009). *Zongmi on Chan*. New York, US: Columbia University Press.

Brown, K. W., Ryan, R. M., & Creswell, J. D. (2007). Mindfulness: Theoretical foundations and evidence for its salutary effects. *Psychological Inquiry, 18*(4), 211–237.

Cummings, N., O'Donohue, W., & Cummings, J. (2009). *Psychology's war on religion*. Phoenix, AZ, US: Zeig, Tucker & Theisen.

Dogen, E., Leighton, T. D., & Okumura, S. (1995). *Dogen's pure standards for the Zen Community: A translation of Eihei Shingi*. Albany, New York: State University of New York Press.

Dogen, E., Nishiari, B., Okumura, S., Suzuki, S., & Weisman, S. M. (2011). *Dogen's Genjo Koan: Three commentaries*. Barkeley, CA, US: Counterpoint.

Dumoulin, H. (2005). *Zen Buddhism: A history volume 1: India and China*. Bloomington, IN, US: World Wisdom.

Gergen, K. J. (1983). Zen Buddhism and psychological science. *Psychologia: An International Journal of Psychology in the Orient, 26*(3), 129–141.

Gilbert, P. (2010). Compassion focused therapy: A special section. *International Journal of Cognitive Therapy, 3* (2), 95–96. doi:10.1521/ijct.2010.3.2.95

Gilbert, P., & Irons, C. (2005). Focused therapies and compassionate mind training for shame and self-attacking. In P. Gilbert & P. Gilbert (Eds.), *Compassion: Conceptualisations, research and use in psychotherapy* (pp. 263–325). New York, NY, US: Routledge.

Grossman, P., Niemann, L., Schmidt, S., & Walach, H. (2004). Mindfulness-based stress reduction and health benefits: A meta-analysis. *Journal of Psychosomatic Research, 57*(1), 35–43. doi:10.1016/S0022-3999(03)00573-7

Gu, J., Strauss, C., Bond, R., & Cavanagh, K. (2015). How do mindfulness-based cognitive therapy and mindfulness-based stress reduction improve mental health and wellbeing? A systematic review and meta-analysis of mediation studies. *Clinical Psychology Review, 37*, 1–12. doi:10.1016/j.cpr.2015.01.006

Hayes, S. C., Barnes-Holmes, D., & Wilson, K. G. (2012). Contextual behavioral science: Creating a science more adequate to the challenge of the human condition. *Journal of Contextual Behavioral Science, 1*(1–2), 1–16. doi:http://dx.doi.org/10.1016/j.jcbs.2012.09.004

Hayes, S. C., Follette, V. M., & Linehan, M. M. (2004). *Mindfulness and acceptance: Expanding the cognitive-behavioral tradition*. New York, NY, US: Guilford Press.

Hayes, S. C., Strosahl, K. D., & Wilson, K. G. (1999). *Acceptance and commitment therapy: An experiential approach to behavior change*. New York, NY US: Guilford Press.

Hayes, S. C., Strosahl, K. D., & Wilson, K. G. (2012b). *Acceptance and commitment therapy: The process and practice of mindful change* (2nd ed.). New York, NY US: Guilford Press.

Hayes, S. C., Villatte, M., Levin, M., & Hildebrandt, M. (2011). Open, aware, and active: Contextual approaches as an emerging trend in the behavioral and cognitive therapies. *Annual Review of Clinucal Psychology, 7*, 141–168. doi:10.1146/annurev-clinpsy-032210-104449

Hofmann, S. G., Sawyer, A. T., Witt, A. A., & Oh, D. (2010). The effect of mindfulness-based therapy on anxiety and depression: A meta-analytic review. *Journal of Consulting and Clinical Psychology, 78* (2), 169–183. doi:10.1037/a0018555

Houts, A. C. (2009). Reformed theology is a resource in conflicts between psychology and religious faith. In N. Cummings, W. O'Donohue, & J. Cummings (Eds.), *Psychology's war on religion* (pp. 257–311). Phoenix, AZ, US: Zeig, Tucker & Theisen.

Japan Buddhist Federation. (1978). *Understanding Japanese Buddhism*.

Jeremias, J. (1963). *The parables of Jesus* (Rev. ed.). New York: Scribner.

Kabat-Zinn, J. (1990). *Full catastrophe living*.

Kabat-Zinn, J. (2003). Mindfulness-based interventions in context: Past, present, and future. *Clinical Psychology: Science and Practice, 10*(2), 144–156. doi:10.1093/clipsy/bpg016

Kasulis, T. P. (1981). *Zen action Zen person*. Honolulu, HI, US: University of Hawaii Press.

Kierkegaard, S., Lowrie, W., & Nelson, B. (1962). *The point of view for my work as an author; a report to history, and related writings*. New York: Harper.

Linehan, M. M. (1993). *Cognitive-behavioral treatment of borderline personality disorder*. New York, NY US: Guilford Press.

Ma, S. H., & Teasdale, J. D. (2004). Mindfulness-based cognitive therapy for depression: Replication and exploration of differential relapse prevention effects [Press release]

Markus, H. R., & Kitayama, S. (1991). Culture and the self: Implications for cognition, emotion, and motivation. *Psychological Review, 98*(2), 224–253.

Menahem, S., & Love, M. (2013). Forgiveness in psychotherapy: The key to healing. *Journal of Clinical Psychology, 69*(8), 829–835. doi:10.1002/jclp.22018

Monteiro, L. M., Musten, R. F., & Compson, J. (2015). Traditional and contemporary mindfulness: Finding the middle path in the tangle of concerns. *Mindfulness, 6*(1), 1–13. doi:10.1007/s12671-014-0301-7

Neff, K. D. (2003). Self-compassion: An alternative conceptualization of a healthy attitude toward oneself. *Self and Identity, 2*(2), 85–101. doi:10.1080/15298860309032

Norcross, J. C., Pfund, R. A., & Prochaska, J. O. (2013). Psychotherapy in 2022: A Delphi poll on its future. *Professional Psychology: Research and Practice, 44* (5), 363-370. doi:10.1037/a0034633

O'Donohue, W. T., & Ferguson, K. E. (2016). Historical and philosophical dimensions of contemporary cognitive-behavioral therapy. In C. M. Nezu, A. M. Nezu, C. M. Nezu, & A. M. Nezu (Eds.), *The Oxford handbook of cognitive and behavioral therapies* (pp. 7–27). New York, NY, US: Oxford University Press.

Okumura, S. (2010). *Realizing Genjokoan: The key to Dogen's Shobogenzo*. Boston MA, US: Wisdom Publications.

Poceski, M. (2015). *The records of Mazu and the making of classical Chan literature*. New York, USA: Oxford University Press.

Reichenbach, H. (1938). *An analysis of the foundations and the structure of knowledge*. Chicago, IL, US: University of Chicago Press.

Robins, C. J. (2002). Zen principles and mindfulness practice in dialectical behavior therapy. *Cognitive and Behavioral Practice, 9*(1), 50–57.

Roemer, L., & Orsillo, S. M. (2005). An acceptance-based behavior therapy for generalized anxiety disorder. In S. M. Orsillo & L. Roemer (Eds.), *Acceptance and mindfulness-based approaches to anxiety: Conceptualization and treatment* (pp. 213–240). Boston, MA, US: Springer.

Segal, Z. V., Williams, J. M. G., & Teasdale, J. D. (2002). *Mindfulness-based cognitive therapy for depression: A new approach to preventing relapse*. New York, NY, US: Guilford Press.

Seligman, M. E. (2011). *Flourish: A visionary new understanding of happiness and well-being*. New York, NY, US: Free Press.

Senzaki, N., & Strout-McCandless, R. (1953). *Buddhism and Zen*. New York, US: North Point Press.

Suzuki, D. T. (1994). *Essays in Zen Buddhism*. New York, US: Grove Press (original work published in 1949).

Suzuki, D. T. (1996). *Zen Buddhism: Selected writings of D. T. Suzuki*. New York, US: An Image Book.

Suzuki, D. T. (2010). *Zen and Japanese culture*. Princeton, NJ, US: Princeton University Press (original work published in 1938).

Timberlake, W. (1995). Reconceptualizing reinforcement: A causal-system approach to reinforcement and behavior change. In W. T. O. D. L. Krasner (Ed.), *Theories of behavior therapy: Exploring behavior change* (pp. 59–96). Washington, DC, US: American Psychological Association.

Timberlake, W., & Allison, J. (1974). Response deprivation: An empirical approach to instrumental performance. *Psychological Review, 81*(2), 146–164. doi:10.1037/h0036101

Tirch, D., Silberstein, L. R., & Kolts, R. L. (2016). *Buddhist psychology and cognitive-behavioral therapy: A clinician's guide*. New York, NY, US: Guilford Press.

Uchiyama, K., & Okumura, S. (2014). *The Zen teaching of homeless Kodo*. Somerville MA, US: Tuttle Publications.

Uchiyama, K., Wright, T., Warner, J., & Okumura, S. (2004). *Opening the hand of thought: Foundations of Zen Buddhism practice*. Somerville MA, US: Wisdom Publications.

Van Gordon, W., Shonin, E., Griffiths, M. D., & Singh, N. N. (2015a). Mindfulness and the four noble truths. In E. Shonin, W. Van Gordon, N. N. Singh, E. Shonin, W. Van Gordon, & N. N. Singh (Eds.), *Buddhist foundations of mindfulness* (pp. 9–27). Cham, Switzerland: Springer International Publishing.

Van Gordon, W., Shonin, E., Griffiths, M. D., & Singh, N. N. (2015b). There is only one mindfulness: Why science and Buddhism need to work together. *Mindfulness, 6*(1), 49–56. doi:10.1007/s12671-014-0379-y

Whitehead, A. N., & Russell, B. (1910). *Principia mathematica*. Cambridge: University Press.

Wright, D. S. (1992). Rethinking transcendence: The role of language in Zen experience. *Philosophy East & West, 42*(1), 113–138.

Zen and Zen Buddhism: An Overview

Shudo Ishii, Akihiko Masuda and Kayla Sargent

Keywords
Zen · Buddhism · History of Zen Buddhism · Chinese Zen · Chan

Zen and Zen Buddhism have a long history. A consensus among Zen Buddhism practitioners and scholars is that Zen Buddhism began with Gautama Buddha, the founder of Buddhism (Dumoulin 2005), who incorporated *dhyana* (i.e., a form of Zen meditation with Indian origins) into his training. As Zen meditation can be traced back to India prior to the time of Gautama Buddha, the history of Zen Buddhism actually began before Buddhism itself. For a moment, imagine the tropical climate of India: It must have been quite natural for the students of diverse spiritual traditions to meditate tranquilly under a tree or on a stone as they explored the meaning of the way.

Translated and Edited by Akihiko Masuda and Kayla Sargent.

S. Ishii (✉)
Komazawa University, Tokyo, Japan
e-mail: soishii@komazawa-u.ac.jp

A. Masuda · K. Sargent
University of Hawaii at Manoa, Honolulu, USA
e-mail: amasuda4@hawaii.edu

K. Sargent
e-mail: kaylansargent@gmail.com

The term Zen (禅) itself sits upon a rich history. It can be used to describe similar but varying concepts or practices depending on the context and culture with which it is used. The term Zen is derived from the Japanese pronunciation of the Chinese word Chan (禪), which came from the Sanskrit word *dhyana* or the Pali word *jhana*. In Japanese Zen Buddhism, the term is often considered synonymous with yoga (瑜伽) or samadhi (三昧, an ultimate state of concentration achieved through meditation). In practice, Zen is often understood as the act of adjusting one's mind by seeing and reflecting the true nature of the universe. As such, Zen is also called *Zenjo* (禅定) because the Sanskrit *dhyana* also emphasizes the *adjustment, settlement, and concentration* of the mind, which is roughly translated as *jo* (定) in Japanese.

Prior to his awakening or enlightenment, Gautama Buddha was said to seek teachings from two sages, Ajara Kalama and Uddaka Ramaputta. According to *Keitoku Dentō-roku* (景徳傳燈録 in Japanese; The Record of the Transmission of the Lamp), one of the most widely read ancient Chan texts, Gautama Buddha sought the samadhi of nothingness (i.e., nondiscrimination) and the samadhi of neither-perception-nor-nonperceptions from these teachers (see Daoyuan and Whitfield

A. Masuda and W.T. O'Donohue (eds.), *Handbook of Zen, Mindfulness, and Behavioral Health*, Mindfulness in Behavioral Health, DOI 10.1007/978-3-319-54595-0_2

2015, p. 76). As noted below, these forms of samadhi were considered the two highest stages of Zen meditation. However, once the Buddha awakened to these states, he questioned the practice of Zen meditation for the purpose of achieving these states. Gautama Buddha then left those teachers and moved to Bodh Gaya of India and attained the enlightenment of the Middle Way (中道; Chudo in Japanese) under the famous Bodhi Tree (Japan Buddhist Federation 1978). The Middle Way describes the profoundly influential Noble Eightfold Path: right view, right resolve, right speech, right conduct, right livelihood, right effort, right mindfulness, and right samadhi. Although transitioning away from zazen for the purpose of attaining the ultimate state of mind, Gautama Buddha continued to practice zazen for the rest of his life.

Earlier Buddhist texts categorize the world into three realms: the world of desire (i.e., physical and material world), the world of form (i.e., energy world), and the world of formlessness (see Shankman 2008). A detailed account of this ancient Buddhist perspective is beyond the scope of this chapter. However, worth noting briefly are the four levels of *dhyana* (zen) as well as the four levels of samadhi in the formless realm described in these texts. It is said that upon mastery of the four *dhayas* in the realms of form, one can move toward the four formless samadhi in the realm of formlessness. The four levels of *dhyana* are said to correspond to the four levels of attainment in the realm of formlessness. According to Shankman, these four levels of *dhyana* are "distinctive meditative states of high concentrations in which the mind becomes unified" (p. 32). The four levels of samadhi in the formless realm are the samadhi of boundless space, of boundless consciousness, of nothingness, and of neither-perception-nor-nonperception.

According to an ancient Buddhist story, when Gautama Buddha attained the highest stage of samadhi in the realm of formlessness (i.e., that of neither-perception-nor-nonperception), he brought himself back to the fourth level of *dhayna*. He did so because the fourth level of *dhayna* represents the optimal balance between meditation practice and samadhi while also capturing the Middle Way of not affirming self-centered desires as well as that of not falling into a pattern of excessive pursuit of samadhi through meditation practice.

Even after the death of Gautama Buddha, zazen training continued in Buddhism and has subsequently been transmitted through generations of Buddhist monks. It is also worth noting that zazen was integrated into various forms of spiritual training in India, including Buddhism, because it was believed to have a mystical power.

Generally speaking, it is said that Zen Buddhism was transmitted to China from India in the sixth century by Bodhidharma (菩提達磨; Bodai Daruma in Japanese) of India. In Zen Buddhism, Bodhidharma is regarded as the founder (i.e., the first patriarch) of Zen Buddhism as well as the 28th patriarch of Buddhism overall. From this perspective, China became the birthplace of Zen Buddhism as a religious organization when the teaching of Bodhidharma was transmitted to his Chinese disciple, Huike (慧可; Eka in Japanese; 487–593), who became the second patriarch of Zen Buddhism.

The philosophy of Zen Buddhism was said to fully develop during the time of the sixth patriarch, Huineng (慧能; Eno in Japanese; 638–713). Subsequently, Baizhang Huaihai (百丈懐海; Hyakujo Ekai in Japanese; 720–814) established the Pure Rules of Baizhang (百丈清規; *Hyakujo Shingi* in Japanese), an early set of rules for Zen monastic discipline, and Zen Buddhism rapidly grew to become a major religious and cultural force. Zen Buddhism faced a significant threat between the years of 845 and 846 when Chinese Emperor Wuzong persecuted and devastated Buddhist schools in an effort to cleanse China of foreign influences. However, some Zen schools survived as their practices did not rely on texts or sutras, and these became the leading sects of Chinese Zen.

Zen Buddhism was also transmitted to Korea from the seventh to ninth centuries, and subsequently to Japan in the twelfth century. In more recent years, Zen was transmitted from Asian areas to the West, and it has become a global phenomenon since. In attempting to understand "what Zen is," we must explore the significance of Chinese Zen in the development and proliferation of Zen worldwide.

Establishment of Zen Buddhism and Its Philosophy

As mentioned above, Zen can be traced originally to India, but Zen Buddhism as a major religious organization originated in China. Although Bodhidharma of India was said to have moved to China, disseminating his teachings through Huike, Zen was actually introduced to China gradually. Prior to the arrival of Bodhidharma, China had already been exposed to Zen meditation since 67 A.D., when Buddhism was first introduced to China. It is speculated that Chinese people were intrigued by Buddhism when it was introduced to them for the first time; this is less so because of its formal teachings and practices and more so a result of the mystic powers that the foreign monks of Buddhism were believed to possess. The Dunhuang manuscripts, a cache of important religious and secular documents discovered in China's Mogao Caves in the early twentieth century, uncovered hidden aspects of the complicated history of Zen Buddhism.

In terms of the history of Zen Buddhism, the Dunhuang manuscripts revealed that Heze Shenhui (荷沢神会; Kataku Jinne in Japanese, 684–758) played a crucial role in the establishment of Chinese Zen as a religious organization. Hu Shih (胡適; 1891–1962), a Chinese philosopher, essayist, and diplomat, studied Shenhui extensively (see McRae 2001). As described in McRae (2001), Hu Shih (1953) gave Shenhui the highest regard as the most successful evangelist in the history of Chinese Buddhism. Hu Shih also described Shenhui as both the persecutor of Indian Zen and the founder of the new type of Chinese Zen. According to McRae (2003), Shenhui fabricated the history of Zen as "a public exponent of the 'good news' of Chan" (p. 107). Seizan Yanagida (柳田聖山; 1922–2006), one the most important Japanese Buddhologists in the twentieth century, also discussed the significance of Shenhui extensively throughout his career (see McRae 1993).

As noted above, the discovery of the Dunhuang manuscripts elicited a revision of the history of Zen Buddhism. For example, Rinzai and Soto sects of Zen Buddhism previously considered the famous encounter between Bodhidharma and Emperor Wu (502–555) as a historical fact (see Ferguson 2011, pp. 14–16). This episode was included both in the Blue Cliff Record (碧巌録; Hekiganroku in Japanese) and in the Book of Equanimity (従容錄; Shōyōroku in Japanese), the fundamental scripts of Rinzai Zen (Linji School) and Soto Zen (Caodong School), respectively. However, this encounter is now considered a fiction created by Shenhui.

The Blue Cliff Record is a collection of koans originally compiled in China during the Song Dynasty in 1125, subsequently expanded into its present form by the Rinzai Zen master Yuanwu Keqin (1063–1135; 圜悟克勤; Engo Kokugon in Japanese). A *koan* (公案) is a story, dialogue, question, or statement, which is used in Zen practice to provoke enlightenment. The book includes Yuanwu's annotations and commentary on 100 Verses on Old Cases (頌古百則), a compilation of 100 koans collected by Xuedou Zhongxian (980–1052; 雪竇重顯, Setcho). The Book of Equanimity was compiled by Soto Zen master Wansong Xingxiu (万松行; 1166–1246), first published in 1224. The book comprises a collection of 100 koans written by the Soto Zen master Hongzhi Zhengjue (宏智正覺; 1091–1157), together with commentaries by Wansong.

In addition to the famous encounter between Bodhidharma and Emperor Wu, Shenhui appears to have created other legends about Bodhidharma, including nine years of wall gazing, Huike cutting off his arm to demonstrate his sincerity in receiving Bodhidharma's teaching, and Huike receiving a robe as the testimonial of the transmission of the True Way.

Hu Shih also emphasized that it was Shenhui who initially considered the robe as a symbol of the transmission of the Way to subsequent leaders, possibly initiating the concept and process of Patriarchal lineage. He also wrote the original text of the Sixth Patriarch's Dharma Jewel Platform Sutra (see Buddhist Text Translation Society 2001). Historically, Shenhui's apparent falsifications played a role in criticisms of Northern School teachings and the proliferation of the Southern School of Zen.

Today, Zen Buddhism generally regards Huineng of the Southern School as the sixth and last patriarch of Zen Buddhism (Dumoulin 2005; McRae 2003), largely as a result of Shenhui's influence in creating a split between the Northern and Southern Schools of Zen. Shenhui, of the Southern School, claimed that Huineng (also of the Southern School) was the legitimate heir of Zen Buddhism. At that time, Shenxiu (神秀; Jinshu in Japanese; unknown-706) of the Northern School was regarded as the heir of the fifth patriarch, Hongren (弘忍; Konin in Japanese; 601–674), and he and his students experienced widespread fame and status through the strong support by China's imperial court.

When Shenhui claimed that Huineng of the Southern School was the heir of the fifth patriarch in 720, he was largely ignored. However, when the An Lushan Rebellion (755–763) devastated northern China in an attempt to weaken the Tang Dynasty, Shenxui and the Northern School's influence was also significantly weakened. At the same time, Shenhui of the Southern School gained the power that the Northern School lost, and his assertions of Huineng as the sixth patriarch were legitimized. Shenhui subsequently proclaimed himself to be the seventh patriarch, the receiver of the robe from Huineng.

Huineng's Dharma Jewel Platform Sutra was one of the most widely read Zen Buddhist texts, particularly the version edited and published in 1291. As a result, many believed that the stories of Huineng cited in the Platform Sutra were historical facts. For example, in the text is a legendary poetry contest between Huineng (Southern School) and Shenxiu (Northern School) at the fifth patriarch's monastery at Huangmei. This episode, which was found to be fictional later in the early twentieth century, symbolized the emergence of the Southern School and the demise of the Northern School. Shenxiu's poem (McRae 2000, p. 20) goes:

> Body is the bodhi tree
> Heart is like clear mirror stand
> Strive to clean it constantly
> Do not let the dust motes land

In response to Shenxiu's poem, Huineng wrote (McRae 2000, p. 22) the following:

> Bodhi is originally without any tree;
> The bright mirror is also not a stand
> Originally there is not a single thing
> Where could any dust be attracted?

A detailed analysis of these poems is beyond the scope of this chapter. However, it is worthwhile to present a brief commentary on this poetry contest. In Zen's Chinese Heritage: The Masters and Their Teachings, a widely read book on Chinese Zen and its heritage, Andy Ferguson (2011) explains this episode:

> To better understand the doctrinal difference between Shenxiu's "Northern" and Huineng's "Southern" Zen, it would be useful to briefly introduce the Buddhist doctrine of "mind." The concept of "mind" is central to Zen, as well as other schools of Buddhist thought and philosophy. A Zen Buddhist teaching holds that there is but one universal "mind" that is constituted by the mind of all living beings. This universal mind is called "Buddha," "Buddha nature," "true self," and so on.
>
> But different schools of Zen and Buddhism had different interpretations about the teaching of mind and how it may be understood. Shenxiu's Northern School believed and advanced the position that there are "impurities" that can cloud the mind. These impurities include an individual's thoughts or interpretations, and any of which necessarily give rise to the illusion of an individual self. Therefore, a "mirror" analogy is applied to this type of understanding. The individual's small mind is likened to a "mirror" that reflects the entire universe. Delusion is an impurity, and the "dust" on the mirror that prevents the individual from maintaining his or her pure, original (and universal) mind.
>
> In contrast, the Southern School advanced the idea that there is no way to realize the nature of mind except through sudden realization, and this must be done quite apart from any ideas of "purity" or "impurity." Even the so-called "dust" on the

allegorical mirror must only be part of mind, so how can it be called "impure"? "Polishing" the mirror, or removing impurities through various practices, does not lead to a genuine realization of the nature of mind. This difference was at the heart of the poems attributed to Shenxiu and Huineng in the contest at Huangmei (pp. 49–50).

Ferguson (2011) also highlights the political significance of this episode in the Platform Sutra as follows:

In that competition, the lowly positioned Huineng proved to have superior spiritual insight, despite the fact that Shenxiu was Hongren's most senior student. This famous episode, well known in the religious folklore of East Asia, is the legendary seed of the growth of Zen into Northern (followers of Shenxiu) and Southern (followers of Huineng) schools. Twentieth-century scholarship has, to a large degree, undermined the evidence that this event really occurred. However, the story of the poetry contest at Huangmei remains informative, for it symbolizes the genuine doctrinal differences that many scholars believe divided the Northern and Southern Zen schools (p. 49).

This episode is also known for highlighting the contrast between the Northern School and the Southern School in their respective accounts of enlightenment. Shenxiu is said to emphasize gradual enlightenment (漸悟), whereas Huineng spoke of sudden enlightenment (頓悟). As such, the story in the Platform Sutra also implies the superiority of sudden enlightenment to gradual enlightenment. According to Hu Shih, Shenhui used this rhetoric to promote the Southern School of Zen and criticized Shenxiu and his lineage as a fundamentally illegitimate practice.

The sudden enlightenment advocated by Shenhui implies an innate nature of enlightenment; that is, we already have the Buddha nature. According to Suzuki (1996, 1997), the suddenness (頓) in the sudden enlightenment (頓悟) is not about the immediacy of time. Rather, it is of a breakthrough in logic and space. The Chinese character 頓 means "sudden," but in Chinese Zen Buddhism, the term also means "as it is" or "thusness." As such, instead of translating it as "sudden enlightenment," Shenhui's position of enlightenment could very well be translated as "original enlightenment," which is synonymous with *honkaku* (本覚; genuine enlightenment). Worth noting is that Hu Shih, who generally disagrees with Suzuki's account of Zen Buddhism, corroborated Shenhui's emphasis on the thusness.

Recent studies on Chinese Zen Buddhism and its heritage suggest that Shenhui's perspective on Zen is not actually distinct from that of the Northern School. In fact, it appears that Shenhui skillfully integrated the teachings of the Northern School into his own. Additionally, whereas Shenxiu was certainly the dominant figure within the Northern School of Zen, the broader teachings of the Northern School reflected diversity and complexity that was traditionally overlooked.

Despite the fictional aspects of Shenhiu's teachings, his influential contributions to Chinese Zen Buddhism remain significant (McRae 2001). His teaching of original enlightenment was considered a core teaching of Chinese Zen Buddhism during the Tang Dynasty (618–907), as well as the key teaching that eventually united all of Chinese Buddhists under the Sudden Enlightenment School.

In sum, the discovery of the Dunhuang manuscripts has offered a more complete history of early Chinese Zen Buddhism. In studying these writings, the focus was largely placed on the investigation of historical facts (e.g., whether episodes in old Zen texts actually occurred). As noted above, many of these episodes are found to be fictional or fabricated. However, as is the case in many religious and influential texts across many cultures, many have strongly advocated that wisdoms within these stories remain profound, despite the fact that the stories themselves are fictional; thus, we should appreciate the influential aspects of these narratives and refrain from shunning them immediately (see McRae 1993).

Chinese Zen Buddhism in Tang Dynasty (750–1000 AD)

Because of Shenhui's influence and the shifting power dynamics following the revolution, the Southern School of Zen emerged as the prominent Chinese Zen organization during the Tang Dynasty. However, Shenhui's line of Southern School teachings did not evolve into the dominant sect of Zen Buddhism. Instead, the lines of Qingyuan Xingsi (青原行思; Seigen Gyoshi in Japanese; 673–741) and Nanyue Huairang (南嶽懷讓; Nangaku Ejo in Japanese; 677–744), Shenhui's fellow disciples, became the major schools of Chinese Zen. Subsequently, Mazu Daoyi (馬祖道一; Baso Doitsu in Japanese; 709–788) and his disciples, such as Baizhang Huaihai (百丈懷海; Hyakujo Ekai in Japanese; 720–814), established the structure of Chinese Zen Buddhism as a major religious organization. Mazu was Nanyue Huairang's dharma heir.

The Bodhidharma line of Zen studied and followed the Lankavatara Sutra, one of the original sutras of Mahayana Buddhism, extensively. Mazu edited the Lankavatara Sutra, emphasizing sudden enlightenment in his teaching (Poceski 2015). In this text, Mazu attempts to make sense of important Zen concepts. For example, one of the most famous questions posed in Zen Buddhism is "What is the meaning of Bodhidharma's coming to China?" This question, canonically asked of Zen students, asks what Bodhidharma taught as well as what Zen teaches. This is how Mazu described the meaning of Zen by quoting the Lankavatara Sutra:

> Each one of you, you should believe that your own mind is the Buddha, that this mind is identical with the Buddha. The great master Bodhidharma came from India to China and transmitted the One Mind teaching of the supreme vehicle in order to cause you to realize awakening. He also quoted the Lankavatara Scripture, in order to imprint the minds of living beings, fearing that they are perturbed and lack faith themselves. The truth of this One Mind is something that each and every one of you possesses. Therefore, according to the Lankavatara Scripture, the Buddha's teaching asserts that the mind is the essential principle, and that the lack of a particular point of entry is the (very essence) of the (true) teaching" (Poceski 2015, p. 83).

The teaching of One Mind in this passage is analogous to the teaching of original enlightenment. Similarly, Mazu also taught that our ordinary, everyday behavior can manifest the Buddha Way. He stated:

> The Way needs no [special methods of spiritual] cultivation—all you need to do is put an end to [engendering all sorts of] defilements. What are defilements? If you have a mind [mired in the circle] of birth and death, and are engaged in deliberate acts and have [self-centered] ambitions, then everything [you do] is defilement. If you want to directly know the Way, then ordinary mind is the Way. Ordinary mind denotes [a state of mind in which there is] no [deliberate] action, no [ideas about] right and wrong, no grasping and discarding, no [notion of] annihilation and permanence, no ordinary and sacred. The scripture says, "Unlike the practice of ordinary people, and like the practice of sages—that is the practice of bodhisattvas." At this very moment, as you engage in walking, standing, sitting, or reclining, and as you respond to [various] situations and deal with [other] people—everything [you do and encounter] is the Way (Poceski 2015, p. 301).

In summarizing Mazu's teachings, it is important to note that what he meant by mind is not what we usually understand as mind. What he means is the act of a whole person interacting fully with his or her surroundings and other individuals in a given moment. For Mazu, the enlightenment or the Way is not somewhere "else," but in the very moment of one's life. It is this mind that blends everyday living and the Way into the original oneness. The following is an episode that summarizes the teaching of Mazu.

> One day Mazu addressed the congregation, saying, "All of you here! Believe that your own mind is Buddha. This very mind is buddha mind. When Bodhidharma came from India to China he transmitted the supreme vehicle teaching of One Mind, allowing people like you to attain awakening. Moreover, he brought with him the text of the Lankavatara Sutra, using it as the seal of the mind-ground of sentient beings. He feared that your views would be inverted, and you wouldn't believe in the teaching of this mind that each and every one of you possesses. Therefore [Bodhidharma brought] the Lankavatara Sutra, which offers the Buddha's words that mind is the essence—and that there is no gate by which to enter Dharma. You who seek Dharma should seek nothing. Apart from mind there is no other Buddha. Apart from Buddha there is no other mind. Do not grasp what is good nor reject what is bad. Don't lean toward either purity or pollution. Arrive

> at the empty nature of transgressions; that nothing is attained through continuous thoughts; and that because there is no self-nature the three worlds are only mind. The myriad forms of the entire universe are the seal of the single Dharma. Whatever forms are seen are but the perception of mind. But mind is not independently existent. It is codependent with form. You should speak appropriately about the affairs of your own life, for each matter you encounter constitutes the meaning of your existence, and your actions are without hindrance. The fruit of the bodhisattva way is just thus, born of mind, taking names to be forms. Because of the knowledge of the emptiness of forms, birth is nonbirth. Comprehending this, one acts in the fashion of one's time, just wearing clothes, eating food, constantly upholding the practices of a bodhisattva, and passing time according to circumstances. If one practices in this manner is there anything more to be done? (Ferguson 2011, p. 75)

When Zen Buddhism was first transmitted from India to China, Chinese people were intrigued by the mystical powers associated with it, rather than its actual teachings. However, as Zen Buddhism became rooted into the Chinese soil, such an image was naturally faded. What made Chinese people attracted to Zen was its teaching of ordinary, and yet wholehearted way of living. A quote by Layman Pang (龐居士; Hokoji in Japanese; 740–808), a nonmonastic student of Mazu, is known to highlight this point. It goes:

> How miraculous and wondrous,
> Hauling water and carrying firewood (Ferguson 2011, p. 109)

According to Layman Pang, there is no act that reflects the Buddha Way more than activities crucial for everyday living, such as hauling water and carrying firewood at his time. Linji Yixuan (臨済義玄; Rinzai Gigen in Japanese; died 866 CE), the founder of the Linji School of Zen Buddhism, further refined the importance of everyday and ordinary living as the core teaching of "人" (*nin* in Japanese; being a person). The teaching of *nin* reflects the continuous practice (the true self) that is not entangled with anything. It is to pee and poo, wear clothes, and eat without being caught up by delusions. Linji used the term "無事人;one who has nothing to do" to describe the fully enlightened person, then stated:

> [He who has] nothing to do is the noble one. Simply don't strive—just be ordinary (see Sasaki and Kirchner 2008, pp. 178–179).

Zen is not based on analysis, differentiation, or logic. In *Genjokoan* (現成公案; sometimes translated as Actualization of Reality), Dogen Zenji (道元禅師; 1200–1253), the founder of the Soto School of Zen in Japan, quoted an episode of Baoche of Mt. Mayu (麻谷宝徹), a student of Mazu, to highlight this point. The episode goes:

> Zen master Baoche of Mt. Mayu was fanning himself. A monk approached and said, "Master, the nature of wind is permanent and there is no place it does not reach. Why, then, do you fan yourself?"
> "Although you understand that the nature of the wind is permanent," Baoche replied, "you do not understand the meaning of its reaching everywhere."
> "What is the meaning of its reaching everywhere?" asked the monk again. The master just kept fanning himself. The monk bowed deeply.
> The actualization of the buddha-dharma, the vital path of its correct transmission, is like this (Dogen and Tanahashi 1985, pp. 72–73).

Then, Dogen continued with his commentary:

> If you say that you do not need to fan yourself because the nature of wind is permanent and you can have wind without fanning, you will understand neither permanence nor the nature of wind. The nature of wind is permanent; because of that, the wind of the buddha's house brings for the gold of the earth and makes fragrant the cream of the long river (Dogen and Tanahashi 1985, p. 73).

Worth nothing is the contribution of Baizhang Huaihai, the dharma heir of Mazu. As noted above, he was said to establish a set of rules for Chan (Chinese Zen) monastic discipline, known as the Pure Rules of Baizhang (百丈清規; *Hyakujo Shingi* in Japanese), and reinforced the independence of Zen Buddhism as a major religious and cultural force. Within the Pure Rules of Baizhang, the most notable is the establishment of group work (普請; *fushin* in Japanese). Fushin meant "to assemble people" for labor. The establishment of this rule was significant because productive labor was strictly prohibited in early Indian Buddhism. The rule of *fushin* with the emphasis on self-sufficiency and daily labor (e.g., farming) became a regular aspect of the monastic life. "Day of no working—a day of no eating" by Baizhang is the most famous quote derived from this outlook (see Sasaki and Kirchner 2008, pp. 320–321).

Furthermore, contemporary to Mazu, there was Shitou Xiqian (石頭希遷; Sekito Kisen in Japanese; 700–790). Shitou was a disciple of Huineng's successor, Qingyuan Xingsi. Later in the line of Shitou, Dongshan Liangjie (洞山良价; Tozan Ryokai in Japanese; 807–869) founded the Caodong School (曹洞宗). The Caodong School of Zen was transmitted to Japan in the thirteenth century by Dogen and developed into the Soto School of Zen.

In his writings, Dogen quoted Dongshan more than anyone else. Dongshan's Zen emphasized the continuous practice without the desire of gaining something, even the experience of enlightenment. This continuous practice is often contrasted with the practice of sudden enlightenment taught in the Linji School of Zen. Consistent with Linji, Dongshan and Dogen stated that every one of us has the Buddha nature, nevertheless. Dongshan and Dogen then said that the students of Zen must not become settled with one-time experience of enlightenment: Instead, they must continue to strive for the Buddha Way.

Zen Buddhism in Song Dynasty (960–1279)

Generally speaking, the development and expansion of Zen Buddhism during the Tang Dynasty is summarized and called "Five Houses of Chan (Zen)." *Bendowa* (辨道話; Discourse on the Practice of the Way), which was completed by Dogen in 1231 AD immediate after his return from China, described the Five Houses of Zen in the context of Zen history. He stated:

> There were two great disciples under the Sixth Ancestor: Ejo of Nangaku and Gyoshi of Seigen. Both of them transmitted and maintained Buddha mandra and were guiding teachings for all beings. As these two streams of the dharma flowed and permeated widely, the five gates opened: the Hogen, Igyo, Soto, Unmon, and Rinzai schools. These days in Song China, only the Rinzai school is present everywhere (see Dogen et al. 1997, p. 21).

Hogen, Igyo, Soto, Unmon, and Rinzai are Japanese names for the five schools of Zen. Following a Chinese pronunciation, these schools are often called the Fayan (法眼), Guiyang (潙仰), Caodong (曹洞), Yunmen (雲門), and Linji (臨濟) schools in English, respectively. As noted above, Linji (Rinzai) became the most dominant house of Zen Buddhism during the Song Dynasty, and it blanched out to the Huanglong line (黄龍派) and Yangqi line (楊岐派). Given these two blanches, Chinese Zen during that time of Song Dynasty is also called The Five Houses and Seven Schools of Zen (五家七宗). Toward the end of Song Dynasty, only Linji (Rinzai) and Caodong (Soto) schools remained in Asia, including China and Japan (Ishii 1987).

Linji and Caodong schools in the Song Dynasty are characterized by Kanna-Zen (看話禅 in Japanese; koan-introspecting Zen) and Mokusho-Zen (黙照禅 in Japanese; Silent Illumination Zen), respectively. Kanna-Zen, which was formalized by Dahui Zonggao (大慧宗杲; Daie Soko in Japanese; 1089–1163), is a koan-based method of Zen Buddhism, and Mokusho-Zen, which was matured by Hongzhi Zhengjue (宏智正覺; Wanshi Shogaku in Japanese; 1091–1157), is known as the practice of just sitting with silence. Of the two, Mokuso-Zen was matured first.

Hongzhi stated that silent illumination was the most authentic expression of Buddha Way. According to the teaching of Silent Illumination Zen, the Buddha nature naturally unfolds through continuous practice, as if a light naturally begins to illuminate in darkness. As such, zazen itself considered the state of enlightenment, the Buddha Way, and the true self. Dumoulin (2005) summarized Hongzhi's Silent Illumination Zen as follows:

> In his view: silent illumination was the most authentic expression of the tradition that had come down from the Buddhas and the patriarchs: To one who forgets the words in silence reality is clearly revealed… Silence is the stillness that grounds the

> enlightened mind, whose natural ability to "shine" is revealed in silence. Reality reveals itself to those sitting in silence mediation without leading them to look on things as objects of intellection. Enlightenment is like the mirror-quality of the enlightened and resplendent Buddha mind (p. 256).

Conversely, Dahui of Kanna-Zen was less enthusiastic about the Silent Illumination Zen. In fact, Dahui is sometimes the best known for calling the Silent Illumination Zen as "silent illumination false Zen (默照邪禪)." Kanna-Zen that he established was his efforts to correct misunderstandings associated with the Silent Illumination Zen. Concerned about the potential pitfalls of Silent Illumination Zen practice (i.e., just-sitting Zen), Dahui criticized the Silent Illumination Zen as follows:

> Recently a type of heterodox Zen… has been grown up in the forest of Zen. By confusing the sickness with the remedy, they have denied the experience of enlightenment. These people think that the experience of enlightenment is but an artificial superstructure meant to attract, so they give it a secondary position, like branches or leaves on the tree. Because they have not experienced enlightenment, they think others have not either. Stubbornly they continued that an empty silence and a musty state of unconsciousness is the original realm of the absolute. To eat their rice twice a day and sit without thoughts in mediation is what they call complete peace (see Dumoulin 2005, p. 257).

Historically speaking, Kanna-Zen of Dahui is said to have established in 1134 when Dahui explicitly criticized the Silent Illumination Zen, particularly the teachings of Zhenxie Qingliao (真歇清了; Shinketsu Seiryo in Japanese; 1088–1151), a senior fellow of Hongzhi (see Ishii 1987, 2016; Schlutter 2010). The core of the controversy was at the *actualization of* enlightenment within the teaching of original enlightenment (Ishii 2016; Schlutter 2010).

Consistent with the Silent Illumination Zen, Dahui acknowledged the original enlightenment (e.g., Buddha nature) in every one of us. However, he argued that having the original enlightenment does not mean that one naturally actualizes it. In Dahui's eyes, the followers of silent illumination confused the actualization of enlightenment with original enlightenment (Ishii 2016). Dahui argued that, to actualize enlightenment, it is crucial for one to wholeheartedly face a great doubt and break through it. To legitimize this point, Dahui pointed out the fact that even the Original Buddha had to undergo the experience of great doubt before he *recognized* his own true nature (Ishii 2016; Schlutter 2010). For Dahui, the Silent Illumination Zen minimized the significance of great doubt as well as importance of practice (i.e., breaking through the doubt) as they confused the original enlightenment with the actualization of enlightenment into one (e.g., "you're already enlightened, so don't worry, and just sit"). Dahui stated that "it is meaningless to talk about an original state of enlightenment before delusion has been overcome and enlightenment realized" (Schlutter 2010, p. 120).

For Dahui, *koan* practice is a crucial way for recognizing enlightenment through overcoming greater doubts. According to Dumoulin (2005), no other Chinese Zen master understood so completely or promoted so vigorously the use of *koan* as Dahui. Many of us today are often gravitated toward *koans* for their literal provocation or deep intellectual paradox. However, the core of a *koan*, according to Dahui, is to make its central point through doubt: Enlightenment draws meaning and value from a great feeling of doubt. Dahui stated:

> Just steadily go on with your *koan* every moment of your life. If a thought rises, do not attempt to suppress it by conscious effort, only renew the attempt to keep the *koan* before the mind. Whether walking or sitting, let your attention be fixed upon it without interruption! When you begin to find it entirely devoid of flavor, the final moment is approaching, do not let it slip out of your grasp. When all of a sudden something flashes out in your mind, its light will illuminate the entire universe and you will see the spiritual land of the Enlightened One fully revealed at the point of a single hair, and the great wheel of the Dharma revolving in a single grain of dust (Dumoulin 2005, p. 257).

He also stated the process of *koan* practice as follows:

> The thousand and ten thousand doubts that well up in your breast are really only one doubt, all of them burst open when doubt is resolved in the *koan*. As

> long as the *koan* is not resolved, you must occupy yourself with it to the utmost. If you give up on your *koan* and stir up another doubt about a word of scripture or about a sutra teaching or about a *koan* of the ancients, or if you allow a doubt about worldly matters to come up—all this means to be joined to the evil spirit. You should not too easily agree with a *koan* solution that you have discovered, nor should you think about it further and make distinctions. Fasten your attention to where discursive thinking cannot reach. Make sure that you do not allow your mind to run off, like on old mouse that ran into the horn of an ox (Dumoulin 2005, pp. 257–258).

The *koan* that Dahui used the most was Zhaozhou's Wu (Ferguson 2011, p. 153). It goes:

> A monk asked Zhaozhou, "Does a dog have Buddha nature?"
> Zhaozhou answered, "Wu! [in Japanese, 'Mu']"

Although Zhaozhou was a Zen master of the Tang Dynasty, Dahui was that of the Song Dynasty, this *mondo* (e.g., Zen dialogue) of Zhaozhou was used as a well-known *koan* during the Song Dynasty. Dahui stated that one must focus on this *koan*, while letting go of all logical and analytic ways of thinking and continue to leap into it. Dahui explained this *koan* further:

> This one character is the rod by which many false images and ideas are destroyed in their very foundations. To it you should add no judgments about being or non-being, no arguments, no bodily gestures like raising your eyebrows or blinking your eyes. Words has no place here. Neither should you throw this character away into the nothingness of emptiness, or seek it in the comings and goings of the mind, or try to trace its origins in the scriptures. You must only earnestly and continually stir it [this *koan*] around the clock. Sitting or lying, walking or standing, you must give yourself over to it constantly. "Does a dong have the Buddha-nature? The answer: "Mu." Without withdrawing from everyday life, keep trying, keeping looking at this koan! (Dumoulin 2005, p. 258)

Finally, Dahui left the following comment to the students of Zen Buddhism.

> Many students today do not doubt themselves, but they doubt others. And so it is said: "Within great doubt there necessarily exists great enlightenment." (see Dumoulin 2005, p. 258)

Conclusions

Many schools of Zen established across the world today have their origins traced back to Chinese Zen developed during the Song Dynasty. For example, Rinzai Zen of Japan is nothing but the Kanna-Zen. Soto Zen of Japan (i.e., Dogen Zen) adheres to the teachings of Mokusho-Zen (Silent Illumination Zen). Core teachings of different Zen schools can be understood in terms of the significance of enlightenment, practice, and its relations (Ishii 2016). As such, the core teachings of Zen discussed in this chapter as well as this entire volume can be summarized as follows:

(A) Zen during the Dang Dynasty: We are inherently Buddhas. As such, all of our activities are the manifestation of enlightenment.
(B) Dogen Zen: One must practice zazen because we are inherently Buddhas. The Buddha nature naturally unfolds when we do zazen.
(C) Kanna-Zen: We are inherently Buddhas, but we must realize it by breaking through the great doubt.

Finally, as the summary above suggests, Zen is often understood as the practice of enlightenment. That being said, I think that Dogen Zen is distinct from other Zen schools in that sense (Ishii 1991). If you are interested in my account of Dogen Zen, please read my paper, titled "Characteristics of Bodhidharma Zen in Japan"(Ishii 2002). Please note that that book is written in Japanese and not yet translated into English.

References

Buddhist Text Translation Society. (2001). *The Sixth Patriarch's Dharma Jewel Platform Sutra*. Burlingame, CA, USA: Buddhist Text Translation Society.
Daoyuan, S., & Whitfield, R. S. (2015). *Records of the transmission of the lamp: Volume I the Buddhas and Indian Patriarchs*. New York: Books on Demand.

Dogen, E., & Tanahashi, K. (1985). *Moon in a dewdrop: Writings of Zen master Dogen*. New York, US: North Point Press.

Dogen, E., Uchiyama, K., Okumura, S., & Leighton, T. D. (1997). *The wholehearted way: A translation of Eihei Dogen's Bendowa with commentary by Kosho Uchiyama Roshi*. North Clarendon, VT, US: Tuttle Publications.

Dumoulin, H. (2005). *Zen Buddhism: A history Volume 1: India and China*. Bloomington, Indiana US: World Wisdom.

Ferguson, A. (2011). *Zen's Chinese heritage: The masters and their teachings*. Somerville MA, US: Wisdom Publications.

Ishii, S. (1987). *The study of Zen Buddhism in Song Dynasty: Caodong School of Zen in China and Dogen Zen, 16*, 123–152.

Ishii, S. (1991). Study on the history of the establishment of Dogen Zen.

Ishii, S. (2002). The characteristics of the Japanese Daruma Sect. *The Annual Report of Researches of Matsugaoka Bunko, 16*, 123–152.

Ishii, S. (2016). Kanna Zen of Dahui Zonggao. Paper presented at *the 4th International Conference Ganhwa Seon*.

Japan Buddhist Federation. (1978). *Understanding Japanese Buddhism*.

McRae, J. R. (1993). Yanagida Seizan's landmark works on Chinese Ch'an. *Cahiers d'Extrême-Asie, 7*, 51–103.

McRae, J. R. (2000). *The platform Sutra of the Sixty Patriarch*. Berkeley, CA USA: Murata Center for Buddhist Translation and Research.

McRae, J. R. (2001). Religion as revolution in Chinese Historiography: Hu Shi (1891–1962) on Shen-Hui (684–758). *Cahiers d'Extrême-Asie, 12*, 59–102.

McRae, J. R. (2003). *Seeing through Zen: Encounter, transformation, and genealogy in Chinese Chan Buddhism*. Berkeley, CA, USA: University of California Press.

Poceski, M. (2015). *The records of Mazu and the making of classical Chan literature*. New York, USA: Oxford University Press.

Sasaki, R. F., & Kirchner, T. Y. (2008). *The record of Linji*. Honolulu, HI, US: University of Hawaii Press.

Schlutter, M. (2010). *How Zen became Zen: The dispute over enlightenment and the formation of Chan Buddhism in Song-Dynasty China*. Honolulu, HI, US: University of Hawaii Press.

Shankman, R. (2008). *The experience of Samadhi: An in-depth exploration of Buddhist mediation*. Boston, MA, US: Shambhala.

Shih, H. (1953). Ch'an (Zen) Buddhism in China its history and method. *Philosophy East and West, 3*(1), 3–24. doi:10.2307/1397361.

Suzuki, D. T. (1996). *Zen Buddhism: Selected writings of D. T. Suzuki*. New York, US: An Image Book.

Suzuki, D. T. (1997). *Eastern Perspective [Toyoteki na mikata]*. Tokyo, Japan: Iwanami Shoten.

Zen and Japanese Culture

Akihiko Masuda

Keywords
Zen · Buddhism · Japanese culture · Epistemology of Zen · Japanese linguistic practices

Overview

Many scholars, both in Japan and in the West, point out the interwoven relation between Zen and Japanese culture. In the West, Japanese culture is often considered the direct opposite of Western culture (Hamaguchi 1985; Markus and Kitayama 1991, 2010; Weisz et al. 1984). Whereas Western culture is viewed as the culture of independent and autonomous self, Japanese culture is considered that of interdependent self, seeing relations with others and what surrounds the self as vital determinants of self (Hamaguchi 1985; Markus and Kitayama 2010). Western culture is said to encourage first-order control coping strategies (e.g., direct attempts to conquer a targeted problem), and Japanese culture values second-order control strategies, characterized by efforts to coexist and harmonize with the events of focus (Weisz et al. 1984). In the West, nature is often perceived as an obstacle to be overcome, and in Japan, it is one with which people identify (Suzuki 1996; Watanabe 1974). Despite globalization and the growing influence of the West, many Japanese cultural practices remain intact. And, these cultural practices in Japan may still be quite peculiar for Westerners.

According to Buddhist scholars (Japan Buddhist Federation 1978), Zen has played a crucial role in forming Japanese culture, and vice versa. In explaining its profound impact on Japanese people, Suzuki (2010) states in *Zen and Japanese Culture* that:

> It is a significant fact that the other schools of Buddhism have limited their sphere of influence almost entirely to the spiritual life of the Japanese people; Zen has gone beyond it. Zen has entered internally into every phase of the cultural life of the people (p. 21).

Even today, Zen teachings are infused in the daily lives of most Japanese people. This is perhaps because Zen has permeated deeply into Japanese cultural wisdoms (e.g., "gratitude toward the very thing offered to you"), being transmitted and valued through generations. At the same time, Zen has shaped itself socioculturally into its present form, one in which Japanese people feel intimately identified (Kasulis 1981; Suzuki 2010).

A. Masuda (✉)
University of Hawaii at Manoa, Honolulu, USA
e-mail: amasuda4@hawaii.edu

A. Masuda and W.T. O'Donohue (eds.), *Handbook of Zen, Mindfulness, and Behavioral Health*, Mindfulness in Behavioral Health, DOI 10.1007/978-3-319-54595-0_3

Knowing Japanese culture is particularly relevant for Westerners who are interested in Zen for several reasons. First, as described in detail elsewhere in this volume, Japanese Zen has been among the earliest influences of Buddhism in the West. Zen became well recognized due to the writings of Japanese Zen teachers, such as D.T. Suzuki (1870–1966) and Shunryu Suzuki (1904–1971) in the 1900s. Interestingly, despite the existence of diverse sects of Buddhism, Zen has become a prominent focus of study for Western scholars and behavioral health professionals (Muramoto 1985, 2002). Although American Zen has evolved into diversified and unique forms, many of its core teachings seem to remain rooted in Japanese Zen.

Second, Japanese cultural practices illuminate an alternative way of experiencing and making sense of the self and the world. Zen states that we must go beyond our habitual ways of thinking in order to embody "the Buddha way" (Suzuki 1996), or what Tanahashi and Levitt call the "original wholeness" (Tanahashi and Levitt 2013). According to Markus and Kitayama (1991), most of what we, as Westerners, know about human nature and our culture is based on the "view of the individual as an independent, self-contained, autonomous entity who (a) comprise a unique configuration of internal attributes (e.g., traits, abilities, motives, and values) and (b) behave primarily as a consequence of these internal attributes" (p. 224). Although a Japanese worldview may not precisely embody the original wholeness, learning an alternative way to experience the self and the world, such as the one in Japanese culture, loosens clinging to one's fundamental assumptions of the self and the world (Wright 1992).

Third, some functional and topographical features of Japan's sociolinguistic environment seem to support a wholehearted way of living. As Skinner (1974), the father of radical behaviorism, argued, the activities of a person can be understood as the function of his or her historical and situational environment (e.g., learning history) combined with his or her genetic endowment. For humans, environments are mainly social and interpersonal, and it is our sociocultural environments that shape and maintain the way we think, feel, and behave (Nisbett et al. 2001). As such, elucidating some key features of Japanese language and cultural practices may point to the way in which a community is built to support the wholehearted way of living. "Wholehearted way," here refers to "the self becoming one with what he or she does, while blending into his or her surrounding."

Fourth and finally, some Japanese cultural practices may be closer approximations of the Zen way of living (Dogen et al. 1997; Suzuki 1970). As the spirit of Zen teachings goes beyond a mediation room, this wholehearted way of living can be expressed in every facet of daily life. While we Westerners tend to apply Zen teachings to limited life domains, such as when we feel stuck with difficult feelings and narratives, Japanese people are taught to strive for a wholehearted way in every waking moment.

The purpose of this chapter is to present some, but certainly not all, features of Japanese cultural context that seem to promote or support the way of living that reflects the heart of Zen. To do so, I will focus mainly on notable features of Japanese sociolinguistic context (e.g., verbal community) that maintain cultural wisdoms linked to Zen. This chapter will focus less on Japanese arts, poems, tea ceremony, and skilled practices (e.g., martial arts), as these cultural practices and their links to Zen are discussed extensively elsewhere (Suzuki 2010; Watanabe 1974).

Japanese Zen and Japanese Culture

Viewing Zen as being monolithic is somewhat misleading, at least formally (Monteiro et al. 2015). In fact, there are diverse sects of Zen in Japan, such as Rinzai, Soto, and Obaku. Despite apparent differences, these sects of Zen coexist somewhat harmoniously without the sectarian or religious conflicts observed elsewhere (e.g., Protestantism vs. Catholicism in Ireland). This trend of diversity and harmony is at least partially attributable to the adaptive nature of Buddhism as well as its worldview of impermanence (e.g., "all things are constantly changing") and the

Dharma of dependent arising (e.g., "all things arise in dependence upon other things"). Young-Eisendrath and Muramoto (2002) highlight this feature of Buddhism below:

> No religion is more able than Buddhism to adjust to, and assimilate, the prevailing ideologies of its adopted cultures. The Buddhism of each country where it is practiced is characteristic of that society and culture: Indian Buddhism was speculative and logical through its interaction with Hindu philosophy; Chinese Buddhism was practiced under the influence of Taoism and Confucianism; and Japanese Buddhism is aesthetic and merged with nature worship under the influence of Shintoism (p. 9).

Transmitting from India to China, and then from China to Japan, Zen has shaped itself into its unique forms through assimilating into Japanese cultural context, which in turn has shaped Japanese culture. What, then, does Japanese Zen look like? Gergen (1983) described Japanese Zen as follows:

> The Zen tradition offers a variety of means toward human well-being. Foremost among these, of course, is meditation, or the practice of za-zen. Although there are variations in mode, za-zen typically requires the devotee to sit for a long periods with legs crossed, hands resting on the lap, body erect, eyes open, and with regulated breathing and the mind peculiarly focused to search unselfconsciously for an unexcelled awaking. Within Zendo, or prayer room, of the Zen monastery, the devotee may further be subject to an occasional thwacking with a large stick carried by his instructor. The presence of the stick keeps one's mind on his task and inhibits drowsing.
> It would be a mistake to equate the Zen means to personal fulfillment with a stringent form of meditation. Not only are there a variety of other types of meditation, far less demanding than what is required for priesthood, but many additional modes of enhancement exist as well. Practices emphasizing harmony with one's environment, control over one's actions, and the suspension of analytic thought have played a highly important role in the Zen tradition. They are more evident in the practice of the formal tea ceremony, the art of calligraphy, flower arranging, pottery making and archery…
> Added to these activities are attempts at the elementalism in the course of one's daily activities. In the food one eats, or its very pattern in the plate on which it is served, in the decoration (or lack of it) with which one surrounds oneself, in the sounds with which one chooses to live, or in the pattern of a day's activities, the attempt is to orient oneself to elemental and essential aspects of nature and oneself within nature. One may discover the universe in a single rock, the lone clap of a bamboo water gong, or in a drop of dew. And finally, we must add to these various means of personal fulfillment the large volumes of philosophy, art, and poetry, which attempt to instruct both through word and sense experience. The "Zen way" is not specifically a way of mediation; it is more adequately viewed as an entire way of life (Gergen 1983, pp. 130–131).

Gergen (1983) made this statement over 30 years ago. However, the contents in this statement parallel the intriguing and yet peculiar image of Zen that many Westerners hold today.

Rinzai Zen and Soto Zen: Two Major Sects of Zen in Japan

As noted above, Zen was brought to Japan from China during the Kamakura period (1185–1338 A.D.). This was the dawn of Samurai, who honored self-discipline, loyalty, and the dharma of impermanence. Today, there are two major sects of Zen in Japan (Japan Buddhist Federation 1978); Rinzai Zen, founded in 1191 A.D. by Eisai, and Soto Zen, brought to Japan in 1224 A. D. by Dogen. Japanese Soto Zen is also called Dogen Zen because his teaching of *shikantaza* (just sitting) is somewhat distinct from the Chinese Soto school of Zen.

Having its root in Mahayana tradition, the goal of Zen is said to be self-enlightenment (i.e., embodiment of true self or nature) or the perfection of self through the self with an earnest endeavor for the benefit of mankind and all sentient beings (Japan Buddhist Federation 1978). Because Zen emphasizes the importance of the details of one's own daily life, its teachings spread among a wide range of secular domains (Japan Buddhist Federation 1978; Suzuki 2010). Traditionally, Rinzai Zen has appealed to many intellectuals and members of the ruling class (Varley 2000). It is Rinzai Zen that has had a profound influence on traditional Japanese arts (e.g., tea and flowers) and swordsmanship. On the other hand, Soto Zen has spread widely among the common people (Hanayama 1978, p. 19).

Interestingly, these features of Rinzai Zen and Soto Zen parallel two well-known Japanese figures influential to the emergence of Zen in the USA: D.T. Suzuki of Rinzai and Shunryu Suzuki of Soto. Following the Rinzai school of Zen, D. T. Suzuki's Zen is dynamic and charismatic. His writing on a sudden breakthrough into enlightenment has mesmerized many Westerners. Masculinity is also a characteristic that is associated with Rinzai Zen. This association is attributable to D.T. Suzuki's writing on Zen and its link to the way of samurai (Suzuki 2010), as well as to Sogen Omori (1904–1994), the founder of Chozen-ji in Hawaii, the first Rinzai headquarters temple established outside Japan. Omori Roshi is well known for his distinct approach to Zen practice integrating insights from his martial and fine arts training with traditional Zen training (Hosokawa 1999; Omori 2001).

On the other hand, Soto Zen is more or less viewed as an ordinary and down-to-earth version of Zen, perhaps because of Shunryu Suzuki and the personal characteristics observed in his writings. His writings (Suzuki 1970, 2002) are profound but also include a number of humorous personal episodes to which many can easily relate.

There are notable stylistic differences between Rinzai Zen and Soto Zen, such as Rinzai's emphasis on the role of *koan* (公案; a paradoxical anecdote or riddle) and Soto's focus on the importance of *zazen* (坐禅; sitting meditation). However, both stress the importance of embodying and experiencing oneness or wholeness. In Zen literature, terms such as enlightenment, Satori, Samadhi, Buddha Way, transcendence, true self, emptiness, and wholeheartedness, to name a few, are used to describe this subjective experience of oneness. According to many Zen practitioners (Dogen et al. 2011; Okumura 2010), there is nothing sensational, liberating, or mystical about the experience of oneness or wholeness. It is as if one simply becomes settled into the here-and-now as a whole person, becoming one with the context (Magid 2002). Suzuki (1996) called this "pure subjectivity" (p. 240). As noted above, the experience of wholeness, or a wholehearted way of living, can be expressed in many behavioral forms, including activities that we engage in every day such as eating, washing your face, talking to a colleague, or watching a child growing.

Unlike our wishful hope, the experience of oneness or wholeness does not make a person wiser or happier. As revealed numerous times in this volume, even experienced Zen practitioners continue to experience pain and suffering throughout their lives. Kodo Sawaki (1880–1965), a prominent Japanese Soto Zen teacher of the twentieth century, stated that "Zen is good for nothing" (Uchiyama and Okumura 2014). Nishiari Bokusan (1821–1910), the father of the modern Soto Sect, described enlightenment in his commentary on a passage in Dogen's *Genjokoan* (現成公案; sometimes translated as Actualization of Reality) as follows:

> We normally talk about enlightenment this and enlightenment that, but what do we actually regard as enlightenment? I want you to fully understand this point (the immovable principle of enlightenment). To regard one person's one-time experience of realization, or an insight leading to a prediction of the future, as enlightenment is absolutely demonic. When we have a true enlightenment there is not even a speck of what you thought was enlightenment (see Dogen et al. 2011, p. 51 for Nishiari's comment).

He then states:

> … to be enlightened is no other than fully experiencing the self and fully experiencing myriad dharma. The self and myriad dharmas are originally one thusness. There is no self apart from myriad dharmas. There is no myriad dharmas apart from the self. Therefore, when dharma is actualized, the ten directions are comprehended. It is essential in the practice to "fully experience one dharma." In whichever practice, it is good to solidly master one dharma. When we fully experience the self, it is not betrayed by myriad dharmas. When we fully experience myriad dharmas, the self drops off spontaneously (Dogen et al. 2011, p. 55).

What Nishiari referred to as myriad dharmas above is what Suzuki (1996) referred to as Nature, "all that constitutes what is commonly known as Man's objective world" (p. 231). Fully experiencing the self and fully experiencing myriad dharma is to become one with what shows up as an experience as if the whole self is melted into the experience.

Zen Account of Linguistic Practice

Rinzai and Soto schools of Zen discuss human *linguistic process* extensively. What is referred to as linguistic process here is also called mind, dualism (dualistic thinking), essentialism, preconception, ordinary habits of thinking, Western worldview, and ego, to name a few, in both classic and contemporary Zen literature. Following D.T. Suzuki's account (1997), the present chapter roughly defines it as the process of cognitively and arbitrarily dividing a collective or whole experience intro pieces, labeling each piece, differentiating it from others, thus resulting in conflicts among them. D.T. Suzuki also stated that these analytical features of linguistic processes are particularly salient in Western cultures. Recent psychological science literature (Markus and Kitayama 2010; Nisbett et al. 2001) corroborates this claim that Suzuki made over 80 years ago.

When reading Zen literature, statements such as "Zen rejects language," or "one must transcend language in order to gain enlightenment," are frequently encountered. Following a conventionally Western way of thinking, we are likely to presuppose that Zen practice is the tool to rid that linguistic obstacle. However, many Zen practitioners and scholars caution us not to draw such a hasty conclusion (Suzuki 1970, 1996; Uchiyama and Okumura 2014). In short, being human means being fully situated within a particular sociolinguistic community (Park 2002; Skinner 1974). As shown in behavioral science literature (Hayes et al. 2001; Wilson et al. 2000; Wright 1992), the complete cessation or avoidance of language, especially trying to do so intentionally, is not possible. To Zen, enlightenment is the embracing of oneness experientially and intuitively, which includes our linguistic practice as well as its product, such as a narrowly perceived sense of self. Enlightenment is to do what one does fully in a given moment (Suzuki 2002), while being relatively less determined by conventional language and cultural practice (Kasulis 1981; Wright 1992). In other words, enlightenment cannot be defined by the absence of these "toxic" linguistic processes.

What does it mean to be less determined by conventional language and cultural practice? Another way to conceptualize this stance is to "relate to our linguistic processes wisely," and to "take them lightly." D.T. Suzuki's words help us to feel the transition from a conventional way of thinking to "pure subjectivity," as well as helping us feel how we relate to our language wisely. He said:

> When I began to study Zen, mountains were mountains: when I thought I understood Zen, mountains were not mountains; but when I came to full knowledge of Zen, mountains were again mountains (Suzuki 1996, p. 240).

In this quote, we can see the transition from how we typically perceive the world (i.e., the first part) and what we typically think of what enlightenment does to us (i.e., the second part) to what D.T. Suzuki means by "pure subjectivity"(i.e., the third part). The first part, "When I began to study Zen, mountains were mountains," describes how we typically relate to the world and ourselves. We tend to perceive and construe an event we see, hear, or touch as what our mind says it is as a distinct and constant entity. When we see mountains, they are "mountains" that are differentiated from "us," the perceivers, as well as other objects we perceive (e.g., rivers).

The second part, "when I thought I understood Zen, mountains were not mountains" is the stance of complete rejection of one's own subjective experience and linguistic processes. Once again, this sentence captures how we typically think of enlightenment (e.g., complete rejection of problems). When we learn the perspective of wholeness and oneness as an alternative to our

Western worldview, we quickly try to reject any perception framed with a word as a delusion (e.g., "everything is empty, so there is no such thing as a mountain or self"). According to D.T. Suzuki, such an attitude is a sign of our attachment to our habitual way of thinking; through this equally incomplete perspective, we continue to see the world from a good-or-bad, right-or-wrong viewpoint.

So, what does it mean by "but when I came to full knowledge of Zen, mountains were again mountains"? In the last part of the quote, Suzuki asks us to experience the mountain as if it is a dimension of the whole, using the word "mountains" accordingly. We do not have to reject our linguistic practices. Instead, we can simply use them from the perspective of the wholeness. In an experiential sense, the mountains are mountains and they are also interdependent entities without any boundaries. From the perspective of the original wholeness, the word "mountain" refers to the point from which we see the whole. This seems to be what he means by "relating to our linguistic process lightly." Suzuki (1970) also touched on this as the most fundamental wisdom of Zen Buddhism. He says:

> … the oneness of duality: not two, and not one. This is the most important teaching: not two, and not one. If you think your body and mind are two, that is wrong; if you think they are one, that is also wrong. Our body and mind are both two and one… Each one of us is both dependent and independent (p. 25).

Japanese Sociolinguistic Context

The Japanese sociocultural community values Zen's worldview of wholeness as well as its view on language. In psychological science literature, Japanese culture is construed as that of *holistic social cognition*, which is contrasted with that of *analytic social cognition*, which flourishes in the West (Nisbett et al. 2001). As noted by Maynard (1997). Cultural contingencies operated in a verbal community shape the way its members think and feel as well as how they communicate with one another (or how its language is used). One of the distinct features of holistic culture is the perceived experience of self and world in *continuity* (e.g., the unity of the self as perceived with the perceived) with the emphasis of context (e.g., where and when the event of interest takes place).

The holistic perspective held by Japanese people differs from the analytic way of thinking, which assumes that the world is a collection of distinct objects with unique properties. In the culture of analytic social cognition, words and phrases (e.g., "cat") are analytical, serving to highlight the unique property of the events, to which they refer (e.g., a hairy, four-legged animal meowing) in order to differentiate them from other events categorized differently (e.g., "dog"). In the field of behavioral health, the Diagnostic and Statistical Manual of Mental Disorders (American Psychiatric Association 2013) is a salient exemplar of this analytic and categorical way of thinking.

Japanese society creates a holistic perspective and encourages its members to use Japanese language accordingly (Maynard 1997). More specifically, the focus of discourse in Japanese language is what Maynard refers to as the *scene* (e.g., time and place) where the topic of discourse takes place, more so than *who-does-what*, as is the case with English. In this linguistic context, the function of Japanese language is to blend the actor or figure into the scene or background, creating a sense of wholeness.

The salience of scene in Japanese language is evident in its grammatical structure. Unlike a conventional English discourse that starts with the actor and then his or her action (e.g., "I went to work yesterday"), a Japanese sentence often starts with the specification of the context, followed by the description of actor and the actor's action taking place in that context. Furthermore, as described extensively below, what is also unique about Japanese language is the way the actor and his or her action are described. Unlike English which centralizes the actor and his or her actions as the cause (e.g., "*I* went to…), Japanese language often describe the actor and his or her actions as *events which happen to emerge from the context*.

This context-focused nature of Japanese verbal community also shapes its unique way of using a word or phrase. That is, the meaning of a word is not within the word, but in the context where it is used, and many Japanese words have different meanings that contradict one another when interpreted without context. Take a word *itooshii* (愛おしい) as an example. In some contexts, it means "dear" and "beloved" as seen in a phrase such as "my beloved daughter." In other contexts, this word means the feelings of "sorrow" and "grief," experiences that we Westerners often consider the direct opposite from "dear" and "beloved." Once again, it is the context (e.g., when-and-where of the scene, the point of the speaker and his or her relations with the listener) that determines the semantic nuance of a given word.

The semantic nuance of a word, such as *itooshii*, is a good example of Japanese style of dialectical thinking and attitudes. As demonstrated above, the Japanese sociolinguistic community seems to encourage its members to become open to a wide range of experiences indiscriminately (Maynard 1997; Nisbett et al. 2001). It is as if one is to see the entire world in a grain of sand, and his or her entire life in a smile of a child. As a Zen saying goes, it is to fully experience myriad dharma through a single experience of here-and-now.

This dialectical attitude is slightly different from that of the West (Miyamoto and Ryff 2011; Peng and Nisbett 1999; Zhang et al. 2015). Take the idiom "Life is sweet and sour." For Westerners, this idiom implies that life is the sum of multiple parts: some aspects of life are sweet and some aspects are sour. Dialectical efforts for Westerners include attempts to synthesize contradicting parts that are fundamentally distinct from one another. For Japanese people, this idiom suggests that life is sweet and sour as *one*, that sweet and sour is life (e.g., the entire universe as a whole). Furthermore, the idiom encourages the perceiver of the idiom to blend into the here-and-now where the person and the idiom meet. The Japanese way of dialectical thinking is not the point of compromise or the coexistence of distinct entities within the perceived field. Rather, it is the experience of one (Suzuki 1970).

Zen and Body

Following the analytic and categorical way of thinking, mind and body are ontologically distinct in the Cartesian paradigm. Accordingly, we Westerners tend to perceive mind and body as separate entities. We also presume that separate principles and remedies are required for each. The field of Western medicine and behavioral health is no exception (O'Donohue and Maragakis 2015). Problems that humans face are categorically sorted into physical or mental domains, subsequently treated separately by different professionals specialized for one or another. Although behavioral medicine and integrated behavioral health movements promote an interdisciplinary approach where medicines and behavioral health are utilized into a coherent treatment system (O'Donohue and Maragakis 2015), the assumption of mind–body dichotomy remains strong in our field (Magid 2002).

A rationalist perspective reinforces the mind–body distinction further in the West (Ozawa-De Silva 2002). For a rationalist, humans are essentially thinking beings, and they should behave based on rational choice (i.e., mind), rather than on emotional or physiological reactions (i.e., body). This is a wisdom transmitted through generations in many spiritual traditions. However, extreme adherence to this Cartesian-rationalist standpoint yields the rejection and trivialization of body.

The fundamental position of Zen is a return to oneness or wholeness. As such, Zen does not view the body and mind as separate entities: these are one. For Zen, all of our activities are viewed as those of a whole person (bodymind), not as physical activities or mental activities. From this standpoint, Zen encourages us to engage in any given activity as that of a whole person.

In *Shobogenzo* (正法眼蔵), the Treasure of the Correct Dharma Eye, Dogen used the term *shinjin* (身心) to denote the oneness of body and mind (Dogen and Tanahashi 1985). The return to *bodymind*, the oneness, is a central theme in Dogen Zen (Shaner 1985; Tanahashi and Levitt 2013) as he expressed enlightenment as "dropping away bodymind." Once again, the oneness here is not to blend two distinct entities into one. What Zen aims to do is to experientially authenticate or return to "the original oneness of bodymind" (Shaner 1985, p. 18). As such, *bodymind* is understood as a *potential* to be cultivated, more so than an entity or a particular state of being in itself. *In Genjokoan* (現成公案), which is included in *Shobogenzo*, Dogen described bodymind as follows:

> When you see forms or hear sounds fully engaging body-and-mind, you intuit dharmas intimately. Unlike things and their reflections in the mirror, and unlike the moon and its reflection in the water, when one side is illuminated, the other side is dark (Dogen et al. 2011, p. 51).

Dogen then stated:

> … When actualized by myriad things, your body and mind as well as bodies and minds of others drop away. No trace of enlightenment remains, and this no-trace continues endlessly (Dogen et al. 2011, p. 55).

Body and Japanese Culture

Generally speaking, Japanese people tend to view mind and body as one more so than Westerners do. According to Nakao and Ohara (2014), this tendency of perceived unity of mind and body is attributable to three core belief systems in Japanese tradition: Shintoism, Buddhism, and ancient Chinese ideology, particularly Confucianism and Taoism. Although the Westernized era of imperialism and democracy has been dominant over the past 150 years in Japan, these traditional views remain influential even today.

In many ways, the unity of body and mind are emphasized in every facet of daily activities in Japanese society. For example, the Japanese education system continues to emphasize the importance of honing the mind and the body equally as described by the idiom *bunbu ryodo* (文武両道; excellence in both scholarship and the martial arts). Many Westerners may feel the idiom of *bunbu ryodo* dualistic. However, if seeing this idiom from the standpoint of Japanese dialectics, we can grasp that body and mind are two sides of the same coin, or a whole. Today, fewer Japanese people practice martial arts. However, a contemporary understanding of this idiom is that the true self is a balanced self and that one cannot neglect either body or mind in order to hone the unity of self.

Traditionally, Japanese society values the processes through which one cultivates the unity of bodymind. Given the pragmatic and realistic nature of Japanese culture (Varley 2000), the term "unity of body-skill-mind (*singitai*; 心技体)" captures the nuance of the "bodymind" unity. Building a skill takes time and requires perseverance, and it is this perseverance (*nintai*; 忍耐) that traditionally many Japanese people value. "*Ishi no ue ni mo san nen*" (石の上にも三年) is a well-known idiom describing the virtue that perseverance prevails. It literally says that "three years on a (cold) stone (will make the stone warm)." Staying on a task with a wholehearted effort, whatever the task one engages in, is an opportunity for a person to confront various subjective experiences; it is like zazen, a sitting mediation. Through a continued practice, one experiences joy, bodily aching, unrelated thoughts, joy, and frustration, to name a few. Given our "microwave society" (i.e., desire to attain what we want quickly), perseverance is decreasingly welcome in recent years. At the same time, it is the very source of personal growth, the unity of mind–skill–body and "dropping off bodymind."

Zen Account of Self and Japanese Culture

One of the most challenging teachings of Zen centers around the nature of self and the meaning of that term. In secular and academic cultures, "no self" is a popular term, with which Zen is often associated with (Mathers et al. 2009).

So what is self for Zen Buddhism? In *Genjokoan*, Dogen stated that:

> To study the Buddha way is to study the self. To study the self is to forget the self. To forget the self is to be verified by all things. To be verified by all things is to let the body and mind of the self and the body and mind of others drop off. There is a trace of realization that cannot be grasped. We endlessly express this ungraspable trace of realization (see Okumura 2010, p. 2).

The self that Dogen talks about in the above passage is not the sense of self as we typically perceive it (i.e., self as an independent and consistent being). Rather, it is the self as an all-interpenetrating being, which is "the reality of life prior to separation into dichotomies such as self/other or subject/object" (Dogen et al. 2011, p. 182). Once again, this self is the experience of original wholeness or oneness described above.

Reflecting his teacher, Kodo Sawaki (1880–1965), Kosho Uchiyama (1912–1998) shares the quote that Sawaki roshi often said to his students, "Zazen is the self selfing the self," or "To practice zazen is to be intimate with the self" (Uchiyama and Okumura 2014, p. 25). Uchiyama explains "Zazen is the self selfing the self," as followed by commenting on the quote by Dogen, which is just mentioned above.

> "To study the Buddha Way is to study the self" means we should study the self, which includes all heaven and earth… Correctly speaking, we should accept everything as the contents of our "self." We should meet everything as a part of ourselves. "To study the self" means to awaken to such a self. For instance, many people visit my house or write me letters. Many of these people talk or write about their problems and anguish and ask for my advice. I never feel troubled by such requests. As soon as I am asked about such troubles, they become my own. As long as I have such an attitude, these problems are my own. And they enrich my life. If I reject other people's problems saying, "That's not my business," my life becomes poorer and poorer. Therefore, to meet everything, without exception, as part of my life is most essential in the Buddha way. This is what Dogen Zenji meant by saying, "To study Buddha Way is to study the self" (Dogen et al. 2011, p. 182)

It is important to clarify Uchiyama's statements above. He does not say that we must *solve* the problems of others for them or that it is our responsibility to take care of others' problems. What he attempts to explain above is the importance of perspective taking and compassion toward the self and others, not necessarily the importance of solving the problems of others. Rather, sharing in life with others and holding that sharing as part of an inherent view of the self is part of the Buddha Way. Uchiyama then explained what Dogen means by "To study the self is to forget the self," as follows:

> … when we forget ourselves in the Buddha Way, we forget ourselves because everything is the contents of "self" and whatever we encounter is part of ourselves. This is not a continuation of egoism. To work as an all-interpenetrating self is merely a thought. Therefore, in Buddhism it is a mistake to say that we have an idea of all-interpenetrating self. It cannot be the Buddha Way as long as we consider the word "all-interpenetrating self" a thought (Dogen et al. 2011, p. 183).

In explaining the "all-interpenetrating self," Uchiyama talked about a mother's attitudes toward her child as an example (Uchiyama and Okumura 2014). He stated that when a mother takes care of her child wholeheartedly, she experientially becomes one with her child and that in her experience in that moment, there is no perceived distinction between herself and her child. When we have a heart-to-heart conversation with our friends or loved ones, we may also experience this forgetting of the self. There is something intimate there, and the experience of it is clear. Uchiyama seems to say that we can simply extend this "forgetting of the self" experience to others and our surroundings.

Self and Japanese Linguistic Practice

Regarding the expression of "self" and "I" in Japanese discourse, one salient feature of Japanese linguistic practice is the absence of a subject, such as "I" in both spoken and written forms (Maynard 1997). While the inclusion of subject is crucial for an English sentence, this is not the case for the Japanese language. For example, a psychotherapist in the USA may ask a client "How do *you* feel?" and in responding to this question, the client may say, "*I* feel sad." In the therapist's question as well as the client's answer, the agent and action are clearly identified.

Alternatively, in Japanese linguistic context, the subject and verb are likely to be omitted. In a similar circumstance as the one just above, a Japanese therapist may ask his or her client "*do nasare mashita ka* (どうなされましたか; how feeling?)," and then the client's answer may be something like, "*kanashii desu* (悲しいです; sadness it is)." In this discourse, the subject is not specified, but implied. Maynard (1997) argues that Japanese discourses do not need to specify who-says-what-to-whom because the dyad (relationship between the speaker and listener) is the basic unit of communication rather than the focus being an individual.

Second, as mentioned above, Japanese linguistic practice emphasizes the context or scene, more so than who-does-what-to-whom (Maynard 1997). This feature of Japanese language also seems to reinforce the experience of self as an interdependent being. Take a typical evening conversation between my wife and myself as an example. My wife is Puerto Rican and I am Japanese. We communicate in English because it is the language that both of us can speak. So, the conversation flows like this:

> My wife: What did you do today?
> Me: I took Kyoko (our youngest daughter) to the zoo this afternoon. We saw pandas. They were so cute and she (Kyoko) really enjoyed seeing them.

This is an ordinary discourse. Now, let us focus on my answer in the discourse. If I respond to her in Japanese, it will be something like this:

> Me: *Kyo no gogo, Kyoko to doubutsu-en ni ittekitayo. Panda ga ite ne, totemo kawai kata. Kyoko ha ooyorokobi data yo* (今日の午後、キョウコと動物園にいってきたよ。パンダがいてね、とてもかわいかった。キョウコは大喜びだったよ).

The word-to-word translation of this Japanese sentence is something like, "this afternoon, with Kyoko, Zoo, (I) went to. Pandas, there were. (they were) so cute, and Kyoko very excited (became)." As can be seen, in a Japanese discourse, the context (when-and-where) is specified first, and "I" as an agent of action is omitted, but implied by finishing the sentence with "went to." The omission of subjects (actors) is also the case in subsequent sentences (e.g., "we saw pandas," "they were so cute"), as if the actions of the agents (I, Kyoko, pandas) happen to emerge from that context.

Third, the Japanese linguistic community utilizes "there is" expressions over who-does-what (Maynard 1997). In English, the phenomenon of interest is often articulated into agent, action, and object as seen in the following sentence, "Aki has two daughters." This straightforward English sentence is translated in Japanese, as "*Aki-san ni ha musume-san ga futari imasu* (あきさんには娘さんが二人います)." The literal meaning of the Japanese sentence is "there are two daughters at Mr. Aki." In Japanese, phenomena that the English language usually expresses as "x has y" tends to be expressed as "there is y in x."

Finally, Japanese language has several ways to de-emphasize the agent and action in a sentence. For example, I recently accepted a faculty position at University of Hawaii at Manoa. In English, I would share this news with my colleague by saying something like, "I recently accepted an offer from University of Hawaii at Manoa." However, I am very likely to share this news with my Japanese colleagues by saying something like "*konotabi Hawaii-daigaku kara itadaita ofa wo shoudaku surukoto ni narimashita.*" The literal translation of this sentence is something like "It turns out that I will become a faculty member at University of Hawaii." In my Japanese expression, myself as an agent is de-emphasized by saying "It turns out…" as if it is the external factor that determines my career in Hawaii, not myself. Pointing out this feature of Japanese discourse, Maynard (1997) calls Japanese a "Be-language" or "Become-language," while English as a "Do-language" or "Have-language." Summarizing the features of Japanese language, Maynard (1997) states:

> … Japanese tends to frame the event as (1) something existing rather than someone possessing something, and (2) something becoming or happening, often beyond the agent's control, and not as something that an agent who has full control

> "initiates and causes to happen." The Japanese are more likely to interpret an event as a situation that becomes and comes to be on its own, while Americans tend to perceive an event resulting from an agent doing something and causing things to happen… Incorporating the concept of centrality of scene, we can conclude that one of the ways that Japanese are characteristically encouraged to see things is as the scene becoming, whereas from the American perspective it is the agent doing. The world that becomes is also a world where elements are held in balance, located in mutual interrelation. Here, instead of recognizing an agent acting on an object, multiple elements constructing the entire scene find themselves in a relational balance (p. 176).

In sum, a verbal community shapes the way its members think and feel (Maynard 1997; Skinner 1957, 1974). The Japanese verbal community seems to socially encourage Japanese people to pay closer attention to the context where their experience unfolds without emphasizing the agent, including themselves. Reinforcing this form of linguistic practice may facilitate one's sense of self as being harmonious with the context and hone his or her sensitivity to the changes unfolding in that context. The Japanese verbal community also seems to punish or at least not encourage linguistic expressions which emphasize the agent (e.g., "I").

Self, Others, and Japanese Culture

A Japanese perspective of others can be understood through the Japanese perspective of self. As noted extensively elsewhere (Hamaguchi 1985; Markus and Kitayama 2010), the perceived sense of self among Japanese people is often referred to as the interdependent perspective of self (Markus and Kitayama 1991). According to Hamaguchi (1985), in Japanese culture, the self is not as constant as the Western notion of ego. It is a fluid and flexible concept that can change through time and situations. Additionally, the sense of identification with others pre-exists prior to the sense of self, and selfness is experienced only through interpersonal relations.

The self as a relational being is also expressed in characters used in Japanese language (Hamaguchi 1985). One of the most commonly used words for self is *Jibun* (自分). In fact, *jibun* literally means "one's share" of something between oneself and another. Furthermore, in some parts of Japan, *jibun* also refers to "you," to whom one feels close: "I" means "you." Hamaguchi (1985) explained this Japanese sense of self as follows:

> … *jibun* as the Japanese consciousness of the self is not an abstract quality which lies within the actor himself, "but rather a reality which is discovered from time to time outside of himself, or more specifically, between oneself and another. In other words, the *jibun* denotes in any given situation the share that is distributed to oneself derived from the life space which is commonly shared by both oneself and other actors… In Japan, who is "I" and who is "you" is not defined absolutely, but is always being redefined according to the nature of "I" and "you" relations (pp. 302–303).

These relational nuances of self are expressed by other idioms. For example, *Hito* (人) in Japanese means both self and others, and English words of "human being" and "mankind" are expressed as *ningen* (人間), which literally means "in-between people." In sum, for Japanese people, the interdependent perspective of self is not a patchwork of multiple individuals. Rather, the self is a contextually navigated interdependence. Once again, we can see the wisdom of Zen within this Japanese perspective of self and others.

Zen, Nature, and Japanese Aesthetic

Japan is an island country located along the Pacific coast of East Asia. Surrounded by the oceans, over 70% of Japan is forested and mountainous. Most regions of Japan are temperate and characterized by four distinct seasons. Because of its wide range of latitude, seasonal winds, and different types of ocean currents, the climate in Japan varies from a cool, humid, and continental climate in the north to warm, tropical, and rainforest climate in the south. Japan is also known for a range of natural disasters. Typhoons occur annually, causing floods and landslides. Due to its location in the Pacific Ring of Fire with over 100 active volcanos, Japan is prone to earthquakes and tsunami, having the highest natural disaster risk in the developed world. The earthquake and tsunami of 2011 are still fresh in recent memory (Normile 2011).

Japanese culture is often characterized by the "love of nature" (Watanabe 1974). However, this love is not what we usually refer to as love. For the Japanese, love is the acceptance, embracement, and even appreciation of whatever nature reveals: that is, the nature is both sweet and sour. More specifically, it teaches us the dharma of impermanence as well as that of dependent origination (Japan Buddhist Federation 1978), two central teachings of Buddhism, which are also followed closely by Zen (Bobrow 2010). Suzuki (1996) stated:

> Nature never deliberates; it acts directly out of its own heart, whatever this may mean. In this respect Nature is divine. Its "irrationality" transcends human doubts or ambiguities, and in our submitting to it, or rather accepting it, we transcend ourselves. This acceptance and transcendence is a human prerogative. We accept Nature's "irrationality" or its "must" deliberately, quietly, and whole-heartedly. It is not a deed of blind and slavish submission to the inevitable. It is an active acceptance, a personal willingness with no thought of resistance. In this there is no force implied, no resignation, but rather participation, assimilation, and perhaps in some cases even identification (p. 234).

The embracement of nature alluded to above also points to the Japanese aesthetic (Suzuki 2010). Simply put, the Japanese aesthetic is the *embracement* of the transience unfolding here-and-now (i.e., the dharma of impermanence), which is heavily influenced by the worldview of Zen (Varley 2000). As many Zen teachings go, Japanese aesthetics is a subjective and relational experience of a person blending into the whole, including nature and some more formal characteristics of arts such as simplicity, harmony, space, and subtlety. In fact, Davies and Ikeno (2002) stated that there are no absolute criteria as to what constitutes the Japanese aesthetic. For Japanese people, aesthetics are subjectively and deeply felt and are experienced as transient. The Japanese aesthetic is considered relational because the experience of transience is said to unfold in the relation between the perceiver (e.g., self as an observer) and the perceived (e.g., cherry blossoms).

Zen, Personal Characteristics, Gender Roles, and Japanese Culture

Zen is sometimes associated with certain gender-specific as well as egalitarian characteristics, such as masculinity and altruism. As noted above, these images are often attributable to personal characteristics of influential Zen teachers in the past, such as Sogen Omori of Rinzai as well as Shunryu Suzuki of Soto. Unlike these images of Zen, Zen training is not designed to shape people into particular personal characteristics. Through Zen practice, one turns out to be however she or he turns out to be. Kosho Uchiyama (Uchiyama and Okumura 2014) described this point very nicely in the context of reflecting on his teacher, Kodo Sawaki, who was known for his dynamic, fearless, and unconventional characteristics. Uchiyama stated:

> Throughout his life, Sawaki Roshi said, "Zen is good for nothing." In 1941, I was ordained and became one of his disciples. Soon after, while walking with him, I asked, "I am such a timid person. If I study under your guidance and practice zazen with you for many years until you pass away, can I become even a little bit stronger?" He immediately replied, "No you can't. No matter how hard and how long you practice, zazen is good for nothing. I didn't become who I am as a result of zazen. By nature I was this kind of person. On this point, I haven't changed at all." As you know, Sawaki Roshi was bighearted, freespirited, and witty, and yet careful and focused. He embodied the image of the ancient Zen master. When I heard his response I thought, "Although Roshi says so with his mouth, if I continue to practice zazen, I must be able to become a better person." With such an expectation, I served him and continued zazen practice until he died. He passed away on December 21 last year. We'll mark the first anniversary of his death soon. Lately I've been reflecting on my past, and I now understand

> that zazen is really good for nothing. I'm still a coward and never became even a little bit like Sawaki Roshi. Finally I came to a conclusion. A violet blooms as a violet and a rose blooms as a rose. For violets, there's no need to desire to become roses (pp. 138–139).

Reflecting on this standpoint within Zen is helpful for understanding gender roles in Japanese culture. Although Japan is known as a patriarchal society, it was originally matriarchal (Reischauer and Craig 1973). Japanese society evolved into a patriarchal culture when the influence of Confucianism permeated into its political and sociocultural practices in the seventh century. As sited in Sugihara and Katsurada (2000), according to Reischauer and Craig (1973), one of the main features of Confucianism is its focus on a hierarchical society whereby strong male dominance is an assumption. Additionally, the establishment of i.e., (house) system in the twelfth century institutionalized gender division of labor and power imbalance between women and men. Following the i.e., system, social and political power and status were given to men on multiple levels (e.g., family, community, and state). The inception of the i.e., system occurred concurrently at a time when Zen was introduced to Japan.

According to Tanahashi and Levitt (2013), Zen is egalitarian in principle. For example, through his writings, Dogen, the founder of Japanese Soto Zen, expressed his attitudes that men and women behave inclusively and avoid discrimination. For example, in *Raihai Tokuzui* (礼拝得髄; Receiving the Marrow by Bowing) of *Shobogenzo*, Dogen stated:

> Why are men special? Emptiness is emptiness. Four great elements are four great elements. Five Skandhas are five skandhas. Women are just like that. Both men and women attain the way. You should honor attainment of the way. Do not discriminate between men and women. This is the most wondrous principle of the Buddha way (cited in Dogen and Tanahashi 2010, p. 77).

The reality for women in Japan is actually quite different than Dogen's vision above. For women, especially Zen nuns, difficulties exist in reconciling religious ideals with their social reality. For example, even today, Soto Zen nuns in Japan face discrimination in the patriarchal institutional hierarchy that continuously considers them to be novices while committing to the Buddha Way (Arai 1999). As is the case in Japanese society, issues related to gender roles and sex inequality are an important, ongoing agenda for those who seek progress in Japan's Zen community.

Zen, Cruelty, and Japanese Culture

While Zen is often associated with the wisdom of peace and compassion, it is also associated with some episodes of cruelty described in koans. The following is one such koan, called "Gutei Raises a Finger," in the Gateless Barrier, a collection of Chan (Zen) koans compiled in the early thirteenth century by the Chinese Zen master Wumen Huikai (Shibayama 2000).

> Master Gutei, whenever he was questioned, just stuck up one finger. At one time he had a young attendant, whom a visitor asked, "What is the Zen your Master is teaching?" The boy also stuck up one finger. Hearing of this, Gutei cut off the boy's finger with a knife. As the boy ran out screaming with pain, Gutei called to him. When the boy turned his head, Gutei stuck up his finger. The boy was suddenly enlightened (p. 42).

Many of us who read this koan are disturbed by the boy's finger and the apparent cruelty inflicted upon the boy. I do not intend to justify Gutei's action here or episodes of cruelty in other koans. However, what seems to be crucial in these koans is the *embodiment of bodymind* (e.g., the original wholeness) through these harsh experiences. It is important to note that the embodiment of the original wholeness is experienced without going through cruelty, but for some people, an episode of cruelty serves as a breakthrough as if it is a "chicken ready to break open the eggshell and its mother hen pecking at it to help the chicken out" (Shibayama 2000, p. 45). Whether Gutei's action is cruel or unethical is up to the boy, depending on how he perceived that experience.

Similarly, Japanese culture is also said to have two sides: one side is politeness and sincerity, and the other side is cruelty. Regarding the latter, Japan is one of the few industrialized nations that still maintain the death penalty. More recently, Japan was identified for its practice of killing whales and dolphins despite bans on commercial whaling and trading of whale products. It is unclear the extent to which Zen contributes to these "cruel" Japanese cultural practices. Even if those who engage in these activities are known to practice Zen, Zen itself should not be used to justify these actions. Rather, Zen should be used as an ethical blueprint for determining whether or not these activities reflect the Buddha nature. As noted above, the fundamental aim of Zen is self-enlightenment (e.g., embodiment of true self or nature) or the perfection of self through the self with an earnest endeavor for the benefit of humankind and all sentient beings.

Greeting, Gratitude, and Appreciation

Politeness and compassion are commonly observed in Japanese culture. In fact, Westerners often describe Japanese people as being "very polite." However, the politeness of Japanese goes beyond simply being well mannered. One of the most valued attitudes in Japanese culture is "*kannsha no kimochi* (感謝のきもち)," a deep feeling of gratitude and appreciation toward others and their surrounding environments. The cultural importance of gratitude also reflects the interdependent worldview infused in Japanese culture as well as that of Zen. For many, gratitude and appreciation are not particular attitudes of isolated beings directed toward other independent beings or objects. Rather, it is the acknowledgment of *shared* relatedness unfolding in a given moment. And it is this sharedness to which gratitude is directed. I recently came across a quote from His Holiness the Dalai Lama (2001). Reflecting the Dharma of Interdependence, His Holiness states:

> We humans are social beings. We come into the worlds as the results of others' action. We survive here in dependence of others. Whether we like it or not, there is hardly a moment of our lives when we do not benefit for others' activities. For this reason, it is hardly surprising that most of our happiness arises in the context of our relationships with others.

He then continues:

> … Here I am not suggesting that the individual whose actions are motivated by the wish to bring others' happiness necessarily meet with less misfortune than the one who does not. Sickness, old age, and mishaps of one sort or another are the same for us all. But the sufferings which undermine our internal peace—anxiety, frustration, disappointment—are definitely less. In our concern for others, we worry less about ourselves. When we worry less about ourselves, the experience of our own suffering is less intense (p. 62).

Once again, the kindness, gratitude, and appreciation that Japanese people express is often directed toward this interrelatedness, which unfolds in a given moment of one's life. It is expressed not for others lessening one's own suffering or for any gain from others in a materialistic or utilitarian sense. It is gratitude toward the Dharma.

Expanding this point, Dogen presented the Bodhisattva's Four Methods of Guidance in *Shobogenzo*. These are giving, kind speech, beneficial action, and identity action (cited in Dogen and Tanahashi 2010, p. 473). Of those, kind speech is the most relevant to this section. Dogen stated this:

> "Kind speech" means that when you see sentient beings, you arouse the heart of compassion and offer words of living care… If kind speech is offered, little by little kind speech expands. Thus, even kind speech that is not ordinarily known or seen comes into being. Be willing to practice it for this entire present life; do not give up, world after world, life after life. Kind speech is the basis for reconciling rules and subduing enemies. Those who hear kind speech from you have a delighted expression and a joyful mind. Those who hear of your kind speech will be deeply touched; they will always remember it (cited in Dogen and Tanahashi 2010, p. 475).

Conclusions

As noted above, many scholars, both in Japan and in the West, point out the interwoven relation between Zen and Japanese culture. The purpose of this chapter is to highlight some, but certainly not all, features of Japanese cultural context that seem to promote or support the wholehearted way of living. Although the influence of Western ideologies has permeated into Japanese cultural practice, Japanese people seem to continue to value the way of living that Zen delineates. Living in this modernized world, we cannot help feeling isolated from others and our surroundings. Visiting the wholehearted way of living and Japanese cultural practice that support such a way of living may illuminate the possibility for nurturing the sense of wholeness shared by many.

References

American Psychiatric Association. (2013). *Diagnostic and statistical manual of mental disorders* (5th ed.). Washington, DC: Author.

Arai, P. K. R. (1999). *Women living Zen: Japanese Soto Buddhist Nuns*. New York: US: Oxford University Press.

Bobrow, J. (2010). *Zen and psychotherapy: Partners in liberation*. New York, NY: W W Norton & Co.

Dalai Lama. (2001). *Ethics for the new millennium*. New York, USA: Riverhead Books.

Davies, R. J., & Ikeno, O. (2002). *The Japanese mind (Eds)*. North Clarendon, VT: Tuttle.

Dogen, E., Nishiari, B., Okumura, S., Suzuki, S., & Weisman, S. M. (2011). *Dogen's genjo koan: Three commentaries*. Barkeley, CA: Counterpoint.

Dogen, E., & Tanahashi, K. (1985). *Moon in a dewdrop: Writings of Zen master Dogen*. New York, USA: North Point Press.

Dogen, E., & Tanahashi, K. (2010). *Tresury of the true Dharma eye: Zen Master Dogen's Shobo Genzo*. Boston, MA: Shambhala.

Dogen, E., Uchiyama, K., Okumura, S., & Leighton, T. D. (1997). *The wholehearted way: A tranlation of Eihei Dogen's Bendowa with commentary by Kosho Uchiyama Roshi*. North Clarendon, VT: Tuttle Publications.

Gergen, K. J. (1983). Zen Buddhism and psychological science. *Psychologia: An International Journal of Psychology in the Orient, 26*(3), 129–141.

Hamaguchi, E. (1985). A contextual model of the Japanese: Toward a methodological innovation in Japan studies. *Journal of Japanese Studies, 11*, 289–321.

Hanayama, S. (1978). Japanese Buddhism from Kamakura through Tokugawa periods. In J. B. Federation (Ed.), *Understanding Japanese Buddhism* (pp. 16–22). Tokyo, Japan: Kyodo Obun Center.

Hayes, S. C., Barnes-Holmes, D., & Roche, B. (2001). *Relational frame theory: A post-Skinnerian account of human language and cognition*. New York, NY: Kluwer Academic/Plenum Publishers.

Hosokawa, D. (1999). *Omori Sogen: The art of a Zen master*. New York: Kegan Paul International.

Japan Buddhist Federation. (1978). *Understanding Japanese Buddhism*.

Kasulis, T. P. (1981). *Zen action Zen person*. Honolulu, HI: University of Hawaii Press.

Magid, B. (2002). *Ordinary mind: Exploring the common ground of Zen and psychotherapy*. Somerville, MA: Wisdom Publications.

Markus, H. R., & Kitayama, S. (1991). Culture and the self: Implications for cognition, emotion, and motivation. *Psychological Review, 98*(2), 224–253.

Markus, H. R., & Kitayama, S. (2010). Cultures and selves: A cycle of mutual constitution. *Perspectives on Psychological Science, 5*(4), 420–430. doi:10.1177/1745691610375557

Mathers, D., Miller, M. E., & Ando, O. (2009). *Self and no-self: Continuing the dialogue between Buddhism and psychotherapy*. New York, NY: Routledge/Taylor & Francis Group.

Maynard, S. K. (1997). *Japanese communication: Language and thought in context*. Honolulu, HI: University of Hawaii Press.

Miyamoto, Y., & Ryff, C. D. (2011). Cultural differences in the dialectical and non-dialectical emotional styles and their implications for health. *Cognition and Emotion, 25*(1), 22–39. doi:10.1080/02699931003612114

Monteiro, L. M., Musten, R. F., & Compson, J. (2015). Traditional and contemporary mindfulness: Finding the middle path in the tangle of concerns. *Mindfulness, 6*(1), 1–13. doi:10.1007/s12671-014-0301-7

Muramoto, S. (1985). Buddhism and psychotherapy in the world today. *Psychologia: An International Journal of Psychology in the Orient, 28*(2), 101–114.

Muramoto, S. (2002). Buddhism, religion and psychotherapy in the world today. In P. Young-Eisendrath, S. Muramoto, P. Young-Eisendrath, & S. Muramoto (Eds.), *Awakening and insight: Zen Buddhism and psychotherapy* (pp. 15–29). New York, NY: Brunner-Routledge.

Nakao, M., & Ohara, C. (2014). The perspective of psychosomatic medicine on the effect of religion on the mind–body relationship in Japan. *Journal of Religion and Health, 53*(1), 46–55.

Nisbett, R. E., Peng, K., Choi, I., & Norenzayan, A. (2001). Culture and systems of thought: Holistic versus analytic cognition. *Psychological Review, 108*(2), 291–310. doi:10.1037/0033-295X.108.2.291

Normile, D. (2011). Devastating earthquake defied expectations. *Science, 331*(6023), 1375–1376.

O'Donohue, W., & Maragakis, A. (2015). *Integrated primary and behavioral care: Role in medical homes and chronic disease management*. Cham, Switzerland: Springer International Publishing.

Okumura, S. (2010). *Realizing Genjokoan: The key to Dogen's Shobogenzo*. Boston MA, US: Wisdom Publications.
Omori, S. (2001). *An introduction to Zen training: A translation of Sanzen Nyumon*.
Ozawa-De Silva, C. (2002). Beyond the body/mind? Japanese contemporary thinkers on alternative sociologies of the body. *Body & Society, 8*(2), 21–38. doi:10.1177/1357034x02008002002
Park, J. Y. (2002). Zen and Zen philosophy of language: A soteriological approach. *Journal of Comparative Philosophy and Religion, 1*(2), 209–228.
Peng, K., & Nisbett, R. E. (1999). Culture, dialectics, and reasoning about contradiction. *American Psychologist, 54*(9), 741–754. doi:10.1037/0003-066X.54.9.741
Reischauer, E. O., & Craig, A. M. (1973). *Japan: Tradition and transformation*. Tokyo: Charles E. Tuttle.
Shaner, D. E. (1985). The bodymind experience in Dogen's "Shobogenzo": A phenomenological perspective. *Philosophy East and West, 35*(1), 17–35. doi:10.2307/1398679
Shibayama, Z. (2000). *The gateless barrier: Zen comments on the mumonkan*. Boston, MA, US: Shambhala Publication. (Originally published in 1974)
Skinner, B. F. (1957). *Verbal behavior*. East Norwalk, CT: Appleton Century Crofts.
Skinner, B. F. (1974). *About behaviorism*. Oxford, England: Alfred A. Knopf.
Sugihara, Y., & Katsurada, E. (2000). Gender-role personality traits in Japanese culture. *Psychology of Women Quarterly, 24*(4), 309–318. doi:10.1111/j.1471-6402.2000.tb00213.x
Suzuki, D. T. (1996). *Zen Buddhism: Selected writings of D. T. Suzuki*. New York, USA: An Image Book.
Suzuki, D. T. (1997). *Eastern perspective [Toyoteki na mikata]*. Tokyo, Japan: Iwanami Shoten.
Suzuki, D. T. (2010). *Zen and Japanese culture*. Princeton, NJ: Princeton University Press. (Original work published in 1938)
Suzuki, S. (1970). *Zen Mind, Beginner's Mind: Informal talks on Zen meditation and practice*. Boston, MA: Weatherhill.
Suzuki, S. (2002). *Not always so: Practicing the ture spirit of Zen*. New York, USA: Harper.
Tanahashi, K., & Levitt, P. (2013). *The essential Dogen: Writings of the great Zen master*. Boulder CO: Wisdom Publications.
Uchiyama, K., & Okumura, S. (2014). *The Zen teaching of homeless Kodo*. Somerville MA: Tuttle Publications.
Varley, P. (2000). *Japanese culture* (4th ed.). Honolulu, HI: University of Hawaii Press.
Watanabe, M. (1974). The conception of nature in Japanese culture. *Science, 183*(4122), 279–282.
Weisz, J. R., Rothbaum, F. M., & Blackburn, T. C. (1984). Standing out and standing in: The psychology of control in America and Japan. *American Psychologist, 39*(9), 955–969. doi:10.1037/0003-066X.39.9.955
Wilson, T. D., Lindsey, S., & Schooler, T. Y. (2000). A model of dual attitudes. *Psychological Review, 107*(1), 101–126. doi:10.1037/0033-295x.107.1.101
Wright, D. S. (1992). Rethinking transcendence: The role of language in Zen experience. *Philosophy East & West, 42*(1), 113–138.
Young-Eisendrath, P., & Muramoto, S. (2002). *Awakening and insight: Zen Buddhism and psychotherapy*. New York, NY: Routledge.
Zhang, B., Galbraith, N., Yama, H., Wang, L., & Manktelow, K. I. (2015). Dialectical thinking: A cross-cultural study of Japanese, Chinese, and British students. *Journal of Cognitive Psychology, 27*(6), 771–779. doi:10.1080/20445911.2015.1025792

Part I

Zen: Overview and Foundations

What Is Zen?: The Path of Just Sitting

Shohaku Okumura

Keywords
Zen · Buddhism · Zazen · Meditation · Behavioral health

I was asked to write a big topic: What is Zen? The word "Zen" is used so vaguely that it is not possible to write an article in a way that fulfills all people's expectations. Zen teaching, in my experience, is what I studied from my teacher, Kosho Uchiyama Roshi (1912–1998). Zen practice is just sitting (*shikantaza*), and this is what I practice. I am going to talk about the particular teaching of my own teacher and the particular practice I have been continuing for more than forty-five years. I hope that my personal path of just sitting will be meaningful for the audience of this book.

Life Is a Koan: My Questions About Life

I was born in Osaka 1948, three years after World War II. My family had been living in the city of Osaka, the second largest city in Japan, working as merchants for more than 200 years and six generations. In March 1945, my family lost all of the wealth they accumulated across generations after an air raid by the U.S. Air Force. My family moved to the countryside in Osaka Prefecture, transitioning briefly into farming until 1952. The family then moved to Ibaraki, a small town between Osaka and Kyoto, where I lived from age 4 through 18.

During and after World War II, Japanese society changed dramatically. More specifically, the people in my parents' generation altered their value systems to incorporate completely different perspectives from what they had been taught. When the war ended, my father was twenty-five years old, and my mother was a few years younger. They were raised in the traditional Japanese culture where family is valued as the most important aspect of one's world. During the war, they were also influenced by the nationalistic ideology of the military government, in which the emperor was worshiped as a god, and the greatest honor achievable for any Japanese man was working hard and dying on the battlefield for the sake of the nation.

After the war, democracy and individualism influenced by the USA became a new foundation for social morality and education in Japan. Given the drastic change in society, my parents' generation lost confidence in how they think,

S. Okumura (✉)
Sanshin Zen Community, Bloomington, USA
e-mail: jiyushohaku@hotmail.com

A. Masuda and W.T. O'Donohue (eds.), *Handbook of Zen, Mindfulness, and Behavioral Health*, Mindfulness in Behavioral Health, DOI 10.1007/978-3-319-54595-0_4

behave, and what they value. Consequently, my generation, the "baby boomers," did not inherit the pre-war way of thinking and behaving from our parents' generation. Not having the role models for the new standards, our generation had to acquire our own way of thinking and behaving. To do so, we became skeptical of almost everything, including the ways Japan used to be and how Japanese people lived after the war. To recover prosperity, Japanese people worked extremely hard. Because Japan had to give up military power, economy became the country's priority.

When I was a high school student, I had many questions about life. As Japan was in a drastic transition, I felt pressure to make many decisions about my future. To do so, I also thought that I needed to understand the basic meaning of life (e.g., "what is my life for?"). Without knowing the true meaning of human life, I felt that I could not make any "right" decision for myself. To find the meaning of life, I often escaped from class and read in the library. I read many books, including those on philosophy, religions, literature, history, science, and many others.

The more I read books, the deeper my question became. I started to see that Japanese society at the time had become one huge money-generating machine. I also began to notice that school systems were serving as factories, manufacturing the components of the machine rather than serving as a place for the young to explore and cultivate the true meaning of life. My parents and teachers, as well as Japanese society, expected me to study hard, attend a prestigious university, have a well-respected job, work hard, and earn money. I could not find any meaning in such a way of life, that is, as being part of the machine. I wanted to escape from this materialistic society, but at the same time, I was not yet aware of alternatives.

I later found out that similar processes occurred in the USA and Europe during 1960s and 1970s. Young people wanted to examine the status quo system of values and escape from the limitations and boundaries of the established society. Some became political advocates while others developed ideas in spirituality. During these periods, many people who were called hippies in the USA and Europe came to Kyoto, Japan, and practiced Zen. Some of them became close friends of mine, and we have remained friends since.

Encountering Zen Teaching

In the process of searching for the meaning of living, I found a classmate who had the same kind of questions. We became very close. He knew someone who went to Antaiji-temple to practice with Kodo Sawaki Roshi (1880–1965) and Kosho Uchiyama Roshi (1912–1998). Antaiji was a small Soto Zen temple. Unlike many other Soto Zen temples and other Buddhist temples, Antaiji did not have community supporters who offer financial contributions in exchange of receiving Buddhist ceremonies (e.g., funeral, celebration for family ancestry). Sawaki Roshi originally borrowed the temple to allow his disciples, including Uchiyama Roshi, to stay and practice. Later, he was asked to be the abbot of the temple. He accepted the role, but he was the abbot in name only. He returned to Antaiji once a month to lead a sesshin, a period of intensive meditation (zazen). Otherwise, Sawaki Roshi traveled all over Japan to teach. Because he did not have his own temple, he was called "Homeless Kodo." In 1963, when he was 83 years old, Uchiyama Roshi took care of his master until his death. In 1965, during a summer vacation, my friend visited Antaiji and practiced with Uchiyama Roshi for a few weeks. That was the time when Uchiyama Roshi published his first book entitled, "*Jiko (Self)*." Uchiyama Roshi gave a copy to my friend, and he lent it to me.

After reading his book, I felt that I wanted to live like Uchiyama Roshi and become his disciple. I knew nothing about Buddhism or Zen. However, I found that he struggled with the same questions about meaning when he was a teenager. Uchiyama Roshi wanted to live the truth of human life. To find his answer, he studied Western philosophy at Waseda University, a prestigious private university located in Tokyo.

He primarily studied German philosophy. After completing his master's degree, he became a teacher at a Catholic seminary in Kyushu, in the southeastern region of Japan, and taught philosophy and mathematics there. At the seminary, Uchiyama Roshi also studied Catholic theology. After six months, he found that he could not become a Catholic because of the institutionalism he observed and studied about. He left the seminary shortly after.

Uchiyama Roshi married a woman while he was a university student, but she died after contracting tuberculosis (TB) a few years into their marriage. He, too, contracted TB, living with it for the rest of his life. After leaving seminary and returning to Tokyo, he re-married, but his second wife also died suddenly while she was pregnant. According to Uchiyama Roshi, these tragic experiences led him to pursue his life as a Zen Buddhist monk. He was ordained by Kodo Sawaki Roshi on December 8th in 1941 (December 7th in the USA). He was 29 years old. Coincidentally, the day he was ordained was Pearl Harbor Day.

During and after the World War II, Uchiyama Roshi practiced Zen under very difficult conditions. Going through difficult times within himself and Japanese society at large for almost 10 years, he began to find the answers that he was looking for. Continuing his practice, he wrote books and shared the answers that he found with others. I had read many books about great individuals in history, but Uchiyama Roshi was the first living teacher whom I encountered in my life.

When I read the book (i.e., "*Self*"), the primary thing I understood was his devotion to searching and his tireless efforts to share wisdom with others. I was not, however, able to discern the answer he had discovered. After reading the book, I began to study Buddhism and Zen more deeply. In 1968, I went to Komazawa University, a well-known Soto Zen Buddhist University located in Tokyo, Japan, where Sawaki Roshi taught as a professor. I studied basic Buddhist teachings and delved more deeply into the teachings of Dogen Zenji, the originator of Japanese Soto Zen. After visiting Antaiji for the first time in 1969 to sit for a five-day sesshin, I was ordained in December 1970. I graduated from Komazawa University in March 1972 and entered Antaiji.

From 1965 to 1971, Uchiyama Roshi published seven books. I read all of them before I entered Antaiji and practiced under his mentorship. Together with what I studied at Komazawa University, Uchiyama Roshi's teachings became the foundation of my practice and understanding of Dharma.

The main points of Uchiyama Roshi's teachings are as follows:

1. What is the self in its true meaning?
2. What is the meaning of Zazen practice?
3. How to live daily lives and the life as a whole as the practice based on the understanding of the true self and zazen practice.

What I read in Uchiyama Roshi's books during that period of time was the actual Zen Buddhist teachings that I received, and it has also become the foundation of my life moving forward. Thus, it is important to elaborate on the main points of his teachings to understand this practice and way of living.

Self

Uchiyama Roshi's search for the way started with inquiring the truth of the self. He wanted to find what the self is and how one lives based on the truth of the self. He found that, from the time of Shakyamuni Buddha, the fundamental point of Buddhism is to inquire about the self and find a peace of mind in settling within the self. Uchiyama Roshi often quotes from old Buddhist scriptures such as follows:

> *Sutta-Nipata*: Walk in the world depending on the self.
> *Dhammapada*: The foundation of the self is only the self.

Mahaparinibbana Sutta: Take refuge in the self; do not take refuge in anything else.[1]

This basic attitude is directly continued in Dogen Zenji's teaching: To study the Buddha Way is to study the self (*Shobogenzo Genjokoan*).[2]

In his book, *Jiko (Self)*, Uchiyama Roshi defined the Buddha-dharma as follows:

Buddha-dharma is, in short, "the self is being in peace reaching the inner most truth of the self," and "within the peace, the self lives and works."

According to Uchiyama Roshi, the self has these two layers. Ultimately, the self is one with all beings without any separation. When we see this interconnectedness, we naturally think of others with a compassionate heart, enacting kindness, and consideration toward others. He also stated that we must have a *parental heart* toward all beings, seeing everything we encounter as our self, connecting our hearts with the universe.

The self is not a fixed, permanent entity that does not change. It is as if we are collections of billions of elements moving and changing within time and space. From the time of our birth, our bodies and minds constantly transition, their shapes and qualities shifting like a flame of the candle. Uchiyama Roshi asked us to see life as the flux of interdependence. It is actually one with everything, and at the same time, each of us has uniqueness distinct from others. Viewing our self from these seemingly conflicting perspectives is important.

Although we are a collection of different elements, we tend to view ourselves as a fixed entity that can exist independently from the rest of the world. This fabricated fixed entity is what we usually recognize as "I," "my," "me," and without a clear reasoning, we attach ourselves to it. Uchiyama Roshi called engagement in this process being "self produced by ignorance." He also stated that this "self produced by ignorance" is not the true self that is interconnected with all things in the universe.

According to a Buddhist teaching, we are a collection of five aggregates (i.e., *skandha: matter, sensation, perception, mental formations, and consciousness*). However, when these five aggregates work together, it somehow produces "I." We consider the "I" as the owner and operator of the five aggregates. In Sanskrit, this is called *panca upadana skandha* (five aggregates of clinging). In other words, this is the karmic self, the self created by various elements and experiences we had in the past. Our psychology works based upon our clinging to the "I," and desires for satisfying this "I" are called karmic consciousness.

When Dogen Zenji says "to study the Buddha Way is to study the self," he does not mean to study the self that is produced by illusory thoughts (i.e., self as the owner and operator). Rather our "true" self is revealed when we deconstruct and become released from such clinging to the karmic self by letting go of the self-centered thoughts that are produced by the karmic consciousness. To study the true self is to study the Buddha way.

Zazen

The transformation of self from the karmic self to the true self is not achieved through thinking. According to a Zen teaching, thinking is the very process of dividing the our experience into pieces. In unison with the desires for satisfaction, it is this "discriminative thinking" that is the core of the problem. Zazen is the posture of forgetting the self that is hardened by illusory conceptual thinking. It is important to let go of the thoughts

[1]In Sutta-Nipata the Buddha said, "They are islands unto themselves. They have nothing. They go from place to place and in every way they are free." (translation by H. Saddhatissa, The Sutta-Nipata, Curzon Press, Richmond, England, 1994) p. 57.

In The Dhammapada the Buddha said, "Only a man himself can be the master of himself: who else from outside could be his master?" (translation by Juan Mascaro, The Dammapada: The Path of Perfection, Penguin Books, London, 1973) p. 58.

In the *Mahaparinibbana Sutta*, the Buddha said, "Ananda, you should live as islands unto yourselves, being your own refuge, with no one else as your refuge." (translation by Maurice Walshe, The Long Discourse of the Buddha: A Translation of the Digha Nikaya, Wisdom Publications, Boston, 1995) p. 245.

[2]Translation by Okumura (Realizing Genjokoan: The Key to Dogen's shobogenzo, Wisdom Publications, Somerville, 2010) p. 2.

that come from the karmic self without making new karma (please see additional discussion below). In zazen, the five aggregates are simply five aggregates without clinging; therefore, we are released from *panca upadana skandha*. In Dogen's expression, this is called dropping off body and mind (*shinjin-datsuraku*). Dogen says in *Fukanzazengi (Universal Recommendation for Zazen)*:

> Let go of all associations, and put all affairs aside.
> Do not think of either good or evil.
> Do not be concerned with either right or wrong.
> Put aside the operation of your intellect, volition, and consciousness.
> Stop considering things with your memory, imagination, and contemplation.
> Do not seek to become Buddha.[3]

When we practice zazen, we let go of everything. We let go of what we studied, what we memorized, and what we thought including any aspiration to become a Buddha. To express what is happening in zazen, Uchiyama Roshi coined the expression "opening the hand of thought." Even when we sit in an upright posture, all different kinds of thoughts come and go. We simply let them come and let them go; we do not pursue them; we do not fight against them; we do not make efforts to eliminate them. We focus on keeping the upright posture as well as deep and quiet abdominal breathing, not through thinking but through our bones and muscles. We entrust everything to this posture. This unique expression later became the title of the book that is the collection of English translations of his several writings.

Zazen is "just sitting." But we can do two more things in addition to just sitting when we are on the cushion in front of the wall: thinking and sleeping. Zazen is neither thinking nor sleeping. Even if we sit in upright posture, if we think, it is the same with thinking at a desk or in front of a computer. If we are sleeping, it is not different from sleeping in a bed. Both are not zazen of just sitting. Whenever we aware we deviate from just sitting, we return to just sitting, by waking up from sleep or letting go of thoughts.

There are important distinctions between "thinking" and "thoughts are coming and going." Even when we sit facing the wall, our stomach continues to digest what we ate and the heart continues to beat and pumps blood. Every organ is still working. There is no reason that only our brain should stop functioning in zazen. Metaphorically speaking, the function of our brain is to produce thoughts. It is as if thoughts are secreted from our brain in exactly the same way as the stomach secretes gastric acid. But as we sit and let go of thoughts, thoughts exist without thinking. When we think, our mind is divided into two parts. One part becomes the subject, and the thoughts that come and go become the objects of thinking. These two parts interact with each other. When we are aware that our mind has such separation and interaction, we return to just sitting, upright posture, deep and smooth breathing. This is what letting go of thought actually means. In zazen, we focus our efforts to just sit, whenever we aware that we are deviating from just sitting and engaging in thinking or sleeping, we return to just sitting.

Within this upright posture and letting go of thoughts, true original self manifests itself. Zazen is experiencing the serene self without being deceived by any kind of karmic thoughts. Dogen says in *Shobogenzo Zuimonki*:

> Sitting itself is the practice of the Buddha. Sitting itself is non-doing. It is nothing but the true form of the Self. Apart from sitting, there is nothing to seek as the Buddha-dharma.[4]

In *Shobogenzo Zanmai-o-zanmai (The Samadhi that is the king of Samadhis)*, he also said:

> Now, we must know clearly that *kekkafuza* (full lotus sitting) itself is the king of samadhis. *Kekkafuza* itself is realizing and entering this samadhi. All other samadhis are the attendants of this king of samadhis. *Kekkafuza* is a straight body, straight mind, straight body and mind, the buddhas and ancestors themselves, practice-enlightenment

[3]This is Okumura's unpublished translation.

[4]Okumura's translation in Shobogenzo-zuimonki: Sayings of Eihei Dogen Zenji recorded by Koun Ejo (Sotoshu Shumucho, Tokyo, 1988) p. 101.

> itself, the essence of buddha-dharma, and Life itself. We sit in *kekkafuza* with this human skin, flesh, bones, and marrow, actualizing the king of samadhis. Shakyamuni Buddha always upheld and maintained *kekkafuza*. He intimately transmitted *kekkafuza* to his disciples, and taught it to lay people. …. This is the essence of the teaching of his whole life. It is lacking nothing. *Kekkafuza* is the essence of all of the sutras. This is when the Buddha sees the buddha. At the very time of sitting, sentient beings attain buddhahood.[5]

For Dogen, zazen is not a method or means to attain some desirable effects, such as awakening, enlightenment, and discovery of one's true nature; zazen is itself true self, true Dharma. In zazen, we gain nothing. We practice without gaining mind. Sawaki Roshi, Uchiyama Roshi's teacher, said that zazen is good for nothing.

Attitude Toward Our Life: Three Minds, Vow, and Repentance

Uchiyama Roshi wrote that there are two paths for human lives. One is to pursue the fulfillment of our desires for satisfaction by working hard and competing with others. We are always dissatisfied with who we are and the conditions we are in. We feel as if there is something lacking and believe that if we gain or accomplish something to fill the empty space, we must become happy. We make efforts to reach it. However, once we obtain it, we know that we are not fulfilled, and we set another goal to fill the next space. The consequence is that our desires grow larger and larger. It is as if we are hungry ghosts. We naturally become competitive with others because what we want to gain is pretty much the same thing other people who have the same kinds of desires want to get. This is how our lives become *samsara*. Even when we become successful and feel we have more power, wealth, fame, social status than others, we are not free from fear of losing them. When we die, everything we have accomplished and gained will be left behind.

[5]Okumura's unpublished translation.

The other path is what Shakyamuni Buddha walked. Even though he was born as a prince, he left his father's palace to pursue the path of liberation. He gave up all of the privileges he had as a young, healthy, strong, and wise prince. In the worldly sense, he became a beggar. After he had awakened, he taught about what he awakened to and gave others the guidance on how to live a wholesome life without being pulled by dissatisfaction and competitive thinking. As the leader of the community of monks and lay followers, he lived the wholesome way through practicing the eightfold correct path as the middle-way for the rest of his life.

The two paths are the opposite ways of approaching life. When we discover the true reality of our self that is connected with all other beings, we cannot avoid aspiring to live harmoniously with all beings. Because we are supported by all beings, we need to support all beings, too. Dogen Zenji described the three minds in *Tenzokyokun* that highlights the mental attitude that we need to maintain if we are aspiring to walk the latter path. The three minds are the magnanimous mind, nurturing mind, and joyful mind. Uchiyama Roshi also often emphasized that we maintain the same attitude in our daily lives based on zazen practice.[6]

Daishin (Magnanimous Mind)

Magnanimous mind is the mind of non-discrimination such as great mountains or the great ocean. Mountains are immovable and embrace different living beings such as tall trees, short trees, grasses, flowers, big and small animals, insects, bacteria, and many others without making discrimination. The great ocean accepts water from different rivers and simply becomes one ocean. As a bodhisattva, we need to embrace all people and living beings, and we need to be free from comparison and evaluations of what is valuable or worthless, what is wonderful or

[6]About the three minds, see *Dogen's Pure Standards for the Zen Community: a translation of Eihei Shingi* (Taigen Dan Leighton and Shohaku Okumura, State University of New York Press, Albany, 1996), and *How to Cook Your Life: From the Zen Kitchen to enlightenment* (translated by Thomas Wright, Weatherhill, Tokyo, 1993).

difficult. We should see various conditions with a single eye without the worldly system of values and judgment.

Roshin (Nurturing Mind)

Dogen stated that a nurturing mind is the mind of parents. Even if they are poor, they protect their children under any circumstances. Childish people want to be taken care of, crying and complaining if they are not. However, matured people find a meaning of life in working hard to protect their children and others. As a bodhisattva, we should consider the three treasures of Buddhism (i.e., Buddha, Dharma, and Sangha) as our children, protecting and nurturing them.

Kishin (Joyful Mind)

Joyful mind is the attitude that finds a joy within working to take care of others. When we are in favorable conditions, we do not need joyful mind because the circumstances are already joyful. We can simply enjoy our life. When we are in difficult situations and cannot find any reason to enjoy them, we need joyful mind for not being overwhelmed by the difficulties and our negative thoughts and emotions influenced by these difficulties.

Vow and Repentance

Another thing Uchiyama Roshi emphasized was that we must take bodhisattva vows and practice repentance. In Mahayana Buddhism, all bodhisattvas have to take four general vows: (1) Beings are numberless, I vow to free them; (2) Delusions are inexhaustible, I vow to end them, (3) Dharma gates are boundless, I vow to enter them; (4) The Buddha way is unsurpassable, I vow to realize it. These are endless vows under the direction of the bodhisattva practice. We must walk toward the direction even one step at a time, but it is not possible to completely accomplish them. Our practice is always incomplete; therefore, as we take these vows we need to make repentance. Repentance in the bodhisattva practice is not simply saying "I am sorry; I will try not to make the same mistake again." Rather, repentance in this context is the awareness of the incompleteness of our practice. This awareness encourages us to take another step forward on the journey.

Specific, concrete, and attainable vows are necessary for each of us. Uchiyama Roshi always said that he had two vows: one was to produce determined zazen practitioners; the other was to write texts of zazen practice for the modern practitioners.

When I began to practice at Antaiji in 1972, I understood that I needed to take the bodhisattva vows, but I had some difficulties in finding my own strong motivation to help all beings. Because my question regarding life originally came from my own desire of escaping from the busy, noisy materialistic society, I was not so much interested in working toward helping others.

Practice at Antaiji

My First Five-Day Sesshin

As mentioned above, I first visited Antaiji in January 1969 to sit for the five-day sesshin, a period of intense meditation (zazen). I was a 20-year-old college student. I had only about half a year of experience practicing zazen after I entered Komazawa University in Tokyo in the previous year. During the sesshin at Antaiji, we sat fourteen 50-min periods of zazen a day. We woke up at 4 a.m., washed our face, brushed our teeth, and went to the zendo (i.e., meditation hall) by 4:10 a.m. We sat two periods before breakfast, which was scheduled at 6:00 a.m. Between the periods of zazen, we had 10 min *kinhin* (walking meditation). After breakfast, we had a short break then sat again from 7:10 a.m. to 12:00 p.m., five consecutive periods. We then had lunch and a short break until 1:10 p.m. We sat five more periods in the afternoon until 6:00 p.m., followed by supper and a short break. Then, we sat from 7:10 p.m. to 9:00 p.m. This extremely simple schedule repeated for five days. On the last day of the sesshin, we sat until 5:00 p.m. instead of 9:00 p.m.

During my first experience of a five-day sesshin, I experienced pain in my feet, ankles, knees, and lower back. To sit in a cross-legged posture was to sit with pain. In Tokyo, I read books until early morning, slept until late morning, and then went to school. I had to wake up around the time I usually went to bed. I was constantly sleepy as if I had jet lag. The zendo at Antaiji was not in good condition. There were spaces between pillars and walls such that cold air entered in freely. We only had two small kerosene stoves. The sesshin was painful, exhausting, and a cold experience. When the sesshin completed, I thought that it would be my last sesshin. Only thing I could enjoy were meals. Even though we had to sit in *seiza*, one of the traditional ways of sitting in Japan, and were required to eat quickly, I was happy to have wholesome, albeit simple foods, as I was a starving student. Several months later, somehow and someway, I returned to Antaiji. To this date, Antaiji style of sesshin has been my main Zen practice.

Antaiji Practice Under Uchiyama Roshi's Guidance

Immediately after I graduated from Komazawa University in 1972, I entered Antaiji. This felt like a natural decision after having spent my years in college constantly reading books and thinking; I was tired of it. I put all of my books in the closet and tried not to read them except for the texts which Uchiyama Roshi gave lectures on, and Dogen Zenji's *Shobogenzo Zuimonki*. Zuimonki is a collection of Dogen's short informal talks recorded by his successor, Ejo. Uchiyama Roshi gave two 90-min lectures on a bimonthly meeting, called Sunday Zazen-kai. He spoke on various texts written by Dogen. I read the entire Zuimonki so many times that I almost memorized the talks.

Sesshin

We had ten sesshin each year except February and August when it was too cold and too hot in Kyoto. June and September sesshin were three days because of humidity and heat. Having a five-day sesshin each month was difficult for me but I was happy to devote myself fully to it.

Daily Practice

For the rest of the month, we sat three periods in the early morning from 5:00 a.m. to 8:00 a.m., and two periods in the evening from 6:00 p.m. to 8:00 p.m. During daytime, we did various necessary work called *samu* (community work), such as cleaning the temple, taking care of the vegetable garden, and chopping firewood. Because we cooked and created warm water with firewood, preparing firewood all year round was one of the most important tasks. Especially at a temple like Antaiji, which was located in a city, collecting firewood was sometimes quite challenging. We had a small garden where we grew vegetables, such as various kinds of greens, cucumbers, eggplants, and tomatoes. We ate them during the summer. From the summer to the fall, we also grew daikon radishes and Chinese cabbages to pickle for the winter and the following year. Cleaning the temple and weeding the temple ground were also important duties. When we did not have community work, I often took a walk in the mountains near the temple while others self-studied.

Takuhatsu

As Antaiji had no family members or particular patrons, monks there had to support their practice by *takuhatsu* (begging), a traditional form of alms common among Zen Buddhist monks in Japan. We went out to do *takuhatsu* two or three times a month to support our practice and purchase foods for the sesshin. Sesshin was also open to the community members. Uchiyama Roshi never required sesshin participants to pay a fee or make donations. He simply asked them to bring one cup of rice for each meal they wanted to have during the sesshin. There were, of course, people who made donations; however, it was never requested of them.

Takuhatsu was a powerful practice. When we walked on the streets wearing traditional

Buddhist robes, bamboo hats, and straw sandals, people bowed to us with *gassho* (both hands putting together) so politely as if they were worshiping the Buddha. Other people insulted us or even shouted at us. Some people simply ignored us. Toward all people who treated us in various ways, we maintained the same sincere and polite attitude. For me, takuhatsu was not simply to receive donation; it was also a practice to be free from our discrimination toward all people regardless of their attitudes toward us.

No Ceremony, No Chanting

One of the most unique aspects of Antaiji, compared to other Zen temples, was that we conducted almost no ceremonies. We had no morning, noon, or evening service except the ones during the two weeks of summer special period in August, which were offered to college students for learning Zen. For the rest of the year, the only time we chanted was when we went to takuhatsu and when we came back from takuhatsu. We chanted the *Heart Sutra,* a famous sutra in Mahayana Buddhism, and *Shosaimyo-kichijo-darani.*[7] We had meals in the dining room using *oryoki*, but we did not chant the meal verses. We, Antaiji monks, had a bad reputation when we went to other monasteries for practice because we could not chant even the *Heart Sutra* without seeing a sutra book.

Antaiji was originally established in 1921 as the study monastery for the selected monks who graduated from Komazawa University and wished to continue to study Dogen's teachings. That was why it did not have family members, and therefore, it was not necessary to do funeral ceremonies or memorial services for lay people. Uchiyama Roshi decided not to have even daily morning, noon, and evening services to make it clear that Antaiji focused on the practice of zazen alone.

[7]*Dharani* is the mystic syllables like a *mantra.* Indian people thoughts the words themselves had the power even to move heavenly gods to bestow them some benefits, therefore dharani and mantra were not translated. We chanted in transliteration of the Sanskrit words. This particular dharani is to praise the blessing of the Buddha to save all beings from suffering.

Cooking

All monks took turns cooking every three days. Our meals were very simple. In the morning, we usually had rice gruel made from the leftover rice from the day before and pickled *daikon* or other vegetables. For lunch, we had brown rice, miso-soup, and some pickled vegetables. For supper, we had either brown rice or white rice, *miso*-soup, one side dish, and pickled vegetables. Cooking is the actual practice of what Dogen taught in *Tenzokyokun (Instruction to Cook).*[8] Uchiyama Roshi wrote a commentary on the text entitled *How to Cook Your Life* and described how we should work in the kitchen as an important practice as zazen in the zendo. Because we did not have a gas or electric stove, we cooked with firewood. Cooking with firewood was completely different from cooking with gas or electricity. It was a practice of concentration and attentiveness. We had to take care of three or four fires simultaneously to cook rice, make soup, a side dish, and boil water for tea. If the fire was too strong, we burned everything; if it was not strong enough, half cooked food was not eatable.

No Bait

As Antaiji was a small temple, we were not qualified to be teachers of Soto Zen School despite having a strict zazen practice. We needed to go to other official monasteries to get qualification to become a temple priest. Uchiyama Roshi stated that the practice at Antaiji had no bait. What he meant was that we needed to just practice for the sake of practice without any expectation of desired outcomes, such as getting the license to become a teacher. In Uchiyama Roshi's teachings, this practice without any expectation, but just practice, was very

[8]See footnote 6.

important. We maintained the same attitude with in zazen in our daily lives without gaining mind.

English

During the monthly five-day sesshin, we usually had about 50–60 people. One-third of the participants were the resident practitioners like myself, another one-third were Japanese from outside Antaiji, and the final one-third were those from the USA, Germany, England, France, Australia, and other countries. Many of them lived in various parts of Kyoto, and they came to sit sesshin regularly. Some of them lived in a neighborhood of Antaiji and came to sit every morning and evening.

In 1960s and early 70s, many Zen centers were established in the USA and Europe. So called "hippies" became very interested in Eastern spirituality including Zen. Many of them came to Kyoto to study Japanese cultures, such as martial arts, tea ceremonies, Noh theater, *sumie* painting, haiku poetry, Japanese traditional carpentry, and vegetarian cooking. They thought that Zen was the spiritual origin of these Japanese arts. Some of them came from Zen centers to practice in a Japanese traditional monastic setting. At that time, there were few Zen Buddhist temples in Japan that were open to the westerners. Uchiyama Roshi accepted and welcomed those young people and allowed them to stay at Antaiji until they found a place to live. Several of them lived at Antaiji and became ordained monks.

Although there were many westerners who regularly came to sit at Antaiji, Uchiyama Roshi himself did not speak any foreign languages. He wanted to teach the true meaning of zazen practice as the Buddha-dharma to those young westerners. He always had a vast perspective of the history of human spirituality, and he thought that the twenty-first century must be the age of spirituality. And he often stated that the world needed people who had thorough experience of zazen practice in order to convey the significance of zazen to other cultures in various languages. I was very much influenced by the depth and breadth of his vision.

When I started to practice at Antaiji, Uhiyama Roshi asked me if I wanted to study English. Even though I was not interested in English, somehow, I could not say "No." My half-hearted "Yes," ultimately changed the rest of my life. After I started studying English, I became one of the "English-speaking" Japanese monks. Many westerners became my friends. Practicing zazen with westerners became very natural to me. My current activity in the USA is a tiny fruit of Uchiyama Roshi's boundless vision. My life would have been quite different had I not met him.

My Practice After Leaving Antaiji

Pioneer Valley Zendo

I practiced in this way until 1975, the year in which Uchiyama Roshi retired. Three of Uchiyama Roshis' disciples who studied English went to Massachusetts in 1975 to establish a small Zen Community, called Pioneer Valley Zendo. I was one of the three disciples.

The purpose of establishing the Pioneer Valley Zendo was to transplant Uchiyama Roshi's style of Zen (i.e., just sitting) in USA soil. We bought roughly six acres of woodland in western Massachusetts. We had nothing but trees, and we built a small house. Three Japanese monks lived together, sat, and worked hard to make the place livable. We still continued the five-day sesshin every month with the same schedule as the one at Antaiji. We cleared the land, made vegetable gardens, and dug a well. Our days consisted completely of sitting and working tirelessly.

Because I was raised in a city (i.e., Osaka, Japan), I enjoyed living in the quiet and peaceful woods in western Massachusetts, practicing zazen, and working tirelessly to establish the zendo. I had almost no access to information about what was happening in the rest of the world for about five years. We did not watch T.V., listen to radio, or read newspapers. I felt that my desire to escape from a busy, noisy society was finally fulfilled.

One day in 1978 or 1979, I had a sesshin at a Zen center in Yew York City. After the sesshin, I had a half-day off before returning to Massachusetts. I took a walk in Manhattan heading south, finally reaching a park where I could see the Statue of Liberty. I did not bring any money, I did not have an ID, neither did I have my driver's license or passport. I simply had robes in my bag and a ticket for a bus ride to return. It occurred to me that if I was hit by a car and killed right in that moment, no one would know who I was. At that very moment, I felt that I did not need to and should not escape any more. From that moment, I felt that I could return to the society not for becoming a part of the money-making machine, but for dedicating myself to the Dharma.

During my earlier days in Massachusetts, I felt the harder I worked, the stronger my body became. It worked really well when I was in my twenties. However, after I turned thirty, my body began to break down from the hard labor of building Pioneer Valley. Because I did not have income to receive medical care, I was forced to return to Japan in the winter of 1981.

Returning to Kyoto: Truly Good-for-Nothing Zazen

Right after returning to Japan, I stayed in my brother's apartment in Osaka. He was traveling to the USA for about six months. I felt that I did not have a place to practice, I had no sangha, I had no money, no job, and my body felt half broken. Given my physical conditions, I could not practice in the way I had previously for the last ten years at Antaiji and Pioneer Valley Zendo. It was difficult for me to live by myself without practice or sangha. In my twenties, I had devoted my life entirely to practice and to working for the Dharma. I did not know what to do.

I was confused and even depressed for a while. I felt that my life was a failure. It was not because I felt that I was in such a miserable situation; I clearly recognized the conditions that I was in and the cause of it. My struggles stemmed from the question of why I was in great agony if I knew that zazen was good for nothing and that I practiced without any expectations. I was very fortunate that, from the beginning of my study and practice of Zen, I encountered Sawaki Roshi and Uchiyama Roshi's teachings. Sawaki Roshi clearly stated that zazen is good for nothing. I thought that I understood it and dedicated myself to the "good-for-nothing" practice. Yet I continued to ask myself why not practicing zazen is a problem if it was in fact good for nothing. This great confusion continued for a while.

One day in a great struggle, I realized that my practice in my twenties was not actually good for nothing. I recognized that I had felt that, because of my zazen practice, my life was good, or perhaps better than others' who worked hard in society to make money. I realized that I actually relied on zazen practice to justify my way of living. I saw that my practice had not been really for the sake of Dharma, but rather for my own self-satisfaction. I felt that I could not continue to practice this way. I also could not stop practicing and go back to an ordinary life in the mundane world. I was stuck at the dead end.

I also realized that, in a deeper part of my karmic self, which was much deeper than my rational thinking, my desire to be a "good" boy had been a strong drive since my childhood.

I was a "good" boy until I became a high school student. It was not easy to keep up with this impression; I always wanted to find out what parents, teachers, friends, and others wanted me to do before doing anything, then I tried to do things in the way I thought they would have liked me to do them. When I became a teenager, I felt this way of choosing my actions was not honest or genuine. When I observed my friends, some of them did things simply because they wanted to do so without considering others. Some of them were considered "bad" boys, and I thought that they were more genuine and honest to themselves than I had been. I remembered having the feeling that I really wanted to change myself. That was one of the major reasons why I wanted to become a Zen monk; I wanted to escape from the influence of society. In a sense, being a Zen monk, I successfully betrayed and rejected all of the expectations I had internalized from my parents, teachers, and the entire Japanese society.

In the midst of this great struggle, I also had the realization that, even after I became a monk, I was controlled by my desire to be a good boy. I wanted to be a good student of the Buddha and a good disciple of my teacher. I had a desire to be a better practitioner than others even though I tried not to express such desires explicitly. The fact was that this realization did not take me to a state of awakening. Rather, it led me to greater disappointment. I felt that I could not continue to live in this way; I could not actually be a good boy as the son of my parents or as a disciple of my teacher. I began to feel that I was really good for nothing, in its worst meaning, not in the meaning of Sawaki Roshi's teaching.

Then, one day, something prompted me to sit on a cushion in my apartment. I had no desire, no reason, and no need to sit, but I found myself sitting by myself. It was very peaceful. I did not sit because of the Buddha's teaching, or my teacher's. No one watched me and saw if I was a good boy or not. I did not need a reason to sit; I simply sat. There existed no need to compare or compete with others or with myself. It was the first time that I felt that I was really doing the "good for nothing" zazen.

It is important to recognize that it was difficult to practice good for nothing zazen. It took me more than ten years of continuous practice. I do not think that I have stopped wanting to be a good boy. However, since I recognized my desire for being a good boy as a disruption, I am less controlled by it. Rather, I can make fun of myself when I behave in ways that focus on pleasing others and being a good boy.

Kyoto Soto Zen Center

In the summer of 1981, I moved to a small temple in Kyoto, called Seitai-an where my friend was the abbot. He graciously allowed me to live there as a caretaker. That was about 6 months after I returned from Massachusetts. Uchiyama Roshi encouraged me to work on the English translation of Dogen's and his writings with one of my American dharma brothers, Daitsu Tom Wright. He also suggested that I establish a place where I could do the translation work and practice mainly with the people from other countries. At that time, there were many people who visited Kyoto to study and practice Zen, but there were not many Soto Zen temples, which accepted them.

In 1983, while I stayed at Seitai-an, I married Yuko. Her father practiced zazen at his family temple. The abbot of the temple practiced with Sawaki Roshi, while he was a student at Komazawa University. Yuko had practiced zazen since she was 16 years old. Later, she went to Komazawa University. Yuko, however, withdrew from Komazawa University before graduation, and then went to the USA to study English and visit Dainin Katagiri Roshi at Minnesota Zen Meditation Center. Minnesota Zen Meditation Center was formed in 1972 by Katagiri Roshi when he was invited to come from California.

After coming back to Japan, Yuko visited Seitai-an with a female disciple of Katagiri Roshi. Three weeks after we married, she went to Antaiji to learn sewing Buddhist robes called *okesa*. She remained there for one year. At Kyoto Soto Zen Center, she did tenzo (cooked) during sesshin until we had children. Our daughter Yoko was born in 1987, and our son Masaki was born in 1991.

In 1984, I started Kyoto Soto Zen Center with the support from Rev. Yuho Hosokawa. He allowed me to live in a temple as a caretaker that he owned outside Kyoto. I decided to take over Uchiyama Roshi's two vows and made them my own: practice zazen with western practitioners and translate the texts of zazen practice to be available for non-Japanese practitioners.

I planned to translate several early writings of Dogen Zenji and Uchiyama Roshi's books with Daitsu Tom Wright and other American practitioners. Five translation books were published from Kyoto Soto Zen Center. I continued to practice five-day sesshin ten times a year. I practiced with many students from other countries there until 1992. Unfortunately, Rev. Hosokawa passed away, and I felt that it was time for me to leave the temple. At the time, our daughter Yoko was four years old and our son Masaki was one year old.

Minnesota Zen Meditation Center

After living with my family in a small house, which belonged to a Catholic convent in Kyoto, I moved to Minneapolis to serve as the interim head teacher at Minnesota Zen Meditation Center (MZMC) in 1993. As mentioned above, MZMC was founded by Dainin Katagiri Roshi in 1972, but he passed away in 1990. They were without a teacher for three years. I taught there for three years as the head teacher and another year as a part time teacher until 1997.

Katagiri Roshi practiced with Eko Hashimoto Roshi at Eiheiji, one of two main temples of Soto Zen in Japan. Hashinoto Roshi was a close friend of Sawaki Rosh, but their styles of practice were quite different. As Hashimoto Roshi emphasized detailed formal practice derived from Dogen Zenji, Katagiri Roshi's style of practice was quite different from what I learned from Uchiyama Roshi.

I then decided to follow Katagiri Roshi's style at MZMC because I was the "interim" teacher for filling in his role. Quite honestly, that was a challenge for me. However, that experience helped me broaden my understanding of practice. Through my experiences at MZMC, I learned many things about Soto Zen practice in the USA.

North America Education Center

In 1996, I was asked to work as the director of North America Soto Zen Education Center that was planned to establish in 1997 in Los Angeles, CA, by Japanese Sotoshu Shumucho (The Administrative Headquarters of Japanese Soto Zen). Then, I moved to Los Angeles from Minneapolis in July, 1997 to work for the Education Center. The center moved to San Francisco in 1999, changing names into Soto Zen Buddhism International Center in 2003. It was founded to bridge Japanese Soto Zen tradition and American Soto Zen centers. Another task of this center was to promote the sense of a larger Soto Zen community in America. Many of the Soto Zen centers were established in 1960s and 1970s by various Soto Zen teachers. However, since then, there have not been many communications and exchanges among the lineages. The director position allowed me to travel frequently between the USA and Japan as well as visit various Zen centers in the USA. I had opportunities to meet many Soto Zen teachers in the USA and practiced together with a number of American practitioners in the various sangha. Once again, these experiences allowed me to have broader perspective about Zen in America. I worked as the full time director of the center for the following five years until 2003.

Sanshin Zen Community

In 1996, I founded Sanshin Zen Community after completing my term as the interim head teacher of MZMC. This was the precursor of Sanshinji temple, where I have served as the founder and guiding teacher since 2003. Sanshin means the three minds that I mentioned above. Because I had to move to California to work at the Education Center, I could not be actively involved in establishing a new Zen center. People worked together even though I was not always with them, establishing Sanshinji in Bloomington Indiana in 2003. My family and I moved there in June of that year. I continued to be the half-time director of the International Center until 2010.

One of the reasons why I decided to relocate Sanshinji in Bloomington was that there had previously been no Soto Zen practice center in the entire state of Indiana. There were many Zen centers and Zen teachers, however, in the West Coast. My teacher, Uchiyama roshi, always encouraged us to pioneer. I found that Indiana was a potential frontier for Soto Zen in America, and I was ready to establish a sangha from scratch. To my surprise, as soon as I moved to Bloomington, several practitioners, including a few priests, came to practice with me. Because

Soto Zen was very new in the area and Bloomington is a small university town, we did not have substantial support from the local community. It must have been challenging for the priests to support their practice, but they still practiced diligently. I deeply appreciated their sincerity. About 20 people became my disciples. Some of them have received transmission and became Zen teachers.

Now I am 66-year old, living in Bloomington with my family and practicing with a small number of dedicated practitioners. We have five Uchiyama Roshi style of sesshin a year. Even though I cannot sit in cross-legged posture anymore because of my knees, I continue to sit the sesshin in the way I practiced with my teacher since I was 20 years old. We have two Genzo-e retreats. Genzo-e is a study retreat to focus on a fascicle of Dogen's *Shobogenzo* each time. We also have the Precepts Retreat once a year in July to study various aspects of the bodhisattva precepts we receive in Soto Zen tradition. Each year, several people receive the precepts at the end of the retreat. More than 70 people have received the precepts and became lay Buddhists.

Yuko, my wife, has been an active member of the sangha as a sewing teacher of *rakusu* and *okesa*, the traditional Buddhist robe and the cooking coordinator of sesshin/retreats. Because we never forced them practice or become Buddhists, our children are not practitioners but they support our practice. Yoko became a filmmaker and has filmed my teaching activities. My son, Masaki, had a difficult time transitioning after the move to Bloomington. However, he recently has been involved in the community as a volunteer cooking meals for sesshin and retreats. My family have been supported by the three Jewel, Buddha, Dharma (i.e., teachings of Buddha), and Sangha (i.e., Zen community).

When I lived at Valley Zendo in western Massachusetts, I hitch hiked to New York once. The driver who gave me a ride was a university student. For some reason, he took me to his apartment. I found an embroidery made by his mother. On the embroidery, there were trees and the words saying, "To love is to give a space to grow." I deeply appreciated this saying. That was why I named our children Yoko (child of leaves) and Masaki (tree of truth) with the hope that they would find something they really want to devote themselves to as I did to my path; my hope is that I gave enough space for them to grow.

I have been working on translation and writing my own books. Because of my limited skill in English, I have been working together with various American writers for each book project. The books published with my name are not only my books. All of them are the fruits of collaborative efforts with my American friends and colleagues who love the Dharma and practice. Several books have been published after I started to practice at Sanshinji.

I have been walking a narrow path of just sitting since I first encountered Uchiyama Roshi's teaching. I was a 17-year-old high school student, and it was more than 45 years ago. I have not done anything else. I have been seeing my life from zazen. In just sitting, we let go of thoughts, meaning that we let them come and go. We try not to prevent any thoughts from coming. Letting go of thoughts is the complete negation of all thoughts either being good or bad, positive or negative. And yet letting go is to embrace all thoughts. We do not pick or choose any thoughts, but we simply let them come and go without judgment. In this way, we can be intimate with all different aspects of our mental activities, in different mental and physical conditions and external situations. We cannot lie to ourselves.

Zazen has been the anchor of my life. Without ongoing zazen practice, I would have gone somewhere else, being pulled by my thoughts, desires, ambitions, or hopes of each stages of my life. Zazen practice allows me to walk stably on the path of vow and repentance.

This is a narrow path, but I have been practicing with many people both in Japan and America. Through my translation work and book writing, I have friends not only in the USA, but also various parts of the world. I am deeply grateful to my teacher, Kosho Uchiyama, and the tradition of Shakyamuni Buddha, Mahayana Buddhism, and Dogen's Soto Zen.

One thing that has become increasingly clear to me by walking this narrow path is that I am connected with all people and beings throughout time and space. I can live only within the relation with all beings and support from them. I should say, instead, there is no such thing called "I" beside the relation and interconnectedness.

Bodhisattva Way and Therapy

Because this book is primarily for various professionals and students in the fled of behavioral healthcare, I would like to say one thing. I do not think that my practice of just sitting as a Mahayana Buddhist or bodhisattva practice is a therapy. In my understanding, a therapy is a method for enabling those who are not able to function well to function in a normal, healthy way. I acknowledge that Buddhism is often considered therapeutic as the teachings of Four Noble Truths are understood as the diagnosis and prescription for the ill by the doctor, Buddha.

I would say that such an understanding of Buddhist teaching is not incorrect. However, it is based on a limited view, I think. At least, for Shakyamuni himself, the practice of the eightfold correct path, which is the fourth of the Four Noble Truths, is not a method for reaching the cessation of suffering. He did not practice the eightfold correct path as the preparation for attaining awakening. He discovered the eightfold correct path as the Middle Way between two extremes, self-indulgence and self-mortification within his awakening. Then, he practiced the eightfold correct path for the rest of his life.

When he taught the five monks at the Deer Park, he taught the same eightfold correct path as the path leading to the cessation of suffering for the people who are in the middle of suffering. Then, the eightfold correct path began to be viewed as a method or a means to be released from suffering. There are two different meanings of the path of practice; one is the meaning for Shakyamuni himself, and the other is for the people transmigrating within samsara.

When Dogen talked about the practice of zazen, he meant his zazen practice in the former meaning of the eightfold correct path. The model of his zazen was Shakyamuni's zazen after he became the Buddha. The Buddha did not practice zazen as a means to attain enlightenment because he was already enlightened. That was why Dogen said that zazen itself is buddhas' practice, not a method to make deluded human beings into enlightened buddhas. To me, this is the difference between the endless bodhisattva practice following the Buddha's way and a therapy that is used to alleviate suffering for those with mental illnesses.

It is fine with the idea that any methods of meditation practice developed in Buddhist traditions can be useful as a therapy to help people who are mentally and physically in trouble to restore a healthy condition. However, if that is the only meaning, then as those people restore their wholesome condition, they have no reason to continue to practice. I believe that Zen practice should be continuous and ongoing.

My practice of zazen is not a temporary "method" to restore mental or physical health. When we are sick, the healthy way of life can be a medicine. But, when we restore health, we still need to continue to practice the same thing as Shakyamuni practiced after he became a buddha until the end of his life. The Bodhisattva way is not simply a method to restore health, but it is a healthy way of life.

Conclusion

To sit 50-min a period 14 times a day may not be possible for most of the clients. However, this practice might be meaningful for the therapists who wish to experience thoroughly who we are as humans and what we are here and now for. I hope that behavioral health professionals and students are also bodhisattvas who take the vow to save all beings, even if they are not "Buddhists."

A Brief Note on Zazen

Tairyu Tsunoda, Akihiko Masuda and Kayla Sargent

Keywords
Zen · Zazen · Buddhism · Meditation · Behavioral health

Today, many think that the posture of zazen (i.e., sitting meditation of Zen) is designed to deliberately produce pain, so that one can become strong by transcending it. For many of us, zazen posture is quite uncomfortable; however, our relative experiences in this form of cross-legged sitting may be the result of lifestyle or culture. Regardless, the assumption that zazen is intended to be painful for the sake of overcoming pain is misguided. The posture of zazen originated in India, supposedly selected because it was actually the most comfortable sitting position for the people of India at that time. More specifically, sitting tranquilly under a big tree was thought of with reverence as a practice associated with ancient wisdom. Many Zen scholars and practitioners believe that zazen posture must have enhanced their survival in the severe climate of India (e.g., heat). During the daytime, the posture of zazen would have been a position in which people could comfortably remain for extended periods of time, saving energy meanwhile.

In *Fukanzazengi* (普勧坐禅儀; Universally Recommended Instructions for Zazen), Dogen Zenji (道元禅師; 1200–1253), the founder of Soto Zen in Japan, stated that Zen is not for enlightenment, but it is simply the dharma gate of joyful ease. Although there are distinctions between Dogen's Zen and a meditative practice native to Indian religions called *dhyana*, these nevertheless overlap at a fundamental level. Zazen utilizes its specific posture for the purpose of settling the self to the here and now; it is by no means intended as a stoic practice of deliberately exposing its participants to pain. Zazen is the posture of tranquility (i.e., joyful ease). As noted elsewhere in this volume, Zen meditation is found to be efficacious for promoting various aspects of well-being (see Chiesa 2009 for a comprehensive empirical review of Zen meditation).

Doing zazen wholeheartedly is the Buddha Way. Gautama Buddha attained the dharma of dependent arising, the Middle Way, and the Four

---

Edited and translated by Akihiko Masuda and Kayla Sargent

T. Tsunoda (✉)
Komazawa University, Setagaya, Tokyo, Japan
e-mail: tsunoda@joen-ji.jp

A. Masuda (✉) · K. Sargent
University of Hawaii, Honolulu, HI, USA
e-mail: amasuda4@hawaii.edu

K. Sargent
e-mail: kaylansargent@gmail.com

A. Masuda and W.T. O'Donohue (eds.), *Handbook of Zen, Mindfulness, and Behavioral Health*,
Mindfulness in Behavioral Health, DOI 10.1007/978-3-319-54595-0_5

Noble Truths through zazen under the Bodhi tree. Later in China, the Tiantai school of Buddhism (天台宗; Tendai shu in Japanese) introduced zazen as a practice of adjusting or correcting one's body and mind, and it was called *shikan* (止観 in Japanese). *Shi* in *shikan* means the stillness or calming of the mind (i.e., samatha), and *kan* means seeing something before you correctly or insight into the true nature of reality. Together, *shikan* means to remain tranquil in response to various external stimuli as well as to see these stimuli openly and correctly from the standpoint of one's wisdom (i.e., true self).

The Tiantai school also established its own meditation based on the principles of *shikan* (i.e., samatha and vipassana). The Tiantai meditation treatises, such as the Concise samatha-vipasyana (小止観) and Maha-samatha-vipassana (摩訶止観), influenced the development of Chinese Zen and its Zen meditation. These two documents were written by Zhiyi (Chinese: 智顗, 538–597), and they also influenced the development of Zen and Zen practice later in Japan.

During the Song Dynasty (960–1279), Chinese Zen was divided into Kanna-zen (看話禅 in Japanese; koan-introspecting Zen), which was formalized by Dahui Zonggao (1089–1163; 大慧宗杲; Daie Soko in Japanese) and Mokusho-zen (黙照禅 in Japanese; Silent Illumination Zen) was matured by Hongzhi Zhengjue (1091–1157; 宏智正覺; Wanshi Shogaku in Japanese). In general, Kanna-zen is a *koan*-based method of Zen Buddhism. A *koan* (公案 in Japanese) is a story, dialogue, question, or statement made by ancient Zen masters that is used in Zen practice to provoke "great doubt" and subsequently the breakthrough into the enlightenment.

The Rinzai school of Zen in Japan is traced back to Kanna-zen in the Song Dynasty. In Rinzai Zen training, student monks meet their teachers individually and learn the Buddha Way in part through dialogues on a given *koan*. As they continue working through koans, students learn the Buddha Way unfolding in everyday living and eventually become true Zen monks.

Conversely, Mokusho-zen is characterized by the practice of just sitting with silence. That is, it is simply the practice of just sitting. This practice of sitting was transmitted from Tiantong Rujing of the Caodong school of Zen (1162–1228; 天童如淨; Tendo Nyojo in Japanese) to Dogen. The zazen of the Soto School, founded by Dogen, is known as *shikantaza* (只管打座), which is to sit single-mindedly. Within Soto Zen, zazen is not a means to achieve a specific end or goal, including the experience or goal of enlightenment. The form of zazen itself is thought to be the form of Buddha, the form of enlightenment. Therefore, zazen in Soto Zen is called just sitting.

According to Dogen, certain personal characteristics and ways of relating to the world can prevent people from attaining enlightenment, namely those with a strong sense of self as a unique being (e.g., ego) or a conventionally Western and analytic perspective will likely experience difficulty integrating zazen into their lives without the concept of the "self" interfering. Because of this, he recommended that we must let go and let ourselves immerse fully into the practice of just sitting. In the practice of wholehearted sitting, one gains everything and loses everything simultaneously. Within such a practice, the Buddha nature naturally unfolds as if a light illuminates naturally in darkness. In *Genjokoan* (現成公案; sometimes translated as Actualization of Reality), Dogen stated as follows:

> To study the Buddha way is to study the self. To study the self is to forget the self. To forget the self is to be verified by all things. To be verified by all things is to let the body and mind of the self and the body and mind of others drop off. There is a trace of realization that cannot be grasped. We endlessly express this ungraspable trace of realization (see Okumura 2010, p. 2).

Furthermore, Dogen stated the significance of *shikantaza* as follows:

> When we sit zazen, what precept is not observed, what merit is not actualized? The ways of practice carried on by the ancient masters have a profound meaning. Without holding on to personal

> preferences, we should go along with the assembly and practice in accordance with those ways (see Dogen et al. 1988, p. 22).
>
> Sitting itself is the practice of the buddha. Sitting itself is non-doing. It is nothing but the true form of the Self. Apart from sitting, there is nothing to seek as the buddha-dharma (see Dogen et al. 1988, p. 103).

Finally, throughout his life, Dogen emphasized the depth of zazen practice. In *Bendowa* (弁道話; Talk on Wholehearted Practice of the Way), he stated the following:

> You should know that even if all the buddhas in the ten directions, as numerous as the sands of the Ganges River, together engage the full power of their Buddha wisdom, they could never reach the limit, or measure or comprehend the virtue of one person's zazen (Dogen et al. 1997, p. 24).

References

Chiesa, A. (2009). Zen meditation: An integration of current evidence. *Journal of Alternative and Complementary Medicine, 15*(5), 585–592. doi:10.1089/acm.2008.0416

Dogen, E., Ejo, K., Okumura, S., & Wright, D. T. (1988). *Shobogenzo-zuimonki: Sayings of Eihei Dogen Zenji*. Tokyo, Japan: Soto-shu Shumucho

Dogen, E., Uchiyama, K., Okumura, S., & Leighton, T. D. (1997). *The wholehearted way: A tranlation of Eihei Dogen's Bendowa with commentary by Kosho Uchiyama Roshi*. North Clarendon, VT, US: Tuttle Publications.

Okumura, S. (2010). *Realizing Genjokoan: The key to Dogen's Shobogenzo*. Boston MA, US: Wisdom Publications.

The Role and the Present Significance of *Koans*

Daiko Matsuyama

Keywords
Rinzai Zen · Koans · Buddhism · Behavioral health · Metaphors

What Is a *Koan*?

In the *Rinzai* school of Japanese Zen Buddhism, the term "koan (公案)" refers to a question or succinct paradoxical statement posed to a student to help him or her seek the truth. A Zen master gives koans to his or her disciples, and they are expected to dedicate themselves to concentrating on these ideas and finding answers. The koans are drawn from collections of ancient masters and have long been considered a fundamental part of training in a *Rinzai* Buddhist monastery. Generally speaking, Soto Zen Buddhism, the other major school of Japanese Zen Buddhism, emphasizes koan practice less so than Rinzai Zen and emphasizes more on zazen (zen mediation) in training.

D. Matsuyama (✉)
Taizoin Zen Buddhist Temple, Kyoto, Japan
e-mail: info@talaoin.com

The History of *Koans*

Zen Buddhism originated in India and was thereafter transmitted to China by Bodhidharma (菩提達磨; Bodai Daruma in Japanese; Also see Dumoulin 2005a for the detailed history of Chinese Zen Buddhism). The practice of Zen already existed, however, before the arrival of Bodhidharma. In the early sixth century, Bodhidharma traveled to China and practiced seated meditation facing a wall for nine years. He later settled in the Shaolin Monastery. A hundred years passed, and a Chinese Zen master, Hongren (601–674; 弘忍; Gunin in Japanese), the fifth Patriarch of Chinese Zen Buddhism, appeared in the late seventh century.

The collective monastacism of Buddhists practicing asceticism began under Hongren. Then, Zen Buddhism became divided into a northern sect, *Hokushu-Zen,* and a southern sect, *Nanshu-Zen*, when the sixth Patriarch, Huineng (慧能; Eno in Japanese; 638–713), appeared.

Zen began to change dramatically when Zen master Mazu Doyi (709–788; 馬祖道—; Baso Doitsu in Japanese) emerged in the eighth century. He emphasized the importance of daily work and life at the monastery (Poceski 2015).

A. Masuda and W.T. O'Donohue (eds.), *Handbook of Zen, Mindfulness, and Behavioral Health*,
Mindfulness in Behavioral Health, DOI 10.1007/978-3-319-54595-0_6

Another Zen master, Baizhang Huaihai (百丈懐海; Hyakujo Ekai in Japanese; 720–814), emerged soon thereafter. He wrote the basic rules of monastic discipline, known as the Pure Rules of Baizhang (百丈清規; *Hyakujo Shingi* in Japanese). Baizhang is also known for the famous quote, "A man who does not work for a day shall not eat for a day." Most certainly, this period gave rise to increasing numbers of Zen masters. Baizhang was followed by many unique disciples during the Tang dynasty, including Huangbo Xiyun (–850; 黄檗希運; Obaku Kiun in Japanese) of the *Hung cho* sect and Linjin Yixuan (–866; 臨済義玄, Rinzai Gigen in Japanese) of *Linji* sect.

As the ideology and culture of Zen Buddhism began to spread widely, its influence spread to poets and artists like Li Bai and Bai Juyi. The conversations of masters, such as Zhaozhou (778–897; 趙州; Joshu in Japanese), Linji, and Dongshan (807–869; 洞山; Tozan in Japanese) of the *Dongshan* sect, have been transmitted as *Zengoroku*—the analects of Zen—from generation to generation.

During the Northern Song dynasty in the eleventh century, the *Linji* sect, the *Yunmen* sect, and the *Fayan* sect gathered strength. Buddhist laymen interested in the memoirs of Zen masters also played an important role in expanding Zen Buddhism. Chinese scholar-bureaucrats in particular acted as receptors and communicators to disseminate Zen culture.

During the Song Dynasty in the twelfth century, Zen Buddhism continued to divide into additional sects, called the Five Houses and Seven Schools of Zen (五家七宗), culminating in the creation of 5 sects and 7 schools derived from the original Zen Buddhism, including the Yang-chi (楊岐; Yogi in Japanese) and *Huang-lung* (黄龍; Oryo in Japanese) schools. By that time, the lifestyle of Zen monks at monasteries had been fully established. It varied depending on the religious school or denomination; however, certain aspects remained stable. For example, a Zen master typically divided his students into two groups, such as east and west, in order to assign tasks and organize a schedule for annual functions and Buddhist ceremonies. As the system developed, the structure for admission to a Zen monastery and training also began to take shape. In the case of a typical Buddhist temple, a person seeking admission to the priesthood was first assigned miscellaneous duties. Later, he would proceed to ordainment by receiving the commandments of Buddhism in order to officially become a monk.

At a Zen Buddhist temple, once a student received the Buddhist commandments, he became an *Unsui* (雲水), a student who undertakes training by visiting notable Zen masters. Such a pilgrimage is called *Kou Un Ryu Sui* (行雲流水), which metaphorically means "floating with the tide." The word *Unsui* is derived from this Zen phrase.

Kou Un Ryu Sui led Zen students to record every encounter and conversation with their masters. This process involves meeting with the master and eventually receiving *Inka* (印可), the authoritative acknowledgement as one of his spiritual heirs. Some students transcribed their conversations and refined the *koans* they received from their Zen masters in order to compile them as *Zengoroku* (禅語録; analects about Zen). As the number of such encounters increased, the records of the conversations also expanded. That enabled students to refer to the past use of the *koans*. Zen masters also began polishing collections of *koans* rather than devising new ones. Thereafter, *Koan-shu* (公案集), a booklet of *koans*, became available.

As time passed, the number of Chinese scholar bureaucrats visiting Zen masters increased. However, the Jingkang Incident in 1126 destroyed the Northern *Song* dynasty, pushing, Chinese traditional culture forcefully into the South. From the end of the twelfth century to the thirteenth century, a movement arose in the southern *Song* dynasty to re-establish aspects of Chinese thought.

Zen Buddhism was no exception as reformation of Chinese culture and traditions began in the South. It, too, saw a return to the classics and basics as it rebuilt denominations in the South. Interacting with the Chinese scholar-bureaucrats who traveled to that part of the country, Dahui Zonggao (大慧宗杲; Daie Soko in Japanese;

1089–1163) settled in *Zhejiang* province. He attracted a thousand students and helped revive the *Linji* School.

Dahui Zonggao cherished the *Zengoroku* and decided to complete *Koan-zen*, a method to learn the secrets of Zen by providing questions to seekers. This led to the emergence of Zen masters, such as Gottan Funei (兀庵普寧; 1197–1276), Muqi Fachang (牧溪法常; 1210–1269), and Mugaku Sogen (無学祖元; 1226–1286), who eventually became well known among Zen Buddhist temples in Japan. As the Mongolian army marched southward under Khubilai Khan, the Zen Buddhists in China began making their way to Japan, as if propelled by the crest of a great wave.

Slightly earlier, Wumen Huikai (無門慧開; 1183–1260) complied a text-based collection of *koans* called *Mumonkan* (無門関; The Gateless Gate). The Zen Buddhism introduced to Japan during the *Kamakura* (or *Muromachi*) era is often described as that of 46 biographies. Disciples inherited the Dharma and established 24 schools of Zen Buddhism. To this date, there are two major styles of Zen practice in Japan, Kanna-zen (看話禅) and Mokushou-Zen (默照禅). *Kanna-zen* is a *koan*-based method of Zen Buddhism that requires a text. By contrast, *Mokushou-zen* utilizes silence without text.

Hakuin Ekaku (白隠慧鶴; 1685–1768) is said to be the founder of what is now the *Rinzai* school of Zen Buddhism in Japan (see Dumoulin 2005b). During the *Edo* era, he referred to a *koan* as a catalyst to lead his disciples to attain enlightenment. Hakuin also produced his own *koans*. *Sekishu Onjo* (隻手音声), the sound of one hand clapping, is perhaps his most famous (see Yampolsky 1971, pp. 163–164).

Gasan Jido (峨山慈棹; 1727–1979) succeeded Hakuin, and he was followed by Inzan Ien (隠山惟琰; 1751–1811) and Takuju Kosen (卓洲胡僊; 1760–1833). The current *Rinzai* Schools of Zen in Japan descended from one or the other of these Zen masters. That explains why Hakuin is regarded as the founder of the *Rinzai* school.

If Hakuin's teaching can be put in one phrase, it would be what he wrote in *Zazen Wasan* (坐禅和讃; Sutra of *Zazen*): "This self is immediately the Buddha nature." The thought relates to Zen master Rinzai's teaching involving realization of the Buddha nature of one's self. In that sense, it also is in line with the Buddha's teachings, such as *Shobou Genzo* (正法眼蔵) and *Nehan Myoshin* (涅槃妙心). *Shobou Genzo* means treasured Buddhism, which is understood through the eyes of the wisdom that see into the truth. *Nehan Myoshin* reveals a calm state of mind by which one emancipates himself from desire and delusion. This is the kind of mind that has attained Buddhist enlightenment. The purpose of the *Rinzai* school of Zen Buddhism is to reach ultimate realization through practicing meditation, *koans,* and engaging in physical activities, such as moving meditation.

The Classic *Koans*

Rinzairoku (The Record of Linji; see Sasaki 2009), *Hekiganroku* (Blue Cliff Record; see Cleary 2002), and *Mumonkan* (The Gateless Gate or Gateless Barrier; see Shibayama 2000) are said to be the three classic *koan collections*. The Gateless Gate consists of 48 *koans*, each accompanied by a commentary and verse. The introduction states, "Those who boldly challenge the 48 *koans* might just as well be able to conquest a demon with three faces and eight arms."

The first *koan* in The Gateless Gate is the most famous, "Joshu's *Mu*" (see Shibayama 2000, pp. 19–31). In this koan, a student asks his Zen master, Joshu, "Does a dog have *Bussho* (the Buddha nature)?" Joshu replies, "*Mu*" (Nothing). That's it. Despite the brevity, this is thought to be one of the most difficult of all *koans*. Wumen Huikai named it *Mumonkan* (the gateless gate) of Zen Buddhism, meaning that this first *koan* acts as the entryway to Zen Buddhism. What, then, does "Joshu's *Mu*" imply?

The basic understanding of this *koan* involves a student applying the most significant and intrinsic aspect or quality of Buddhism, *Bussho* (仏性), to a dog by asking his Zen master whether the two are associated. However, this kind of understanding is completely wrong. Rather, it should be interpreted as the student asking: If a dog has *Bussho*, *might* a person like me one day come to his senses and achieve enlightenment? However, Joshu simply says, "Nothing."

This reply makes the *koan* even more intense, and a spiral of speculation begins. Does it mean a dog has no *Bussho*? Or does the meaning of *Mu* imply that there is nothing between Joshu and the student? Why does Joshu say, "Nothing?" Or is the question too ridiculous to warrant an answer? Which is it? Even if any of these thoughts leads to an answer, what does it have to do with a dog? The more one thinks, the less one understands.

Nevertheless, that pondering process is an integral part of Zen. It is important to have no idea of how to cope with the problem and therefore set logic aside. Zen challenges us to eradicate discrimination, and this generalizes to important aspects of our lives in obvious ways. If one makes a distinction against others based upon his or her ego, how can one be unified with the others?

In Joshu's *Mu*, Wumen first leads us to stumble, focusing on the one word, "*Mu*" (nothing), thinking of it all day long, and persevering with it. Wumen also says *Mu* should be associated with neither the presence nor the absence of nothingness. Rather, it can be thought of as a hot iron ball. It is as if one cannot swallow it or remove it completely even if she or he tries to do so. Eventually, the hot iron ball would eradicate logic and dualism as it ultimately explodes and disappears into the whole.

This is rather a dangerous *koan*; it helps renounce the distinction that separates subjectivity and objectivity. In that space, one breaks out of his shell, surrenders logic and experience, and even breaks free of confining circumstances eventually, as Joshu's *Mu* opens the first gate. This is not nihilism. It is not telling one to be selfless or to empty the mind. Rather, it points to something that unites what is within and without, causing everything to explode. In order to apprehend it, one must roar and repeat "Mu" over and over for a year or two.

Next, I will discuss the 14th *koan*, "Nansen Zanmyo" (see Shibayama 2000, pp. 107–113), which at first glance may appear to be extremely cruel. The koan begins with a fight over a cat between eastern and western groups of Buddhist students. Nansen picks up the cat and says, "If you can speak up, this cat will be saved. If you can't, I will kill it." Neither group has any idea what to say. Nansen then completes his threat.

The koan may sound brutal, but it begs the important question of why the students are fighting over the cat; what purpose did that quarrel have? Surely, it is not something so mundane as to who will keep the cat, or where. Whatever the reason, the problem remains. One must first realize that for Nansen, the cat is not the primary issue. If so, you may think that Nansen need not actually kill the cat. However, this idea arises from taking his words literally. Moreover, Nansen does not have to kill the cat if the students had not been sparring over the cat. Perhaps the point is that the students were so influenced by the thought that the cat might be killed that they did not make time to accomplish what was presumably more important. The cat, therefore, was sacrificed in the end.

Stories like this may leave the impression that Zen is rather cruel and unreasonable. Yes, Zen *is* unreasonable and is intentionally so. Returning to the example of Joshu *Mu*, even if the students are arguing whether a cat has *Bussho*, Joshu would only reply "*Mu*," "nothing."

Be it a cat, dog, or bamboo stick, this *koan* implies that Zen challenges one to depart from the matter, to come back to it all at once, and to quickly become selfless at that moment. In Zen Buddhism, this is called *Koji Kyumei* (己事究明), meaning the process of examining the self. In this moment, one must let go of unnecessary concerns; otherwise, they stand in the way and block him in surpassing the superficial. He will continue to keep company with worthless things, ideas, or desires. "Stop it," Nansen threatens, or else "the cat will be killed."

What Nansen means by this is that he would eliminate the problematic self that the students hold on to as they sit on the cushion doing zazen. If not, they may never succeed in the process of examining themselves. Nansen uses a cat as a metaphor to refer to the self that students hold onto and as an approach to purposefully confront them. Wumen thinks that something meaningful may arise once practicing this *koan* has erased everything.

The story is not over, though. Joshu comes back at night. As Nansen relates what happened, Joshu puts his sandals on his head and departs. Nansen mumbles, "If Joshu had been there, the cat would still be alive."

This is how The Gateless Gate is presented. *Unsui* will not necessarily encounter *koans* in the sequence listed in the *Zengoroku*. Each Zen master decides which *koan* to offer, based upon the student's level. This is called *Taiki-seppo*, the most suitable expression of the teaching for the particular student.

Koans for Zen Training at the Monastery

Working with *koans* is the most important part of Zen training at a *Rinzai* monastery. The training would not be complete without *it*. In order to gain permission to enter a monastery, one must endure three days with his or her forehead lowered to the floor of the entrance. The applicant then proceeds to spend another four days meditating in a dark room with no sunlight at all. This room is called *Tangaryo* (旦過寮). The purpose of this process is to test the applicant's determination. Once his or her intent has been confirmed, the applicant may be permitted to enter the Zendo as a trainee monk, *Unsui*, and meet the Zen master. That same day, he may be allowed to take a lesson in the master's room.

Once the new student enters that room, she or he receives a *koan*. A bell signals to enter. The bell is called *Kansho* (喚鐘) and is usually rung in the hallway. When the bell is sounded, *unsui* run to queue up. One by one, they ring the bell twice before entering the master's room. The proper manners for entering begin with *Gassho Reihai* (合掌礼拝), meaning joining hands in prayer and bowing. The *tatami* mat near the entrance door shines black, a somewhat intimidating residue of the finger marks and sweat of all those who have sought entry.

The rule at a monastery is that students must engage in koan practice twice a day, morning and evening. The term for this practice is *Chosan-boshin* (朝参暮請). The master allows only one student at a time to enter. The *unsui* (student) offers his or her answer to the koan and asks for the master's judgment. The room is sometimes described as a battlefield with no one else around. Whether the *unsui* is a novice or a veteran, he or she receives the same type of extreme challenge. Those who persevere through this training are often described as metal that has been thrown into a fireplace, had its impurities removed to become 100% pure iron, and then forged by hammering. In this way, the pure human nature of the student is said to be revealed.

Koans are the means for coming in contact with the doctrines of Zen Buddhism as well as understanding that the Buddha represents a purified human being. They are a ladder to climb in order to reach the rooftop of enlightenment. Once one has reached the destination, he or she must come down. The training at the monastery seeks supreme enlightenment and helps achieve self-realization; this realization, however, is not for the purpose of self-satisfaction. The truth attained by risking one's own life at the monastery will only become meaningful once it is used to bring salvation to mankind.

Koans transcend common sense. For example, one *koan* asks, "Listen to the sound of one hand clapping." As a matter of physics, clapping with one hand to create a sound is impossible. However, an old saying posits that it is possible to listen to the sound of one hand clapping, which is described as the voice of a student whose heart has been purified. When such an enlightened voice is heard, she or he has realized and accomplished the *koan* of "one hand clapping." But then, another *koan* will follow.

The Role and Purpose of *Koans*

A *koan* is often described as a finger pointing at the moon. If the full moon could represent enlightenment, the finger pointing at the full moon is said to be the *koan*. Looking at the finger itself does not help see the moon. What counts is the direction of the finger. This approach may be similar to treatment goals in behavioral health care in that often the knowledge of a diagnosis or a particular treatment is not the mechanism of change for people who are suffering. Alternatively, it is the process by which the treatment unfolds, the journey that unfolds in the direction of the full moon, that results in meaningful change.

There are pros and cons for both *Kanna-zen*, the type of meditation that utilizes *koans,* and *Mokusho-zen,* another type that does not. A *koan* merely turns into knowledge instead of experience if a student is swayed too much by the *koan* itself. Describing the taste of tea, for example, requires expressions such as bitter, mild, and hot. However, no expression can help another person understand the taste unless the person tries it herself or himself. The same goes for Zen.

Even if one has extensive knowledge of tea, discussing it is rather dangerous without having actually tried it. A painter in Japan once set out to draw a picture of a tiger. However, he had never seen one. Relying solely on what he had heard from the experiences of others, he ended up producing a picture of a cat. If *koans* become nothing more than concrete and impersonal knowledge, they may lead to results that are equally misguided. On the other hand, the *koan*-less practice of *Mokusho-zen* also has its downsides. If one becomes too caught up in the meditation itself, he or she may become isolated from the world in which enlightenment exists. A person who tells about the taste of the tea without trying it is actually causing harm due to lack of actual experience and firsthand knowledge.

The 30th *koan* in The Gateless Gate is called *Sokushin Sokubutsu*, meaning "The self is immediately the Buddha nature" (see Shibayama 2000, pp. 214–222). Nanyue Huairang asked his student, Basho, "What is the purpose of your daily meditation?" Basho answered, "I meditate in order to become Buddha." Nanyue Huairang picked up a tile from the ground, placed it on a rock and began polishing it. Basho asked him, "Master, what are you doing?" Nanyue Huairang replied, "I am trying to make it into a mirror." Basho replies him, "That is impossible. Polishing a tile will not help to make it turn into a mirror." Nanyue Huairang says, "Having known that, why are you trying to become Buddha through meditation? Meditation will not help you become Buddha."

Basho asked, "Then what can I do?" Nanyue Huairang countered with another question, "When a cart does not move, is it right to hit the cart or the cow?" Basho could not come up with an answer, so Nanyue Huairang continued, "Your approach to daily meditation is basically to learn about Buddha conceptually. But if Buddha could be conceptually learned, Buddha would have no truth. You are not meant to become Buddha. You are Buddha yourself, and the self is immediately the Buddha nature. Do not think that mediation and Buddha are two separate things. Meditation means to forget about Buddha and to forget about your own self. You must realize that you have to renounce such duality."

Simply meditating will not enable one to attain realization. Meditation and *koans* are just methods to help bring about realization. If a student becomes too caught up in doing meditation or solving *koans*, he may be unable to move toward enlightenment itself. Similarly, meditating for the purpose of becoming aware of the Buddha nature will not enable one to attain the realization as long as he or she is caught up with the dualism, such as treating meditation and Buddha nature as two separate events.

In *Mokusho-zen*, checking whether the student has achieved realization is difficult, even if he believes he has. *Koan-zen* on the other hand, provides a means for a Zen master to evaluate the progress of his or her student frequently as they work through the *koans* together. This is the major difference between the two approaches.

A *koan* acts as a catalyst to attain realization, helping the master to confirm the student's progress. A catalyst is a catalyst, nothing more. It should not be the main purpose; it is not the goal. Therefore, since ancient times, students have been prohibited from sharing information about the *koan* they are working on or their answers for it. This rule reduces the likelihood of *koans* being reduced to nothing more than knowledge.

The Present Significance of *Koans*

The prevalence of western ideas and philosophy in the modern world has not diminished the value of Zen and the role of *koans* in Zen practice. Koans help a person to transcend logic and commonsense mental habits (e.g., judgment of right and wrong, worldview, and preconception) and unfold the Buddha nature as it is within the person. This transcendence is the key, and practice without it falls short no matter how authentic and genuine it seems.

In recent years, various meditation and mindfulness practices have attracted attention in western countries, becoming part of the mainstream culture. While some of these practices parallel Zen, many of them do not. Nevertheless, many people often misunderstand these practices with Zen. This is not intended to criticize these practices, as the path that Zen takes is not superior to the path of others. However, what Zen seeks is not what we usually want from a mediation and mindfulness practice. It is simply a choice, and koans serve as a guiding light on the path, navigating one to the heart of Zen.

Many mediation and mindfulness practices in the West are often bound to utilitarianism, a commonsense mental habit. Even though some of them advocate the transcendence of utilitarianism, they seem to do so while remaining in this utilitarian mindset. In these practices, mindfulness is the goal to be achieved, or a means to a particular end. In other words, people practice with the expectation of gaining something although it is not stated explicitly. For example, in the field of behavioral health, some pursue mindfulness as the ultimate state of psychological well-being, and others practice it for saving their marriage or alleviating suffering. Note that utilitarian-like desire never runs out, and there is nothing wrong with having such a desire; we cannot help having utilitarian-like desires which reflect one's clinging to a narrowly defined self (e.g., self as a distinct and essential entity separated from the surrounding) and desire to protect it. However, once we begin to cling to and act on it excessively, efforts to fulfill it become quite detrimental.

Transcending common sense and preconception, Zen does not seek any gain in this utilitarian-like sense. Nor does Zen service as an antidote for logic and common sense. Zen is "doing" without knowing whether it leads to anything. This position is rooted in the original wisdom of Buddhism. Zen is to do whatever one does in a given moment seriously and wholeheartedly, and this doing itself is the gain.

It is difficult for us, modern people, to grasp this "doing Zen" as we are caught up with common sense and preconception of what is valuable. For some of us, "doing" is almost too trivial to devote our time and energy into it. For others, this "doing" of Zen seems very discouraging in the absence of a mystical element. And yet others believe that there are hidden wisdoms behind this "doing" and wish to find them (e.g., "Once I am enlightened, I can find the true meaning of *doing*"). These reactions stem from our shared worldview (i.e., common sense) that there is something absolute and unchanged. For example, many of us are monotheists who believe in the existence of one God. According to this view, God is an absolute who transcends the human reality, and people seek salvation from her. Similarly, many of us assume that there are aspects of ourselves that are absolute and unchanged. For example, many of us believe that there exists a "soul" and "true self" within us that is distinct and perpetual, while things around us are constantly changing. Holding this worldview, we naturally differentiate the self from others and view it as something each of us owns (e.g., "this is my body", "this is my life"). As the sense of ownership becomes excessive, we become satiated with it and are driven to protect it. As such, for many of us, practicing mindfulness and meditation for a utilitarian-like purpose is a result.

By contrast, through transcending logic and common sense, Buddhism does not divide the world. It does not posit the absolute existence or absolute rightness of God, self, or even Buddha. Buddha was simply a person who engaged in reflection and attained enlightenment. Anyone with a strong will may be able to do the same. What Buddhists believe is neither a miracle nor salvation from the absolute. Rather, Buddhists believe that Buddha achieved enlightenment, and enlightenment is the path that they choose to take. No one can prove that the Buddha actually was enlightened. For Buddhists, it does have to be proved. Buddhists simply believe that those who reach enlightenment will discover the heart of his realization. The mathematical expression for realization would be an X. X is intangible, and Buddhists believe in intangibility. The Buddha nature does not demand any particular form of existence or any substance to be added to or removed from living.

The same goes for enlightenment. Enlightenment is often viewed as the absolute truth in Zen and meditation as a means to achieve this sense of realization. However, according to Zen, meditation offers no guarantee for it. It is like polishing the tile that cannot turn into a mirror no matter how well it is buffed. Realization is not something one aims to achieve; it is more likely a natural consequence of one's devotion.

Relevant to seeing Zen as intangibility, another major difference I find is that the recent mindfulness movement in the West is perhaps too logical, linear, and reductionistic. The world overflows with absurdity and contradiction, and it is far more complicated than one can imagine. Consider love as an example. Scientists and scholars have studied love for centuries, and yet we cannot grasp it simply by logic. Unfortunately, logic falls short at the most critical moment. Zen is rather unreasonable and illogical, intentionally. Thus, it is necessary to transcend the mental habit of logical reasoning so that one can be versatile, taking the most natural and original actions without being caught up with preconception. This is often called *Hataraki* in Rinzai tradition.

A flexible mind is more versatile and works better at any time and in any situation. This is Zen. Modern society celebrates logic and scientific theory, but we slow down and closely see the reality of our life, we find it not that linear. For this reason, the Zen approach has much to offer. Confronting problems with logical thinking may not lead us to the answers that truly reflect the reality of our life. Once again, K*oans* help a person to become more versatile, grasping the nature of a problem and leading him or her to enlightenment.

I came across an example of this versatility just the other day in the temple where I serve as a priest. Zen priests often receive requests for calligraphy. One day, a master called his student and told him, "The writing brush is worn out because I have used it quite a bit." The student asked, "Should I go get a new one?" The Zen master then said, "Don't be silly. Untie the writing brush, pick up the long strands, and make a new brush with them." The dialogue between the master and his student captures Zen quite nicely. The commonsense solution in this circumstance would be to purchase a new brush as the student asked, because it is easier and more time-efficient to do so. It was likely that the student had never experienced making a writing brush.

Zen transcends logic and commonsense preconceptions. Logical reasoning has advanced societies over time, resolving barriers to progress. Zen, however, says that the dominance of logical thinking and attachment to preconception often obscures the moment of living fully here-and-now. Through Koans and Koan-like practice, Zen tests deliberately whether a person is only capable of solving a problem using logic, or whether he or she is flexible enough to willingly take an action under unconventional circumstances. In the example above, the student was told to get involved in a seemingly absurd task. However, he complied with the longer and more complex task and created a writing brush himself in the end. I will not forget the accomplishment and vitality he expressed. Through this task, the student had gotten in touch with the reality he otherwise missed and expanded a new possibility.

Conclusion

At the dawn of Western Zen, Suzuki (1994, 1996) highlighted the importance of transcending logical thinking and preconceptions pervasive in our cultures (e.g., dualism, essentialism, and reductionism). This transcendent quality is at the heart of Zen, and *koans* have played a crucial role for elucidating it. The application of koans or koan-like practice is not limited to Zen practice because there are logic and preconceptions no matter where humans go. The field of behavioral health is no exception. I believe that Koans practice may shed the light of transcendence in behavioral health professionals and patients, allowing them move more freely in the flux of human conditioning.

References

Cleary, T. (2002). *Secrets of the Blue Criff Record: Zen comments by Hakuin and Tenkei*. Boston MA: Shambhala.

Dumoulin, H. (2005a). *Zen Buddhism: A history volume 1: India and China*. Bloomington, Indiana US: World Wisdom.

Dumoulin, H. (2005b). *Zen Buddhism: A history volume 2: Japan*. Bloomington, Indiana US: World Wisdom.

Poceski, M. (2015). *The records of Mazu and the making of classical Chan literature*. New York, USA: Oxford University Press.

Sasaki, R. F. (2009). *The record of Linji* In T. Y. Kirchner, x16b, & x14d (Eds.), University of Hawaii Press.

Shibayama, Z. (2000). *The gateless barrier: Zen comments on the mumonkan* Boston, MA: Shambhala Publication (originally published in 1974).

Suzuki, D. T. (1994). *Esseys in Zen Buddhism*. New York, US: Grove Press (original work published in 1949).

Suzuki, D. T. (1996). *Zen Buddhism: Selected writings of D. T. Suzuki*. New York, US: An Image Book.

Yampolsky, P. B. (1971). *The Zen Master Hakuin: Selected writing*. New York, USA: Columbia University Press.

Zen and Body

Kenshu Sugawara, Akihiko Masuda and Kayla Sargent

Keywords
Zen · Body · Behavioral health · Zazen · Koan

The body plays a central role in Zen (Dogen et al. 2010). In this chapter, three major themes regarding Zen and body will be presented. Briefly, these themes are (a) the relation between mind and body in Zen, (b) the significance and implications of body in Zen, and (c) proper conduct in Zen training and sangha, a monastic community of ordained Zen practitioners.

Relations Between Mind and Body in Zen

Etymologically, the term "Zen (禅)" in Japanese seems to refer to a particular mental state or mental activity (e.g., a focused mind), not necessarily the body. The term was originated from the Chinese term Chan (禪), an abbreviated form of Channa (禪那). Channa was derived from Sanskrit dhyāna, meaning "meditation" or "cultivated states of mind." Likewise, some of the original Zen teachings and scriptures, such as the Four Sacred Verses of Bodhidharma (Ferguson 2011) and the Platform Sutra of the Sixth Patriarch (see Buddhist Text Translation Society 2001) used the term referring to mind but not the body. For example, the Four Sacred Verses of Bodhidharma say:

> A special transmission outside the scriptures
> Not founded upon words and letters;
> By pointing directly to one's mind
> It lets one see into one's own true nature and thus attain Buddhahood

Taken together, it is not surprising that Zen Buddhism is sometimes viewed as a sect of Buddhism in which the primary focus is the training of mind.

Nevertheless, in Zen (at least in the Japanese sects of Rinzai and Soto Zen), the body is considered essential for studying the Buddha Way (Buddhahood; Dogen et al. 2010, 2011). It is important to note that what is referred to as body in Zen is not limited to the body as a physical entity. The body also means an *act* of a whole

Translated and Revised by Akihiko Masuda and Kayla Sargent.

K. Sugawara (✉)
Aichi Gakuin University, Aichi, Japan
e-mail: tenjin1975@gmail.com

A. Masuda (✉) · K. Sargent
University of Hawaii at Manoa, Honolulu, USA
e-mail: amasuda4@hawaii.edu

K. Sargent
e-mail: kaylansargent@gmail.com

A. Masuda and W.T. O'Donohue (eds.), *Handbook of Zen, Mindfulness, and Behavioral Health*,
Mindfulness in Behavioral Health, DOI 10.1007/978-3-319-54595-0_7

person. This important understanding of how the body is conceptualized in Zen is illustrated nicely in the chapter *How to Breathe in Zazen* of *Eihei koroku* (永平広録; The Extensive Record of Teacher Dogen's Sayings). Dogen (1200–1253), the founder of the Soto school of Zen in Japan, presented the following regarding the role of body-action in regulating and correcting mind:

> … first you should sit correctly with upright posture. Then regulate your breath and settle your mind (Dogen et al. 2010, p. 348).

Keizan (1268–1325), the second great founder of the Soto school of Zen in Japan, described the link between body-action and mind in a similar fashion in *Zazen Yojinki* (Points to Keep in Mind when Practicing Zazen):

> Put your right hand on your left heel and your left hand on top of your right, thumbs together and close to the body at the level of the navel. Sit straight without leaning to left or right, front or back. Ears and shoulders, nose and navel should be aligned. Place the tongue on the palate and breathe through the nose. The mouth should be closed. The eyes should be open but not too wide nor too slight. Harmonizing the body in this way, breathe deeply with the mouth once or twice. Sitting steadily, sway the torso seven or eight times in decreasing movements. Sit straight and alert (retrieved from http://antaiji.org/en/classics/english-zazen-yojinki/).

As such, the two founders of Soto Zen in Japan explicitly emphasized the significance of body-action for realizing tranquility (e.g., the experience of original wholeness) through zazen practice; that is, one must first correct body-posture and breathing, and doing so naturally corrects the mind.

Furthermore, ancient and contemporary Zen literatures postulate that it is impossible to correct the mind through the mind (Dogen et al. 2010; Dogen and Tanahashi 2010; Uchiyama et al. 2004). In studying the Buddha Way, one must not consider his or her own mind as the teacher; instead, one must become the teacher of his or her own mind. According to Soto Zen in Japan, through becoming a teacher of one's own mind, one can correctly practice Zen. In *Shobogenzo Zuimonki* (The Treasury of the True Dharma Eye: Record of Things Heard; Dogen et al. 1988), Dogen commented on how Zen is experienced via and with the body:

> Is the Way attained through mind or body? …it is said that since body and mind are not separate, the Way is attained through the body. Yet, it is not clear that we attain the Way through the body, because they say "since" body and mind are not separate. In Zen, the Way is attained through both body and mind. As long as we only think about the Buddha-dharma with our minds, the Way will never be grasped, even in a thousand lifetimes or a myriad of eons. When we let go of our minds and cast aside our views and understandings, the Way will be actualized. One sage clarified True Mind (Reality) when he saw peach blossoms, and another realized the Way when he heard the sound of a tile hitting bamboo. They attained the Way through their bodies. Therefore, when we completely cast aside our thoughts and views and practice *shikantaza*, we will become intimate with the Way. For this reason, the Way is doubtlessly attained through the body. This is why I encourage you to practice zazen wholeheartedly (pp. 109–110).

Shikantaza is simply sitting mediation in Soto Zen in Japan. Dogen explained mind further by stating that we cannot grasp the Buddha Way through our mind (i.e., our analytic way of thinking), and that we can realize the Buddha Way only through transcending body–mind (see Shaner 1985 for transcendence of body and mind). Finally, Dogen stated:

> Students of the way, let go of body and mind, and enter completely into the Buddha-dharma. An ancient said, "At the top of a hundred foot pole, how do you advance one step further?" In such a situation, we think that we would die if we were to let go of the pole, and we cling firmly to it. Saying "advance one step further" means that same as having resolved that it would not be bad and so let go of bodily life. We should give up worrying about everything, from the art of living to our livelihood. Unless we give up such things, it will be impossible to attain the Way even if we seem to be practicing earnestly as though trying to extinguish a fire evolving our heads. Just let go of body and mind in a decisive manner (Dogen et al. 1988, p. 111).

"At the top of a hundred foot pole, how do you advance one step further?" means that one must choose to jump as a leap of faith, metaphorically speaking of course. As we can easily imagine, doing so is quite difficult as the conception of life and death freezes our bodies. However, Zen values precisely this level of commitment for studying the Buddha Way (Dogen and Tanahashi 2010). Letting go of body and mind includes the transcendence of a narrowly identified self (i.e., self as an independent and constant entity) as well as the analytic preconception of right and wrong. In the past, this degree of commitment attracted many samurai as the way of letting go of self-oriented doubts, crucial for the moment of life and death within them (Suzuki 2010).

"Body and mind dropped away" is a phrase that Dogen often used for his practice of Buddha Way (see Dogen et al. 2011; Dogen and Tanahashi 2010). For Dogen, the Buddha Way is simply dropping off body and mind, transcending the distinction of body and mind as well as letting go of body and mind. As noted extensively elsewhere in ancient and contemporary Zen literatures (Dogen and Tanahashi 2010; Suzuki 1970; Uchiyama et al. 2004), we cling to many different things such as profit, fame, physical appearance, and financial security. According to Zen, this tendency is due to our *attachment* to the narrowly defined sense of self (i.e., self as a unique and independent entity). If our mind is rooted within this sense of self, we cannot escape clinging no matter how much we practice Zen. Dogen stated that arriving at a state of freedom from the body and mind naturally requires that we must first correct our body through proper conduct (see Dogen and Tanahashi 2010 for English Translation of Shobogenzo). Therefore, "advancing one step further at the top of a hundred foot pole" points to the practice of Dogen's body and mind dropping away.

According to Zen, a perceived sense of self as a unique and separate entity is a confused self (Dogen et al. 2011; Suzuki 1964, 1970). The confused self is referred to as a state of *mumyo* (*ignorance* in English; *avidyā* in Sanskrit), which is also known for a lack of grasping the transient nature of life, excessive pursuit of happiness, and belief that everything goes one's own way. Zen states that we must let go of this confused sense of self for studying the Buddha way. Dogen elaborated in *Gakudo Yojin-Shu* (Guideline for Studying the Way):

> … when you understand discontinuity the notion of self does not come into being, ideas of name and gain do not arise… Just forget yourself for now and practice inwardly—this is one with the thought of enlightenment (Dogen and Tanahashi 1985, pp. 31–32).

Discontinuity in this passage refers to the transient and interdependent nature of life (Uchiyama et al. 2004), and *name and gain* refers to the fames and profits that we often seek throughout our lives. According to Zen, when an individual fully realizes impermanence, he or she naturally becomes detached from the egocentric self, embodying nirvana. The dropping off body and mind is also the standpoint of practice from which the individual experiences nirvana.

Significance of Body in the Worldview of Zen

Buddhism and Zen state that we live exceedingly short lives; during our short lives in this world, we are tossed back and forth by the concepts of life and death (Japan Buddhist Federation 1978). According to Dogen, the body is the best teacher to direct us to *mujo* (impermanence). For example, he stated in *Shobogenzo* that paying attention to one's body, such as seeing a gray hair, helps us realize that our life is not perpetual (see Dogen and Tanahashi 2010, p. 801 for experiencing the impermanence through pay attention to one's own body). Such realizations may also help us see an alternative perspective that the body does not have to an object to which we cling excessively (Uchiyama and Okumura 2014).

Our bodies are transient, and they simply unfold in the here and now due to the principle of interdependence (e.g., the dharma of interdependent co-arising). From this perspective, there is nothing concrete or unchanging about our bodies; realizing this fact of life ceases our excessive clinging. Dogen described the importance of realizing the transient nature of the body in *Gakudo Yojin-Shu* (Guidelines for Studying the Way):

> Just forget yourself for now and practice inwardly —this is one with the thought of enlightenment…

> Is there a real basis inside or outside body now? Your body with hair and skin is just inherited from your father and mother. From beginning to end a drop of blood or lymph is empty. So none of these are the self… How could you be attached to any of them. Deluded people are attached to them. Enlightened people are free from them (Dogen and Tanahashi 1985, pp. 32–33).

Rinzai Zen and Body

In Record of Linji (臨済語録; *Rinzai Goroku* in Japanese), an essential text of Chinese and Japanese Zen Buddhism for nearly a thousand years, Linji Yixuan of China (–866; 臨済義玄, Rinzai Gigen in Japanese) described the transient nature of the body (i.e., body of the Buddha Way) as follows:

> Virtuous monks, the physical body [composed] of the four great elements is impermanent; [every part of it,] including the spleen, stomach, liver, and gallbladder, the hair, nails, and teeth as well, only proves that all dharmas are empty appearances. The place where your one thought comes to rest is called the bodhi tree; the place where your one thought cannot come to rest is called the avidyā tree. Avidyā has no dwelling place; avidyā has no beginning and no end. If your successive thoughts cannot come to rest, you go up the avidyā tree; you enter the six paths of existence and the four modes of birth, wear fur on your body and horns on your head. If your successive thoughts can come to rest, then this [very body] is the pure body (see Kirchner and Sasaki 2008, p. 23).

In the passage just above, Linji contrasted the pure body (the body of Buddha Way) with a conventional perception of body, also emphasizing the importance of letting go of the conventional sense of body through considering a transient being. Finally, in the passage above, Linji implied that he could see his disciples achieving enlightenment by seeing whether they let go of their bodies and regulated their minds accordingly. The pure body above refers to the body that is boundless and whole.

Linji stated that if we cling to the body, we cannot grasp the pure body that reflects the dharma of impermanence (see Kirchner and Sasaki 2008). He also stated that realizing the pure body is possible if we open the hand of thought (e.g., the transcendence of verbal categorization), doing so for one thought at a time.

Physical Body and Dharma Body

Discussion on the distinction between the physical body and pure body (i.e., Dharma body, body of Buddha Way) is traced back to the dialogue between Master Huineng of China (638–713), the Sixth and Last Patriarch of Chan Buddhism, and one of his students, Bhikshu Chih Tao. This dialogue is cited in The Sixth Patriarch's Dharma Jewel Platform Sutra (Buddhist Text Translation Society 2001). This is how it goes:

> Bhikshu Chih Tao, a native of Nan Hai in Kuang Chou, asked a favor: "Since leaving home, your student has studied the Nirvana Sutra for over ten years and has still not understood its great purport. I hope that the High Master will bestow his instruction."
>
> The Master said, "What point haven't you understood?"
>
> Chih Tao replied, "All activities are impermanent, characterized by production and extinction; when production and extinction are extinguished, that still extinction is bliss. My doubts are with respect to this passage."
>
> …
>
> The Master said, "What are your doubts?"
>
> "All living beings have two bodies," Chih Tao replied, "the physical body and the Dharma-body. The physical body is impermanent and is produced and destroyed. The Dharma-body is permanent and is without knowing or awareness. The Sutra says that the extinction of production and extinction is bliss, but I do not know which body is in tranquil extinction and which receives the bliss.
>
> "How could it be the physical body which receives the bliss? When this physical body is extinguished, the four elements scatter. That is total suffering and suffering cannot be called bliss. If the Dharma-body were extinguished it would become like grass, trees, tiles, or stones; then what would receive the bliss?" (pp. 299–302)

According to Huineng, the perspective that the pure body exists as a unique entity distinct from the physical body is an ill-advised one. Such a way of understanding and experiencing the body is analytic and intellectual. He also stated that one must transcend the distinction between physical body and Dharma body, impermanence and permanence, life and death, and happiness and sorrow if the body and the Buddha Way are to converge as one.

Xuansha Shibei of China (玄沙師備; 835–908) highlighted pure body, Dharma body, world, the Buddha Way, and emptiness as one. In the following passage, he used the Buddhist term emptiness to refer to an undivided *wholeness* or *oneness* that cannot be described formally and topographically. He also cautioned his students not to get caught up with the *idea* of transcendence.

> Buddha's way is vast and serene. There is no path on which to travel there. There is no gate of liberation. There are no thoughts about a person of the Way. There are no "three worlds." Therefore, one cannot transcend or "fall into." Setting something up runs counter to the truth. Negation is a formation. Movement gives rise to the root of birth and death. Stillness is the province of falling into delusion. When movement and stillness are extinguished, one falls into empty negation. When movement and stillness are both accepted, Buddha nature is concealed. With respect to worldly affairs of states of mind, you should be like a cold dead tree. Then you will realize that great function and not forfeit its grace. All forms will be illuminated as if in a mirror. Brightness or obscurity will not confuse you. The bird will fly into emptiness, and it will not be apart from empty form. Then in the ten directions there will be no form and in the three words, there will be no trace (see Ferguson 2011, p. 298).

Dogen described a similar process in the chapter of *Shinjin gakudo* (身心学道; Body and Mind Study of the Way) of *Shobogenzo* (正法眼蔵):

> To study the way with body means to study the way with your own body. It is the study of the way using this lump of red flesh. The body comes forth from the study of the way. Everything that comes forth from the study of the way is the true human body. The entire world of the ten directions is nothing but the true human body. The coming and going of birth and death is the true human body. To turn this body around, abandoning the ten unwholesome actions, keeping the eight precepts, taking refuge in the three treasures, and leaving home and entering the homeless life is the true study of the way. For this reason it is called the true human body. Those who follow this must not be like outsiders who hold the view of spontaneous enlightenment (Dogen and Tanahashi 2010, pp. 426–427).

In the passage just above, consistent with the teaching of Xuansha Shibei, Dogen stated that the true body and the Buddha Way are essentially indistinguishable. The students of the Buddha Way practice the Buddha Way through the body (Dogen and Tanahashi 1985). Studying the Buddha Way in this way actualizes the true body. Through the practice of Buddha Way, one's body becomes the true body, and this is the body that is not dictated by the sense of self as a unique, independent, and perpetual being (Uchiyama et al. 2004). Therefore, the true body realized through the study of Buddha Way is no longer one's possession. It is part of all myriad beings with no boundary, and it is the Buddha Way. The Buddha Way is realized through continuous practice (Dogen et al. 2010).

The Association Between Body and Zen Training

As described above, Dogen pointed to the significance of the physical body in Zen practice. According to Dogen, the physical body, Zen practice, and the Buddha Way are inseparable from one another. However, Zen also seems to caution the students of Zen not to cling to the teaching of physical body, Zen practice, and the Buddha Way as one literally and excessively. Zen does so by presenting contradicting statements. For example, in the dialogue between Yunyan Tansheng of China (780–841; 雲巌曇晟, Ungan Donjō in Japanese) and Dongshan Liangjie (807–869; 洞山良价, Tōzan Ryōkai in Japanese), Yunyan stated that sitting (i.e., zazen) is the Buddha Way, and that not sitting is not Buddha Way. Conversely, Dongshan stated that not sitting is the Buddha Way, and that sitting is not the Buddha Way. The point of the dialogue is not to decide which form of practice is right. Rather, it points to the importance of going beyond conventional problem-solving processes such as classification, analysis, and judgment in order to practice the Buddha Way.

Similarly, Dogen also cautioned his students not to become caught up with the idea of becoming a Buddha by correcting the physical body through zazen. Clarifying this point, he also used the dialogue between Nanyue Huairang (677–744; 南嶽懐譲, Nangaku Ejo in Japanese) and Mazu Daoyi (709–788; 馬祖道一, Baso Dōitsu in Japan) as an example. In *Eihei Koroku* he stated:

> Nanyue asked Mazu, "Great worthy, what is your intention in seated meditation (zazen)?"
> Mazu said, "I intend to become a Buddha."
> Nayue picked up a tile and, in front of Mzu's hermitage, began to polish it with a rock.
> Mazu asked, "What are you doing, teacher?"
> Nanyue said, "I'm polishing it to make a mirror."
> Mazu said, "How can you make a mirror by polishing a tile?"
> Nanyue said, "How can you become a buddha though zazen?"
> Mazu said, "What shall I do?"
> Nanyue said, "Like someone riding a cart that won't go, which is right, to hit the cart or to hit the ox?"
> Mazu did not reply. [Nanyue] further gave instruction saying, "Do you study sitting meditation, or study sitting Buddha? If you study sitting meditation, meditation has nothing to do with sitting or lying down. If you study sitting Buddha, Buddha has no fixed form. Within the Dharma of non-abiding, you should not pick or choose. If you do sitting Buddha, this is simply killing Buddha. If you cling to the form of sitting, you will never reach the truth." (Dogen et al. 2010, p. 561)

Through the dialogue of Nanyue and Mazu, Dogen taught his students not to become caught up in the *idea* of equating the Buddha Way to zazen. Such way of understanding the Buddha Way paradoxically squeezes the formless and boundaryless (the Buddha Way) into a form. Nanyue's emphasis on non-clinging to forms and ideas is seen in the dialogue with his teacher, Huineng, the Sixth and Last Patriarch of Chan Buddhism.

> Huineg said to Nanyue, "Where did you come from?"
> Nanyue said, "From Mt. Song."
> Huineng said, "What is it that thus comes?"
> Nanyue couldn't answer.
> After eight years, Nanyue suddenly attained enlightenment. He informed the Six Ancestors of this, saying "I have an understanding."
> The Sixth Ancestor said, "What is it?"
> Nanyue said, "To say it's a thing misses the mark."
> The Sixth Ancestor said, "Then can it be made evident or not?"
> Nanyue said, "I don't say it can't be made evident, but it can't be defiled."
> The Sixth Ancestor said, "Just this that is undefiled is what is upheld and sustained by all buddhas. You are thus, and I also am thus." (Ferguson 2011, p. 53)

Another implication of Nanyue's approach to Zen is that Zen goes beyond formal sitting meditation. That is, the Buddha Way is practiced in every single moment of our everyday activities.

To date, there are two major styles of Zen practice in Japan, *Kanna-Zen* (看話禅) and *Mokusho-Zen* (黙照禅). *Kanna-Zen* is a *koan*-based method of Zen Buddhism that requires a text. By contrast, *Mokusho-Zen* utilizes silence without text. The former style of practice is emphasized in Rinzai Zen, more so than Dogen's Soto Zen. Although Rinzai and Soto sects of Zen do not negate the significance of zazen, the Rinzai school of Zen in Japan makes use of koans (a Zen question or succinct paradoxical statement posed to a student) methodologically to help students seek the truth more so than Dogen's Sōtō Zen. Conversely, Sōtō Zen emphasizes zazen as the act of Buddha Way, calling it *Shikantaza* (只管打坐 in Japanese). *Shikandaza* is often translated as "just sitting," "nothing but precisely sitting," and "doing only zazen wholeheartedly." Although the difference between *Kanna-Zen* and *Mokusho-Zen* has been discussed somewhat emotionally in terms of the extent to which the practice emphasizes the act of body or mind, the difference is simply the matter of style and preference.

Additionally, as described below, Dogen's Zen focuses on *gyo* (行; the act of body) more so than Buddhist texts. Dogen and Keizan, two founders of Sōtō Zen in Japan, established a series of Shingi (清規). *Shingi* are the precepts or regulations that students should observe when practicing in Zen monasteries. *Eihei Shingi*

(永平清規; Pure Standards for the Zen Community), which was written by Dogen, is an example of this precept (Dogen et al. 1995).

Zen and Body: Summary

In Zen practice, the body is often viewed dialectically. Whereas the body and its significance are fully acknowledged and centralized in practice, students of the Buddha Way are encouraged to be free from the idea of their bodies. While acknowledging the importance of the latter, the present chapter has focused primarily on the former. In the former, it is the body through which one can become fully settled to the present moment (i.e., unfolding the Buddha Way). More specifically, correcting the act of one's physical body (i.e., the function of behavior as a whole person) corrects the mind. To promote correct conduct, Dogen et al. (1995) wrote *Eihei Shingi* that contains Dogen's principal guidelines and instructions for everyday life and rituals in the monastic training centers (i.e., Eihei-ji Temple) that he established.

Dogen's thoughts on the role of *shingi* in practice are also described in *Shobogenzo Zuimonki* (正法眼藏隨聞記; The Treasury of the True Dharma Eye: Record of Things Heard). *Shobogenzo Zuimonki* (Dogen et al. 1988) is a collection of informal Dharma talks given by Dogen, recorded by his primary disciple Koun Ejo. In one of his teachings, Dogen said:

> You should maintain the precepts and eating regulations (one meal a day before noon, etc.). Still, it is wrong to insist upon them as essential, establish them as a practice and expect to be able to gain the Way by observing them. We follow them just because they are the activities of Zen monks and the life style of Buddha's children. Although keeping them is good, we should not take them as the primary practice. I don't mean to say, however, that you should break the precepts and become self-indulgent. Clinging to such an attitude is an evil view and not that of a Buddhist practitioner. We follow the precepts or regulations simply because they form the standard for a Buddhist and are the tradition of Zen monasteries. While I was staying at Chinese monasteries, I met no one who took them as the primary concern.
>
> For true attainment of the Way, devoting all effort to zazen alone has been transmitted among the buddhas and patriarchs. For this reason, I taught a fellow student of mine, Gogenbo, a disciple of Zen-Master Eisai, to abandon his strict adherence of keeping the precepts and reciting the Precept Sutra day and night.
>
> Ejo asked, "When we practice and learn the Way in a Zen monastery, we should keep the pure regulations made by Zen Master Hyakujo (Baizhang), shouldn't we? In the beginning of the Regulations (Haykujo-Shingi), it says that receiving and maintaining the precepts is prerequisite. In this tradition, the Fundamental Precept has also been handed down. In the oral and face-to-face transmission of this lineage, the students are given the precepts transmitted from the West (India). These are the Bodhisattva Precepts. Also, it says in the Precept Sutra that people must recite the Sutra day and night. Why do you have us discontinue this practice?"
>
> Dogen replied, "You're right. Practitioners of the Way certainly ought to maintain Hyakujo's regulations. The form of maintaining the regulations is receiving and observing the precepts and practicing zazen, etc. The meaning of reciting the Precept Sutra day and night and observing the precepts single-mindedly is nothing other than practicing *shikantaza*, following the activities of the ancient masters. When we sit zazen, what precept is not observed, what merit is not actualized? The ways of practice carried on by the ancient masters have a profound meaning. Without holding on to personal preferences, we should go along with the assembly and practice in accordance with those ways (Dogen et al. 1988, pp. 21–22).

Dogen encouraged his disciples and the practitioners in the way to model proper conduct outlined in a *shingi*. This is mainly because, according to Dogen, such behavior would facilitate the practice of Buddha Way while minimizing the intrusion of egocentric desires and because the true students of Zen had practiced Zen in this way.

Focusing on the conduct of the body also undermines the categorical and analytic worldview derived from our minds. Not being caught up with our mind means letting go of categorization, differentiation, or evaluation, including the differentiation between physical body and Dharma body. In the chapter of *Katto* (葛藤; Twining Vines) of *Shobogenzo*, Dogen exemplified the significance of body that goes beyond the ideas of body in practice:

> Bodhidharma once said to his students, "The time has come. Can you express your understanding?" Once of the students, Daofu, said, "My present view is that we should neither be attached to letters nor be apart from letters, and allow the way to function freely."
>
> Bodhidharma said, "You have attained my skin."
>
> The nun, Zongchi, said, "My view is that it is like the joy of seeing Akshobhya Buddha's land just once and not again."
>
> Bodhidharma said, "You have attained my flesh."
>
> Daoyu said, "The four great elements are originally empty, and the five skandhas do not exist. Therefore I see nothing to be attained."
>
> Bodhidharma said, "You have attained my bones."
>
> Finally, Huike bowed three times, and stood up, and returned to where he was.
>
> Bodhidharma said, "You have attained my marrow." Thus, he confirmed Huike as the Second Ancestor and transmitted dharma and the robe to him. (see Dogen and Tanahashi 2010, p. 479)

The passage above really delineates the significance of body in the Buddha Way. In the passage, Bodhidharma, the transmitter of Chan Buddhism to China, and regarded as its first Chinese patriarch, highlighted his students' awakening by pointing to his bodily parts metaphorically. His teachings on the practice through the body also highlight that the Buddha Way cannot be described wholly in words. From this standpoint, the body is the standpoint of no discrimination and differentiation (Suzuki 1996), where the Buddha Way can unfold. This is the significance of body in Zen.

References

Buddhist Text Translation Society. (2001). *The Sixth Patriarch's Dharma Jewel Platform Sutra*. Burlingame, CA, USA: Buddhist Text Translation Society.

Dogen, E., Ejo, K., Okumura, S., & Wright, D. T. (1988). *Shobogenzo-zuimonki: Sayings of Eihei Dogen Zenji*. Tokyo, Japan: Soto-shu Shumucho.

Dogen, E., Leighton, T. D., & Okumura, S. (1995). *Dogen's pure standards for the Zen community: A translation of Eihei Shingi*. Albany, New York: State University of New York Press.

Dogen, E., Leighton, T. D., & Okumura, S. (2010). *Dogen's extensive record: A translation of the Eihei Koroku*. Somerville, MA, USA: Widsom Publications.

Dogen, E., Nishiari, B., Okumura, S., Suzuki, S., & Weisman, S. M. (2011). *Dogen's genjo koan: Three commentaries*. Barkeley, CA, USA: Counterpoint.

Dogen, E., & Tanahashi, K. (1985). *Moon in a dewdrop: Writings of Zen master Dogen*. New York, USA: North Point Press.

Dogen, E., & Tanahashi, K. (2010). *Tresury of the true Dharma eye: Zen Master Dogen's Shobo Genzo*. Boston MA, USA: Shambhala.

Ferguson, A. (2011). *Zen's Chinese heritage: The masters and their teachings*. Somerville MA, USA: Wisdom Publications.

Japan Buddhist Federation. (1978). *Understanding Japanese Buddhism*.

Kirchner, T. Y., & Sasaki, R. F. (2008). *The record of Linji*. Honolulu, HI, USA: University of Hawaii Press.

Shaner, D. E. (1985). The bodymind experience in Dogen's "Shobogenzo": A phenomenological perspective. *Philosophy East and West, 35*(1), 17–35. doi:10.2307/1398679.

Suzuki, D. T. (1964). *An introduction to Zen Buddhism*. New York, NY, USA: Grove Press.

Suzuki, D. T. (1996). *Zen Buddhism: Selected writings of D. T. Suzuki*. New York, USA: An Image Book.

Suzuki, D. T. (2010). *Zen and Japanese culture*. Princeton, NJ, USA: Princeton University Press (original work published in 1938).

Suzuki, S. (1970). *Zen Mind, Beginner's Mind: Informal talks on Zen meditation and practice*. Boston, MA USA: Weatherhill.

Uchiyama, K., & Okumura, S. (2014). *The Zen teaching of homeless Kodo*. Somerville MA, USA: Tuttle Publications.

Uchiyama, K., Wright, T., Warner, J., & Okumura, S. (2004). *Opening the hand of thought: Foundations of Zen Buddhism practice*. Somerville MA, USA: Wisdom Publications.

Zen and Language: Zen Mondo and Koan

Takashi Ogawa, Akihiko Masuda and Kayla Sargent

Keywords
Zen · Buddhism · Behavioral health · Koan · Mondo

A common definition of Zen Buddhism found in Japanese dictionaries is "a religion that seeks enlightenment through zazen (Zen meditation)." Although zazen is a crucial component of Zen Buddhism, it is misleading to imply that Zen Buddhism consists of nothing but meditation practice. Although zazen is often associated exclusively with Zen Buddhism, other schools of Buddhism emphasize zazen as a crucial part of their practices and teachings. In Mahayana Buddhism, to which Zen Buddhism belongs, zazen is one of the Six Perfections (e.g., culmination of certain virtues). Furthermore, it is important to note that zazen actually predated Buddhism. As noted elsewhere, zazen existed prior to the birth of Gautama Buddha, and Buddhism is said to have begun when Gautama Buddha attained enlightenment through zazen.

This sentiment regarding the dawn of Buddhism can be misleading, too, as its precise origin varies. Recently, a Rinzai Zen master said to me that Buddhism did not begin when the Gautama Buddha attained enlightenment; instead, it began when he got up from zazen and began teaching the Way to others. Buddhism would not have existed if Gautama Buddha had not shared his wisdom and compassion of the Way with others.

For Buddhism to be Buddhism, it must involve two processes: the teachings themselves as well as the people who are committed to those teachings. Furthermore, there must be a *language* that connects Buddhism's teachings with its followers. Gautama Buddha's enlightenment would not have become what is known as Buddhism today if there had been no followers, and these followers would not have existed without language to transmit his teachings. This position is congruent with D.T. Suzuki's perspective on the history of Buddhism and Zen Buddhism. In his writings, Suzuki repeatedly stated that wisdom and compassion are at the core of Buddhism and that there is no Buddhism without them (e.g., Suzuki 1994). According to Suzuki, wisdom is the Buddha Way

Translated and Edited by Akihiko Masuda and Kayla Sargent

T. Ogawa (✉)
Komazawa University, Tokyo, Japan
e-mail: ogawat@komazawa-u.ac.jp

A. Masuda (✉) · K. Sargent
University of Hawaii at Manoa, Honolulu, USA
e-mail: amasuda4@hawaii.edu

K. Sargent
e-mail: kaylansargent@gmail.com

A. Masuda and W.T. O'Donohue (eds.), *Handbook of Zen, Mindfulness, and Behavioral Health*,
Mindfulness in Behavioral Health, DOI 10.1007/978-3-319-54595-0_8

that one can direct toward or find within him or herself, and compassion is the Buddha Way that one directs toward others.

Like any other cultural or spiritual human activities, Zen Buddhism is interpersonal and social in nature. If a person merely enlightens through zazen alone, the practices of zazen and Zen teachings do not have to be established as a religious system. As is the case for other schools of Buddhism, language (e.g., discourse) plays a crucial role in learning and transmitting the Way in Zen Buddhism.

What may be unique to Zen language are its styles (e.g., *mondo* and *koan*) and its purpose. A *mondo* (問答) refers to a verbal exchange between a disciple and his or her master, and a *koan* (公案) is a paradoxical anecdote or riddle, used in Zen Buddhism to demonstrate the shortfall of logical and analytic reasoning and to provoke enlightenment. Discourse between a teacher and a disciple is generally literal and linear in other religions and other schools of Buddhism. That is, when a speaker asks a listener a question (e.g., "Where do we go after we die?"), the listener responds to the speaker by answering the question the speaker asks in a logically consistent and direct manner (e.g., "We all will go to heaven"). Similarly, many religious systems use this structure of discourse to exchange, learn, and teach information (i.e., teachings, attitudes, and beliefs) in a literally and logically coherent manner. On the other hand, Zen *mondos* appear relatively illogical or disorganized in content and structure. For example, in some *mondos*, a master does not respond to a student's question but asks the student a seemingly irrelevant question instead. Other times, Zen discourse abandons the purpose of uncovering unknown truths altogether. In these cases, the purpose of the teacher–student dyadic conversation is left to the listener or reader to interpret.

Tetsuharu Kawakami (川上 哲治; 1920–2013) is known as Japanese baseball's first Zen master; he presented the nature and purpose of Zen dialogue eloquently. Kawakami was a professional baseball legend in Japan, known for his exceptional batting skills and later, his legendary coaching skills which led the Tokyo Giants to nine consecutive championships, the longest streak in Japanese pro-sports history. In his book *Zen to Nihon Yakyu* (Zen and Japanese Baseball), Kawakami described the nature of Zen as follows:

> [Baseball] skills are not simple "things" that are taught by others. Rather, these skills require personal discipline and must be seized by the people who seek to develop them. This is also the case with Zen. Zen *mondo* is not a practice that seeks to merely hand enlightenment over students. For an enlightened master, it is actually a process of guiding his or her students to a state of enlightenment without directly pointing to where it can be found. Although the master may help the student attain enlightenment, he or she never teaches the student what enlightenment is directly. Rather than being taught by others, enlightenment must be grasped by students on their own. That is Zen (the translation is made by the translators).

Zen dialogues, such as *mondo* and *koan*, appear illogical and disorganized. However, they do so deliberately so that the student learns the Buddha Nature *personally* and *experientially*. In this sense, Zen dialogue is intentionally inconvenient. It is used not for expedience or comfort but so that students may attain enlightenment through themselves. In Zen, we are not able to simply receive enlightenment directly from others as a gift. Through discourse, a master deliberately prohibits him- or herself from directly revealing what enlightenment is for his or her student. "Enlightenment" taught by others is better conceptualized as attaining knowledge as opposed to the full and whole experience that is enlightenment.

Zen Dialogues in the Tang Dynasty (750–1000 AD)

Zen Buddhism grew as an independent religious organization in China during the Tang Dynasty (750–1000 AD). During that time, many dialogues among Zen monks and students were recorded and assembled as a collection. These collections were further edited with the additions of commentaries by Zen masters during the Song

Dynasty (960–1279). Many of the popular Zen dialogues of our current times were actually compiled during the Song period. One example of such a dialogue is the one between Mazu Daoyi (709–788; 馬祖道一; Baso Doitsu in Japanese) and another monk. Mazu is the dharma heir of the sixth patriarch of Zen Buddhism, Huineng (慧能; Eno in Japanese; 638–713), and together they are the most famous of the ancient Chinese Zen masters. This *mondo* is cited in the Records of the Transmission of the Lamp (景德傳燈錄; Keitoku Dento-roku in Japanese), a voluminous work consisting of biographies of the Zen patriarchs and other prominent Buddhist monks. The *mondo* goes:

> A monk asked, "What is the essential meaning of Buddhism?"
> Mazu said, "What is the meaning of this moment?" (see Ferguson 2011, p. 76)

This dialogue can be described as disorganized and illogical as Mazu responded to the monk's question by asking him another question rather than answering the monk's original question. Responding to a question by asking a question occurs in our daily discourse as well. Between life partners, a routine conversation may include responses in the form of questions; for example, a wife may respond "What do you wanna eat for dinner?" to her husband asking "Where is the TV remote?" This dialogue between the wife and the husband is illogical if its aim is to exchange the concrete information implied by the original questions. In response to the husband's question, the wife changes the topic. As such for the husband, the goal of asking the question (i.e., finding the remote controller) is not achieved. If the purpose of the dialogue between Mazu and a monk is similar to that of the discourse between the couples, it is also extremely incoherent. However, would it be the case? Let's try another discourse of everyday life.

> Person A: Do you like Yankees?
> Person B: Where do you think I'm from?

In reading the dialogue, it is unclear whether the person B is from and what the person B means by "Where do you think I'm from?" However, B's intension seems very clear to person A. If the person B is from the Bronx, New York, his answer "Where do you think I'm from?" means "Yes, I like the Yankees." If the person B is from elsewhere, let's say Boston, his response means "no," as there are many die-hard Boston Red Sox fans in Boston, and this cultural link would imply that Person B's question is in reference to being a Red Sox fan. Unlike the dialogue of the couple above, the exchange between the person A and person B in this second scenario is established as a complete dialogue, despite person B responding to person A's question by asking another question.

The conversation between person A and person B is established as a complete dialogue if the two participants share the implied knowledge (i.e., where person B is from). In this symbolic exchange, person B is able to respond with a question so that person A can understand the answer himself. The answer that person A seeks emerges naturally within her by the prompt response question. Psychologists often call this an "aha moment" or insight learning.

Similarly, we can apply our understanding of this type of learning to *mondo* and *koan* practice. The dialogue between the monk and Mazu above embodies the same sense of nuance. Mazu asked the question from the standpoint of the first Zen patriarch's (Bodhidharma) teaching. Mazu described the core of Bodhidharma's teaching as follows:

> Each one of you, you should believe that your own mind is the Buddha, and that this mind is identical with the Buddha. The great master Bodhidharma came from India to China and transmitted the One mind teaching of the supreme vehicle in order to cause you to realize awakening (see Poceski 2015, p. 83).

Mazu asked the monk the question from the standpoint of the One mind teaching (i.e., one's own mind is the Buddha). Mazu's intention was to direct the monk's focus to the present moment, where the monk's mind could unfold as the Buddha. This was the teaching that Bodhidharma brought from India.

The dialogue between Mazu and the monk is said to be complete if that question from Mazu prompted him to become fully aware of the One mind teaching of Bodhidharma. If the monk did not have an "aha moment" of realization, the dialogue is illogical and disorganized such that its purpose is not yet realized. For the monk, it was crucial to find out the teaching of Buddha on his own, the teaching from which Mazu asked him that question. Mazu has another episode:

> A monk asked (Mazu): "What is the meaning of (Bodhidharma's) coming from the West?"
>
> Mazu then hit him. Thereafter he said, "If I did not hit you, (people) everywhere would laugh at me" (see Poceski 2015, p. 290).

Mazu hit the monk in response to his question (i.e., "What is the meaning of Bodhidharma's coming from the West?"). If teachers or physicians of the present time in Japan or the USA do the same thing to their own students or patients, it will be an extremely serious problem. So what would be his intention? Mazu's intention comes from the standpoint of wisdom and compassion. He hit the monk in the hope that the monk would feel his Buddha mind (i.e., the body-mind) fully. Unfortunately, despite Mazu's intention, the monk did not find the Buddha mind in his experience.

However, another episode of Mazu presented that the same action yielded the awakening of a monk, named Shuilao (水老). The *mondo* in this episode goes as follows:

> Reverend Shuiliao of Hongzhou came to see Mazu for the first time. He asked, "What is the true meaning of (patriarch Bodhidharma's) coming from the west?"
> Mazu said, "Bow down!"
> Just as Shuilao was bowing down, Mazu gave him a kick. Thereupon Shuilao had great awakening. He rose up, clapping his hands and laughing heartily.
> Shuilao exclaimed, "How wonderful! How wonderful! The source of myriad samadhis and limitless subtle meanings: they can all be realized on the tip of single hair." He then paid his respects to Mazu and went away.
> Later, Shuilao told the assembly (at his monastery), "Ever since the day Master Ma kicked me, I had not yet stopped laughing." (Poceski 2015, p. 54–55)

It is important to highlight that not all Zen *mondos* include hitting or responding to questions with questions. There are, in fact, many gentle Zen *mondos*. A *mondo* of Zhaozhou (趙州從諗; Joshu Jushin in Japanese; 778–897) is an example. The *mondo* goes:

> A monk asked Zhaozhou, "The ten thousand things return to the one. Where does the one return?"
>
> Zhaozhou said, "When I lived in Qingzhou I made a cotton shirt weighing seven pounds." (Dogen et al. 2010, p. 331)

This is a well-known mondo, cited in some of the well-known Zen texts, such as the Records of the Transmission of the Lamp, the Blue Cliff Record (碧巌録; Hekiganroku in Japanese), and *Eihei Koroku* (永平広録; The Extensive Record of Teacher Dōgen's Sayings). Similar to other *mondos* mentioned above, the *mondo* of Zhaozhou appears illogical and incoherent. However, if the monk knew the background of Zhaozhou as well as the teachings of Mazu, Zhaozhou's master, the intention of Zhaozhou from his answer might make sense.

Zhaozhou was from Qingzhou. A cotton shirt was a cloth that people at the time of Zhaozhou wore every day. There was nothing formal or special about it, and it symbolized the ordinary way of living. Seven pound in the Chinese metric system is about the weight of a new born baby. "A cotton shirt made in Qingzhou" symbolized Zhaozhou himself. For Zhaozhou, all myriad dharmas return to him, and for the monk, all myriad dharmas return to the monk himself. Zhaozhou's intention was to have the monk realize the importance of the monk himself in that very moment.

The mondo of Zhaozhou is similar to that of Fuxi (福谿; Fukukei in Japanese). This dialogue is also cited in the Records of the Transmission of the Lamp.

> A monk asked, "Karma scatters and returns to emptiness, but where does emptiness return to?"

"Fellow!" shouted the master.
"Yes," answered the monk.
"Where is emptiness?"
"May the master please tell!" replied the monk.
"The Persians eat spices," said the master. (see Daoyuan and Whitfield 2015, p. 244–245)

A focal point of the discourse is the monk's "Yes." More specifically, it is within the monk that emptiness (i.e., the Buddha Way) returns in the very moment when he wholeheartedly said "Yes." Fuxi then asked him "where is emptiness?" in the hope that the monk might realize that the emptiness returns to the monk himself. Unfortunately, the monk did not realize that the emptiness was in him in the moment he said yes. Perhaps, being slightly disappointed, Fuxi said, "The Persians eat spices." During the time of Zhaozhou and Fuxi, spices were imported from Persia to China through the Silk Roads, and they were as valuable as golds. "The Persians eat spices" implies that the monk did not realize himself as the locus of emptiness, as if the Persians waste their own spices by eating them. Although the entire dialogue presents Fuxi as somewhat sarcastic, he showed the monk where the emptiness goes.

Zen Koans During the Song Dynasty (960–1279)

As shown above, Zen *mondos* during the Tang Dynasty appear illogical, but they include the event to be realized (e.g., self as the locus of emptiness in the *mondo* of Fuxi). In other words, all of these *mondos* point to the very person who asked a question as the locus of what he was looking for.

Conversely, when Zen Buddhism entered into the Song Dynasty, Zen dialogues became inherently illogical and unsolvable. These were called *koans* (gong'an). Koans strip all meanings from words, disrupt logical flows, and transform a conversation into mere chunks of sounds. They were used to remove all analytic and logical mindsets from the practitioners and have them leap into the realization of enlightenment. In *Muchu mondoshu* (夢中問答集; the Dialogues in a Dream), Muso Soseki (夢窓 疎石; 1275–1351), a great Japanese Rinzai Zen master, described the development of koan-based practice within the history of Zen Buddhism as follows:

> Students in former times were not shallow in their desire for the Way. Unconcerned with physical discomfort and prepared to travel any distance, they sought far and wide for good teachers. Zen masters, in their compassion, would utter a word or two to help them. These words were intended only as direct pointers to Original Nature—the meaning was not in the words themselves. Superior students were able to perceive this meaning apart from the actual statements. What need, then, was there to engage in further discussions regarding other words and phrases?
>
> Even those slower students who got caught up in the master's utterances soon saw that the words were like iron spikes, impenetrable to ordinary thought. However, their aspiration for the Way being strong, their hearts were filled with deep questioning. Forgetting to eat and sleep, they pursued this questioning until, after one or two days, or after one or two months, or, in some cases, after ten or twenty years, they finally broke through. Although the time required depended on their karmic propensities from previous lives, none of them failed to breakthrough within the span of their lifetimes. This is what an ancient master meant when he said, "Where there is great doubt, there is great enlightenment."
>
> In this way, no one was even told by the ancient masters to take their words and use them as koans to contemplate upon. Nor did the ancient masters ever advise anyone either to doubt or not to doubt what they said. However, people nowadays lack strong karmic propensities for practice and their aspiration for the Way is shallow. Hearing a master's words, they contrive intellectual interpretations and then quit Zen, convinced that they have already attained enlightenment. Others, too dull-witted to devise such explanations, simply lose interest. It is out of compassion for such people that Zen masters from the time of Yuanwu Keqin and Dahui Zonggao developed koan practice as an expedient means (Muso and Kirchner 2015, p. 237–238).

"Former times" in the passage above refers to the times of famous Zen masters during the Tang Dynasty, such as Huineng and Mazu. Yuanwu

Keqin (圜悟克勤; Engo Kokugon in Japanese; 1063–1135) was a Chinese Zen monk, who was best known as the compiler of the Blue Cliff Record, a collection of one hundred famous Zen *koans* in their present form. Dahui Zonggao (大慧宗杲; Daie Soko in Japanese; 1089–1163) was a student of Yuanwu. He was best known for his contribution to systematizing Kanna-Zen (看話禅), a *koan*-based Zen practice. Muso placed a great emphasis on *koans* in his Rinzai Zen practice. He explained a *koan* as follows:

> Koans are not assigned so that one may be born in the Pure Land or realize Buddhahood and the Way. Nor is a koan some kind of strange puzzle or an expression of Zen doctrine. It is simply that which cannot be grasped by the ordinary mind—that is the nature a koan. It can be likened to a dumpling made of iron. Faced with that which the "tongue" of ordinary consciousness cannot taste, you chew away and chew away, and finally you chew right through. Then, for the first time, you realize that this iron dumpling has nothing to do with the five tastes and six flavors of the world. Nor is it the flavor of the Dharma or the taste of the doctrine (Muso and Kirchner 2015, p. 169).

Ordinary mind in the passage above refers to our conventional analytic and logical ways of thinking. Muso stated that one cannot make sense of a *koan* through a careful analysis or logic. Instead, one must stay focused on the *koan*, and doing so inevitably removes his or her own thoughts and feelings from it, eventually yielding the great enlightenment. As mentioned above, this *koan*-based practice was systematized as Kanna-Zen by Dahui. The *koan* that Dahui used the most was Zhaozhou's Wu. It goes:

> A monk asked Zhaozhou, "Does a dog have Buddha nature?"
> Zhaozhou answered, "Wu! [in Japanese, 'Mu']"

Although Zhaozhou was a Zen master of the Tang Dynasty, this mondo of Zhaozhou was used as a well-known *koan* during the Song Dynasty. Dahui stated that one must focus on this *koan*, while letting go of all logical and analytic ways of thinking and continue to leap into it.

Gaofeng Yuanmiao (高峰原妙; Koho Genmyo in Japanese; 1238–1295) is also well known for his *koan*-based teaching. His disciple, Zhongfeng Mingben (中峰明本; Chuho Myohon; 1263–1323) described his teaching as follows:

> Looking back, my master Gaofeng Yuanmiao lived deep in the mountains for thirty years. Throughout these periods, he only used the *koan* of "all myriad things returns to the original one, and then where the original one returns to" for teaching his disciples. He left his disciples to face it quietly and yet dynamically, study it continuously without being caught up by external affairs or various karmas (e.g., like-dislike, joy-sorrow). He then said that as one continued to focus on the *koan* in every single moment, one reached the point where no thought could intrude, and then break-through unfolds. Then one for the first time feels the Buddha Way.

The *koan* practice by Gaofeng Yuanmiao was identical with that of Dahui. Both Dahui and Gaofeng told their disciples to chew away and chew away a *koan* until they finally chewed right through. By focusing wholeheartedly on the *koan*, they could reach the great breakthrough. This is the experience of enlightenment through Kanna-Zen practice systematized during the Song Dynasty, and this Kanna-Zen practice has continued to this date.

Finally, it may be worthwhile to recapitulate the theme of this chapter. I think that Ruth Benedict (1887–1948), an American anthropologist and folklorist, eloquently summarized *koan* practice in her *the Chrysanthemum and the Sword*. This book was originally published in 1946 as an anthropological study of Japanese cultural practices, including Zen Buddhism, and it remains influential to this date. Benedict (2005) stated:

> The most favored technique for inducing the novice's desperate attempt "to know" were the *koan*, literally "the problems." There are said to be seventeen hundred of these problems, and the anecdote books make nothing of a man's devoting seven years to the solution of one of them. They are not meant to have rational solutions. One is "to conceive the clapping of one hand." Another is "to feel the yearning for one's mother before one's own conception." Others are, "Who is carrying one's lifeless body?," "Who is it who is walking toward me?," "All things return into One; where does this last return?" Such Zen problems as these were used in China before the twelfth or thirteenth century, and Japan adopted these techniques along with the cult. On the continent, however, they did

> not survive. In Japan they are a most important part of training in "expertness." Zen handbooks treat them with extreme seriousness. "Koan enshrines the dilemma of life." A man who is pondering one, they say, reaches an impasse like "a pursued rat that has run up a blind tunnel," he is like a "man with a ball of red-hot iron stuck in his throat," he is "a mosquito trying to bite a lump of iron," he is beside himself and redoubles his efforts. Finally the screen of his "observing self" between his mind and his problem falls aside; with the swiftness of a flash of lightening the two—mind and problem—come to terms. He "knows." (p. 245–246)

As noted by Benedict, Koan is crucial in Kanna-Zen, which was formalized by Dahui Zonggao of China during the Song Dynasty (1089–1163; 大慧宗杲; Daie Soko in Japanese). This *koan*-based method of Zen was transmitted to Japan in the twelfth or thirteenth century, and it was further systematized by Hakuin (白隠; 1686–1768) during the Edo period. In his *koan* practice, Hakuin encouraged his students to interact with multiple *koans*, one after another, along with additional questions attached to each *koan*. Today, Kanna-Zen practiced by Rinzai Zen is that of Hakuin.

Zazen, or Zen meditation, is crucial in Zen Buddhism. However, Zazen itself is not Zen Buddhism. It is inevitable for the students of Zen as well as Zen masters to awaken on their own through Zen *mondos* and *koans,* a set of language practice unique to Zen Buddhism. The heart of Zen is not in a single person. Zen is interpersonal, and it is in a communication between two individuals. Whereas Zen Buddhism does not worship its founder or sutras, it cherishes the records of over thousands dialogues between a Zen master and a student. This fact may symbolize the interpersonal nature of Zen Buddhism and its acknowledgment of the significance of language.

References

Benedict, R. (2005). *The chrysanthemum and the sword.* New York; US: Marinar Books (original work published in 1946).

Daoyuan, S., & Whitfield, R. S. (2015). *Records of the transmission of the lamp: Volume II The early masters*. New York: Books on Demand.

Dogen, E., Leighton, T. D., & Okumura, S. (2010). *Dogen's extensive record: A translation of the Eihei Koroku*. Somerville, MA, US: Widsom Publications.

Ferguson, A. (2011). *Zen's Chinese heritage: The masters and their teachings*. Somerville MA, US: Wisdom Publications.

Muso, S., & Kirchner, T. Y. (2015). *Dialogues in a dream: The life and Zen teachings of Muso Soseki.* Somerville, MA, US: Wisdom Publications.

Poceski, M. (2015). *The records of Mazu and the making of classical Chan literature*. New York, USA: Oxford University Press.

Suzuki, D. T. (1994). *Essays in Zen Buddhism.* New York, US: Grove Press (original work published in 1949).

Part II

Zen: Everyday Living and Current Evidence

Zen and Desire

Kiyozumi Seijun Ishii, Akihiko Masuda and Kayla Sargent

Keywords
Zen · Buddhism · Behavioral health · Desire · Bonno

Zen offers a unique account of desire, discussing desire itself as well as attachment to specific desires (煩悩; *bonno* in Japanese), sometimes referred to as earthly desire. Zen is based upon the absolute validation or affirmation of the self and reality, fostering a fundamental assumption that desires are not a separate entity, and they do not inherently prevent people from becoming a Buddha. From a Zen perspective, individuals are essentially pure, and the Buddha Nature exists in every sentient being.

Before going into more detail about Zen's account of human desires, let us present the story of Tanzan Hara (原坦山; 1819–1892), which was said to have happened in Japan in late nineteenth century:

> Tanzan Hara was a famous Zen monk of the Meiji Period (1868–1912). He was also a Buddhist scholar who became the first lecturer of Indian philosophy at Tokyo University. When Tanzan was a young pilgrim monk, he traveled country roads with a close friend. One day, the two of them came to a shallow and narrow river. However, there was no bridge, and they were going to have to wade across. They saw a beautiful young woman who was hesitating to wade through the stream. Tanzan said to her, "Here, I'll carry you across. Hold on to my shoulders tightly. All right?" and lightly held her and carried her across.
>
> The girl blushingly thanked Tanzan, but he, in his haste to catch up with his friend, did not hear her. The two monks walked about a mile in silence, and Tanzan's friend appeared to be displeased. Suddenly the friend could contain himself no longer and bluntly said, "You're a disgrace. Do you think monks should embrace girls?" He looked angry.
>
> Tanzan, pretending not to understand, looked round about him and said, "What? Where is a girl?"
>
> Don't go on pretending. You held a beautiful girl just a short while ago.
>
> Ha, ha, ha, ha, ha—you mean that girl. I carried her across the river and put her down. Have you been carrying her in your mind all this way?
>
> Hearing this, the friend was at a loss for words.

Historically, it is unclear whether this episode actually happened as very similar episodes are cited in other Zen Buddhism records. Nevertheless, Hara's behavior in this episode captures the ideal conduct of a Zen monk, and his choice to

Translated and edited by Akihiko Masuda and Kayla Sargent

K.S. Ishii (✉)
Komazawa University, Tokyo, Japan
e-mail: seijun@komazawa-u.ac.jp

A. Masuda · K. Sargent
University of Hawaii at Manoa, Honolulu, USA

A. Masuda and W.T. O'Donohue (eds.), *Handbook of Zen, Mindfulness, and Behavioral Health*,
Mindfulness in Behavioral Health, DOI 10.1007/978-3-319-54595-0_9

carry the woman can be analyzed from many perspectives. At the time, physical contact with the opposite sex was prohibited in Zen Buddhism as doing so might have inflamed sexual desires. Instead, however, it was the fellow monk who was corrected for his rigid adherence to the rule of conduct that advises monks to refrain from touching women. The wisdom within this episode is that we should choose the best, within the context, freely and flexibly, and then move forward. A choice that is deemed to be inappropriate in one context may not be inappropriate in another.

Furthermore, it is also unclear whether Tanzan actually experienced an egocentric desire during the encounter with the woman. Perhaps his friend reacted strongly to this incidence because of this lack of clarity. However, Tanzan had already let go of the encounter with the woman when he was disrupted by his friend. Regardless of whether he felt an egocentric desire or not, he refrained from forming an attachment to the potential desire and the choice, whereas his friend remained attached to both. The way Tanzan acted in this episode captures the heart of Zen and the Zen way of responding to human desire (Uchiyama et al. 2004).

The significance of flexibility and adaptation to one's circumstances is traced back to the precept of formlessness taught by the Huineng (惠能; 638–713), the sixth patriarch of Zen Buddhism. The precept of formlessness is also known as the precept of Buddha Nature. Formlessness does not include statements of what *not* to do. This is because there is no need for listing such statements if there were nothing fundamentally tainted in us.

Huineng also stated that precepts are aspirational; they are striving for and expressing the Buddha Nature in us rather than punishing us for wrong doings. Once we become fully connected to the Buddha Nature, we naturally direct our behavior along with the Buddha Nature. Once we become cognizant of how the Buddha Nature manifests in us in every awaking moment, that itself becomes the precept of Buddha Nature. Hara's decision to carry a woman was not criticized by the Zen community mainly because of the way in which he manifested the Buddha Nature (e.g., compassion) according to the precept of formlessness, transcending the rigid attachment to the "rules" of Zen at the time.

Teachings of Huineng

Many Zen Buddhist monks and scholars consider Huineng a preeminent figure of Chinese Zen heritage (see Dumoulin 2005a; Ferguson 2011). All of the five traditional schools of Chinese Zen during the Tang Dynasty (750–1000 AD) trace their origins through Huineng. Ferguson (2011) stated that:

> The traditional story of Huineng's life reveals an iconoclastic personality whose defiance of religious convention sharpened the unique cultural flavor of Chinese Zen (p. 43).

The teachings of Huineng are summarized eloquently by his famous verse cited in the Platform Sutra of the Sixth Patriarch (see McRae 2000). The verse goes:

> Bodhi is fundamentally without any tree;
> The bright mirror is also not a stand.
> Fundamentally there is not a single thing—
> Where could any dust be attracted? (McRae 2000, p. 22).

Huineng was said to make this verse in response to a verse made by Shenxiu (神秀; Jinshu in Japanese; unknown–706). Shenxiu was Huineng's fellow disciple, and they studied Zen under the fifth patriarch, Hongren (弘忍; Konin in Japanese; 601–674). At that time, many considered Shenxiu to be the Dharma heir of Hongren, not Huineng. Shenxiu's poem (McRae 2000, p. 20) goes:

> The body is the bodhi tree;
> The mind is like a bright mirror's stand.
> Be always diligent in rubbing it—
> Do not let it attract any dust.

The bodhi tree and the mirror in Shenxiu's verse symbolize the experience of enlightenment, and for Shenxiu, the body and mind are like the tree and the stand that hold the experience of enlightenment. Finally, dust represents worldly, egocentric desires. As such, Shenxiu's verse implies that we must strive to remove egocentric desires in order to unfold the experience of enlightenment in us.

When Huineng heard the verse, he found it incomplete and presented his own verse that was mentioned above. As shown above, his verse completely negates the Shenxiu's verse. The first two lines of Huineng's verse state that the body and mind are not the tree or a mirror stand that holds bodhi. The third line of Huineng's states the Buddha Nature is a whole, and there is no separation of self from the things that one should react to or act upon, including the Buddha Nature or human desires. The fourth Huineng then concludes that in the realm of wholeness, there is no particular place where a speck of dust lands; that is, there is no worldly desire as a separate entity. In sum, the fundamental teaching of Huineng is that our body and mind are essentially pure, encompassing the Buddha Nature already, and even egocentric desires are not to be eliminated.

As described extensively elsewhere (Dumoulin 2005a), Shenxiu's teachings became popular and dominant after Hongen's passing. That is, a belief persisted that one must get rid of worldly desires in order to pursue a state of enlightenment. In the history of Chinese Zen, P'u-chi (普寂; Fujaku in Japanese; 651–739), Shexiu's disciple, flourished Shenxiu's teaching further and established the Northern School of Zen.

Conversely, Huineng's Zen is now known as the Southern School of Zen. The shift in power occurred when the An Lushan Rebellion (755–763) devastated northern China in an attempt to weaken the Tang Dynasty where the Northern School of Zen based. Shenxui and the Northern School's influence was also significantly weakened accordingly. Around the same time, Shenhui (荷沢神会; Kataku Jinne in Japanese, 684–758), a disciple of Huineng, expanded the Southern School of Zen as the dominant religious organization and thrived since then. Zen Buddhism transmitted to Japan during the Kamakura period has its root in the Southern School of Zen, and this Zen is the Zen Buddhism transmitted to the West from Japan in the early and mid-twentieth century.

Guifeng Zongmi's Classification of Zen Buddhism

Various schools of Zen Buddhism today can trace their origins to those branched out from the Zen Buddhism of the Sixth Patriarch Huineng, and the practice of zazen itself predated Buddhism. As such, the understanding of zazen (*dhyana*) varies greatly across different spiritual traditions as well as various schools of Buddhism. Simply put, this diversity is attributable to different perspectives in practice, enlightenment, and both. Within the context of a practice–enlightenment relationship, different forms of worldly desires are identified.

In response to the diverse ideas of zazen (*dhyana*), Guifeng Zongmi (圭峰 宗密; Keiho Shumitsu in Japanese; 780–841), a Buddhist scholar-monk of the Tang Dynasty, categorized a range of Zen practices into five groups in his Collection of Expressions of the Principle and Practice of Dhyana (禅源諸詮集都序). Guifeng stated:

> The true nature is neither stained nor pure, neither common nor noble. Within dhyana, however, there are different grades, ranging from the shallow to the deep. To hold deviant views and practice because one joyfully anticipates rebirth in a heaven and is weary of the present world is outsider dhyana. Correctly to have confidence in karmic cause and effect and likewise practice because one joyfully anticipates rebirth into a heaven and is weary of the present world is common-person dhyana. To awaken to the incomplete truth of voidness of self and then practice is inferior-vehicle dhyana. To awaken to the true principle of the dual voidness of self and dharmas and then to practice is great vehicle dhyana. [All four of the above types show such distinctions as the four (dhyanas of the realm of) form and the four (concentrations of the) formless (realm).]. If one's practice is based on having all-at-once awakened to the realization that one's own mind is from the outset pure, that the depravities have never existed, that the nature of the wisdom without outflows is from the outset complete, that this mind is buddha, that they are ultimately without difference, then it is dhyana of the highest vehicle. This type is also known by such names as tathagata-purity dhyana, the one-practice concentration, and the thusness concentration. It is the basis of all concentrations. If one can practice it from moment to moment, one will naturally and

> gradually attain the myriad concentrations. This is precisely the dhyana that has been transmitted down from Bodhidharma. Before Bodhidharma arrived, all of the scholars from early times had understood only the four dhyanas (of the realm of form) and the eight concentrations (that is, those four plus the four formless concentrations of the formless realm). Various illustrious monks had effectively practiced them, and they had all obtained results (see Broughton 2009, p. 103).

In sum, as presented above, Guifeng Zongmi classified zazen (*dhyana*) practices into five categories based on the presence of particular desires and awareness. These are as follows:

1. Outsider Dhyana (外道禅; *gedo zen* in Japanese): Zazen while holding deviant views and practicing, because one joyfully anticipates rebirth in a heaven and is weary of the present world.
2. Common-person Dhyana (凡夫禅; *bonpu zen* in Japanese): Zazen practice while correctly having confidence in karmic cause and effect, and doing so because one joyfully anticipates rebirth into a heaven and is weary of the present world.
3. Inferior-vehicle Dhyana (小乘禅; *shojo zen* in Japanese): Zazen practice while awakening to the incomplete truth of voidness of self (e.g., the self as a transient being).
4. Great-vehicle Dhyana (小乘禅; *daijo zen* in Japanese): Zazen practice while awakening to the true principle of the dual voidness of self and dharmas.
5. Dhyana of the Highest Vehicle (最上乘禅; *saijojo zen* in Japanese): Zazen practice with awareness that one's own mind is from the outset pure and that this mind is Buddha.

In Guifeng's classification, the *dhyana* of highest vehicle is that of Zen Buddhism systematized by the Sixth Patriarch Huineng. According to many Zen Buddhists, it was the authentic Zen practice transmitted from the founder of Zen Buddhism, Bodhidharma (菩提達磨; *Bodai Daruma* in Japanese). Once again, Huineng's Zen is based on the standpoint that all sentient beings are from the outset pure; therefore, there would be no "dust" (i.e., no worldly desire) in need of elimination. Mazu Daoyi (709–788; 馬祖道一; Baso Doitsu in Japanese), a well-known Chinese Zen monk of Huineng's lineage, then later summarized the teaching of Huineng as "mind is Buddha" (Poceski 2015).

Following Guifeng's classification, Zen and mindfulness practices incorporated into Western behavioral health can be considered the common-person *dhyana* or *bonpu zen*. As described elsewhere, there is nothing wrong with considering and practicing mindfulness and Zen as a remedy for personal gains, such as the alleviation of pain and suffering (Uchiyama et al. 2004). Kosho Uchiyama (1912–1998), one of the most influential Japanese Soto Zen monks in disseminating Zen to the West, used the term *bonpu zen* (i.e., utilitarian Zen) to refer to such Zen-like practice. However, Uchiyama also made a clear distinction between practicing Zen unconditionally for unfolding the Buddha Way (e.g., practicing Zen with an attitude of letting go of all thoughts of how Zen could benefit "self") and Zen that is practiced for utilitarian purposes.

Dahui's Kanna Zen

Zen Buddhism bases its practice on the assumption that the self is at the outset pure, and there is no problematic worldly desire to be ceased from the self. It is important to note that the complete validation and affirmation of the self as a Buddha does not mean that one should relax and do nothing. It also does not mean that one can do whatever he or she likes to do by following one's egocentric desire. These are common misunderstandings of Zen Buddhism pervasive throughout time and place. In fact, Zen Buddhism became the practice of passivity during the Tang and Song dynasties.

The "Seven Perfecta" (七去; *shichikyo* in Japanese) is an example of a Zen teaching at that time that might have unintentionally encouraged passivity in Zen practice. The Seven Perfecta is a verse composed by Shishuang Qingzhu (石霜慶諸; Sekiso Keisho in Japanese; 807–888), and it was said to capture the ideal image of a Zen monk. The verse goes:

Have been totally ceased;
Have been totally extinguished;
Have become a cool land of desolation;
Have had only one awareness for ten thousand years;
Have become cold ashes and a withered tree;
Have become a fragrant censer in an ancient shrine;
Have become a vertical stripe of white silk.

As shown just above, this verse gives the impression that the ideal state of Zen is passivity. Dahui Zonggao (大慧宗杲; Daie Soko in Japanese; 1089–1163) of Linji school, the founder of Kanna Zen (koan-based Zen; see below), was extremely concerned about the perceived passivity and the absence of efforts to attain enlightenment in Zen practice at that time. Dahui also believed the misunderstood tranquility was encouraged further by Mokusho Zen (黙照禅; Silent Illumination Zen). Dahui stated as follows:

> In recent years, heretical teachers sprang up within the sangha like wild weeds, and blinded the eyes of numerous sentient beings. When one does not use the koans of the ancients in meditation, he will be like a blind man without a walking stick and cannot advance even one step…. [Some people] think that Buddha Dharma and Ch'an cultivation are not dependent upon written words. Therefore they denigrated all koans as ready-made. They just sit in a ghostly cave on a dark mountain after their meals. They call this practice "silent illumination," "dying the great death," "the state before the birth of one's parents." They sit there until calluses appear on their bottoms, yet they still do not dare to move. On the contrary, they regard this as the gradual maturation of their effort.
> On the other hand, there were also other types of heretical teachers who only had an intellectual understanding of koans.
> Nowadays there are people who have never personally experienced enlightenment, but only know how to play intellectual tricks. Before they ascend the high seat in the morning, they would stay up all night, memorizing two phrases from this pamphlet [koan collection] and two phrases from that one. After pasting them together they present the end product like a bouquet. They can talk with great fluency, but people with clear eyesight know this is a ridiculous parody (cited in Yu 1979, pp. 225–226).

In order to correct these misunderstandings, Dahui established and systematized his own style of teaching, called Kanna Zen (看話禅). Kanna Zen is a koan-based practice (Yu 1979). A *koan* (公案) is a story, dialogue, question, or statement, which is used in Zen practice to provoke enlightenment. Kan (看) in Kanna (看話) means "see and think wholeheartedly," and *na* (話) in Kanna refers to a "story" (i.e., koan).

It is also important to note that the use of koans in Zen practice predated Dahui. Nevertheless, his Kanna Zen practice was considered unique as it placed a great emphasis on the assumption of a "confused self" as the outset of practice. According to Dahui, all sentient beings are confused, so those who pursue the Buddha Way must practice thoroughly and persistently. Dahui believed that in order to benefit from a koan practice, a person must be willing to make a sincere commitment and let it penetrate into every part of his or her life. This attitude starkly contrasted the approach of passivity, which had been associated with Zen Buddhism at that time.

In his Kanna Zen practice, Dahui used ready-made koans of famous Tang masters. One of the most frequently recommended koans was Zhaozhou's "Wu" ("Joshu's Mu" in Japanese). The koan was cited in the *Mumonkan* (無門関; Gateless Barrier), a collection of koans complied in the Song Dynasty. The koan goes:

> A monk once asked Master Joshu, "Has a dog the Buddha Nature or not?" Joshu said, "Mu!"(see Shibayama 2000, p. 19)

Dahui told his followers to concentrate on this "Wu" ("Mu") all the time. He encouraged them to concentrate on this koan perpetually, even while eating and drinking, while carrying out official duties or fulfilling social obligations. All these activities could be treated as the proper occasions for concentrating on "Wu." They were taught to focus on all of these tasks as ideal opportunities "to work on the koan, to dwell constantly on it and finally to gain an awakening from it" (Yu 1979, p. 227). In order to do so, Dahui stated that one must be willing to make a sincere commitment and let it penetrate into every part of his or her life. Dahui stated:

> Please concentrate on the feeling of doubt and do not give it up whether walking, standing, sitting or lying down. This one word "Wu" is no other than the knife which can clear away this great doubt of

> life and death. The handle of this knife is right in your own hand. No one else can take hold of it for you, but you must do it yourself. If you are willing to lay down your life, you will be able to begin the task. However, if you are not willing to lay down your life, you should concentrate on the feeling of doubt and do not let it slip by (Yu 1979, p. 227).

In sum, Dahui's teaching still has its base in the fundamental assumption of Zen Buddhism, that all sentient beings have Buddha Nature. However, in response to the misguided passivity pervasive in Zen practice during his time, Dahui placed the "confused self" at the outset of practice to revitalize the active and dynamic nature of Zen practice. Worldly desires were part of this "confused self," and Dahui encouraged his followers to break into the state of enlightenment from the state of "confused self."

Zen Buddhism in Japan

Zen Buddhism in the Song Dynasty of China was brought to Japan during the Kamakura (鎌倉時代; 1185–1333) and Muromatchi (室町時代; 1336–1573) periods. The majority of Zen teachings transmitted to Japan at that time were those of Dahui and his Linji School lineages. Dogen Zenji (道元禅師; 1200–1253) was one of many Zen monks who contributed to the transmission of Zen to Japan during the Kamakura period. However, he did not bring Dahui's Kanna Zen. Instead, he brought the Caodong School of Zen (曹洞宗; Soto Zen in Japanese) and transformed it into his unique form of Zen, which is often called Dogen Zen.

Dogen is one of the most influential figures in Japanese Buddhism and Japanese philosophy. Dumoulin (2005b) described Dogen and his contribution to Japanese Buddhism as follows:

> No other religious personality in the history of Japan has so stirred contemporary interest and admiration as the Zen Master Dogen Kigen (1200–1253). Buddhists-members of the Soto school and numerous members from the various other Buddhists schools alike—hold him in reverence. Philosophers are attracted to "the depth and precision of his thought… which early on perceived and penetrated what is the starting point for the systematic thought of contemporary philosophy." They regard Dogen as a "religious person." During the first half of this century in Japan this unique blend of lofty religious achievement and uncommon intellectual gifts awakened a strong interest in the Zen master, whom not a few Japanese take to be one of their strongest and most spirited intellectual figures. At the same time, Dogen is not without his critics. Researchers are turning up new data that makes a definitive judgment impossible at this time. Yet the two main components of his personality—a religious expression inspired by genuine inner experience and his early contribution to a Japanese philosophy grounded in Mahayana Buddhism—assure him an important place in the religious and intellectual history of his country (p. 51).

Similar to the Sixth Patriarch Huineng, Dogen's Zen is out of the assumption that all sentient beings are pure and that they all have the Buddha Nature. His core teaching, which is distinguished from that of Dahui's Kanna Zen, is *shikantaza* (只管打坐; just doing zazen wholeheartedly, nothing but precisely sitting). For Dogen, there is no distinction between practice and enlightenment, and practice (i.e., just doing zazen wholeheartedly) is enlightenment. As such, instead of prioritizing the "confused self" in order to motivate student monks in the case of Dahui's Kanna Zen, Dogen highlighted the importance of practice by equating it to the state of enlightenment.

For Dogen, a given person does not unfold as a Buddha if he or she remains stagnant. Dogen stated that despite the innate nature of being a Buddha, one must actively engage in practice to reveal the Buddha Nature as the true self. For Dogen, practice is not merely a method of attaining enlightenment that exists in some other distinct place. Rather, it is the expression of the true self residing in the here and now. Instead of trying to cease worldly desires, Dogen's Zen places active practices on the standpoint of Buddha Nature. Below is the dialogue between Dogen and his teacher Tiantong Rujing (天童如淨; Japanese: Tendo Nyojo; 1162–1228). This dialogue seems to capture Dogen's thoughts on zazen and its association with worldly desires.

sum, the core of Dogen's teaching is that "all sentient beings are Buddha from birth; therefore, all of us practice the Buddha Way." This perspective of Dogen is not seen in the recorded teachings of Ruijin, yet it appears that Dogen reached this perspective though his discourse with Ruijin.

Hakuin and Zazenwasan

Hakuin Ekaku (白隠 慧鶴; 1686–1768) is another influential figure in Japanese Buddhism. Dumoulin (2005b) described his significant contribution below:

> Hakuin (1685–1768) is one of the greatest figures of Japanese Buddhism. His significance is most evident in the impact he had on subsequent history. After him, nearly all Japanese Rinzai masters belonged to his line and practiced what may be called "Hakuin Zen." His achievements represent a turning point in the history of Japanese Zen as inasmuch as he put an end to the decline that had set in the Zen movement since the end of the medieval period. He also laid new foundations for the Rinzai school. He was the first to develop a system for applying the practice of koan to enlightenment, a system that his disciples would bring to perfection. At the same time, he invigorated and consummated the work that Bankei and Munan had begun in expanding Rinzai Zen among the common people (p. 367).

Hakuin Zen is a koan-based Zen. As mentioned above, Kanna Zen was brought to Japan by many monks prior to Hakuin. Nevertheless, Hakiin's koan-based Zen is considered unique in that it differs from that of Dahui. More specifically, its core assumption is that all sentient beings are pure from the birth, which was a similar perspective to that of Dogen. However, unlike Dogen, Hakuin emphasized the systematic use of koan. "Listen to the Sound of the Single Hand" is Hakuin's most well-known *koan*. He presented it to his students as the first koan in his particular method of Zen training. In Sekishu no Onjo (隻手の音声), Hakuin commented on the role of this koan in his Zen training as follows:

> Five or six years ago I made up my mind to instruct everyone by saying, "Listen to the Sound of the Single Hand." I have to come to realize that this koan is infinitely more effective in instructing people than any of the methods I had used before. It seems to raise the ball of doubt in people much more easily and the readiness with which progress in meditation is made has been as different as the clouds are from the earth. Thus I have come to encourage the meditation on the Single Hand exclusively.
> What is the Sound of the Single Hand? When you clap together both hands a sharp sounds is heard: when you raise the one hand there is neither sound nor smell… This is something that can by no means be heard with the ear. If conceptions and discriminations are not mixed within it and it is quite apart from seeing, hearing, perceiving, and knowing, and if, while walking, standing, sitting, and reclining, you proceed straightforwardly without interpretation in the study of this koan, then in the place where reason is exhausted and words are ended, you will suddenly plunk out the karmic root of birth and death and break through the cave of ignorance (see Yampolsky 1971, pp. 163–164).

As such, Hakuin established his teaching method in hopes that his disciples would grasp the original self (i.e., true self) that goes beyond conventional logic and analysis. Fully experiencing "Listen to the Sound of One Hand" is intended to elicit an experience equivalent to what Dahui called the state of enlightenment. Hakuin taught his disciples to continue practicing even after their first experiences of enlightenment, subsequently going through other koans one by one while maintaining complete affirmation of the self as being as pure as a Buddha. For Hakuin, the self, who does not have *bonno*, practices to realize his or her true nature, and the self does so through *koan* practice. Finally, another notable teaching of Hakuin is his emphasis on zazen, summarized below in *Zazen Wasan* (坐禅和讃):

> All sentient beings are essentially Buddhas. As with water and ice, there is no ice without water; apart from sentient beings, there are no Buddhas. Not knowing how close the truth is we seek it far away—what a pity! We are like one who in the midst of water cries out desperately in thirst. We are like the son of a rich man who wandered away among the poor. The reason we transmigrate through the Six Realms is because we are lost in the darkness of ignorance. Going further and further astray in the darkness, how can we ever be free from birth-and-death? As for the Samadhi (zazen) of the Mahayana, there are no words to

> Rujing said "Zazen is to drop off body and mind. It is to sit wholeheartedly with burning incense, following rituals, or chanting sutras."
> Dogen asked, "What is dropping off body and mind?"
> Rujing answered, "Dropping off body and mind is zazen. When you sit, you remove yourself from hindrances" (e.g., confusion, greed, and aversion).
> Dogen continued to ask Rujing, "If it is to remove these hindrances, your zazen is no different from methods practiced by other sutra-based schools of Buddhism. Would this mean that I am a practitioner of both Mahayana and Theravada schools of Buddhism?"
> Ruijin answered, "The follower of the Gautama Buddha (the original Buddha) should not discriminate the Mahayana from Theravada. If you are against sutras, how could you call yourself the student of Buddha?"
> Dogen continued to ask, "Recently, I heard pseudo Buddhists saying that the three unwholesome roots (i.e., confusion, desire, and hatred) are the Buddha Way, and that if one is trying to end them, that is the sign of discrimination and differentiation, and such act is no different from Theravada Buddhism."
> Ruijin then answered, "If you are possessed by these unwholesome roots, you're no different from savages in ancient India. For the student of Buddha, it would be beneficial if one could remove one or two of these. When you are able to do so, that is the time you meet the Gautama Buddha." (translated by the translators of this chapter)

The dialogue above was recorded by Dogen in *Hokyoki* (宝慶記). *Hokyoki* was the collection of Dogen's journals during his study in China, including the teachings of his conversation with Ruijin. As such, Ruijin's statements in *Hokyoki* were Dogen's account of Ruijin's teachings, and these are slightly different from Ruijin's actual perspectives. That being said, the dialogue itself is extremely interesting from a Zen perspective as it includes the topics of desire and defilement, which are not common or central themes in Zen Buddhism. In the dialogue above, Ruijin suggests that we are able to remove desires and defilements. Yet, Zen practice for the purpose of ceasing desires and defilements is in the direct contrast with the heart of Zen practice. Therefore, Dogen questioned Ruijin further by asking if such a way of practice is no different from a sutra-based practice, which emphasizes the removal of desires. It was not surprising that Dogen asked Ruijin this question as he bas practice on the assumption that there is no to remove because all sentient beings are b be pure.

In response to Dogen's question, Ri cautioned Dogen not to become caught u arbitrary differentiation of Mahayana and avada Schools of Buddhism. But this respo Ruijin did not answer Dogen's question di Ruijin neglected the association betwee practice and the cessation of desires. As a Dogen asked him a more direct question the three unwholesome roots and five ments. His intention behind this questio that if desires and defilements are, in a themselves, the manifestation of Buddha N making a effort to cease them becomes *h* (e.g., acting on desires), and this very ac direct contrast to Zen teaching. This way practice can be considered *bonpu Zen* o tarian Zen (Broughton 2009; Uchiyama 2004). According to Dogen, utilitarian Ze quite pervasive in Chinese Zen during his the Song Dynasty, and Dogen strongly op this form of Zen practice (Dumoulin 2005b).

The final response in the dialogue m actually be from Reijin, but from Dogen' ization of the Way. The goal of Zen is eliminate desires or defilement; however, t nothing wrong with the cessation of through Zen practice, and perhaps this ces can be a good thing. Either way, it is simp way it is. Adhering to the complete affirmat the self as being pure does not mean that w ignore or act in service of desires and defile when they occur. Instead, we must learn to them wisely.

Whereas some schools of Buddhism co desires and defilements to be poisons that be eliminated, Dogen Zen considers them part of our everyday lives. Because the nothing inherently wrong with desires or d ments, these aspects of our experiences s not be ignored; rather, they should be w heartedly experienced. Experiencing them, ever, does not always entail acting upon the praise it fully; the six paramitas, such as giving, maintaining the precepts, and various other good deeds like invoking the Buddha's name, repentance, and spiritual training, all finally return to this. Even those who have experienced it for only a single sitting will see all karma erased. Nowhere will they find evil paths, and the Pure Land will not be far away. If we listen even once with open heart to this truth, then praise it and gladly embrace it, how much more so then if on reflecting within ourselves we directly realize Self-nature, giving proof to the truth that Self-nature is no nature. We will have gone far beyond idle speculation. The gate of the oneness of cause and effect is thereby opened, and not-two, not-three, straight ahead runs the Way. Realizing the form of no-form as form, whether going or returning we cannot be any place else. Realizing the thought of no-thought as thought, whether singing or dancing, we are the voice of the Dharma. How vast and wide the unobstructed sky of samadhi! How bright and clear the perfect moonlight of the Fourfold Wisdom! At this moment what more need we seek? As the eternal tranquility of Truth reveals itself to us, this very place is the Land of Lotuses and this very body is the body of the Buddha.

Conclusion

In sum, *bonno* (煩悩; worldly desires) is significant in various forms of Zen teachings. Following the Mahayana tradition, Zen Buddhism does not reject worldly desires. For Zen Buddhism, worldly desires are not events to be eliminated deliberately. Instead, they are the internal events to which one must learn to relate to wisely. To unfold the Buddha Nature, one must continue to practice.

References

Broughton, J. L. (2009). *Zongmi on Chan New York*. US: Columbia University Press.

Dumoulin, H. (2005a). *Zen Buddhism: A history volume 1: India and China*. Bloomington, Indiana US: World Wisdom.

Dumoulin, H. (2005b). *Zen Buddhism: A history volume 2: Japan*. Bloomington, Indiana US: World Wisdom.

Ferguson, A. (2011). *Zen's Chinese heritage: The masters and their teachings*. Somerville MA, US: Wisdom Publications.

McRae, J. R. (2000). *The platform Sutra of the sixty Patriarch*. Berkeley, CA USA: Murata Center for Buddhist Translation and Research.

Poceski, M. (2015). *The records of Mazu and the making of classical Chan literature*. New York, USA: Oxford University Press.

Shibayama, Z. (2000). *The gateless barrier: Zen comments on the mumonkan* Boston, MA, US: Shambhala Publication (originally published in 1974).

Uchiyama, K., Wright, T., Warner, J., & Okumura, S. (2004). *Opening the hand of thought: Foundations of Zen Buddhism practice*. Somerville MA, US: Wisdom Publications.

Yampolsky, P. B. (1971). *The Zen Master Hakuin: Selected writing*. New York, USA: Columbia University Press.

Yu, C. F. (1979). Ta-hui Tsung-Kao and Kung-an Chan. *Journal of Chinese Philosophy, 6*(2), 211–235. doi:10.1111/j.1540-6253.1979.tb00084.x.

Zen, Self, and Personality

Hidetaka Shuryu Okajima, Akihiko Masuda and Kayla Sargent

Keywords
Zen · Self · Personality · Jiko · Humanity

Personality and Present Era

Self is one of many English terms that have different meanings across scholars and literatures. Translating the term self into Japanese is also challenging. For example, *jiko* (自己) usually refers to self (e.g., "I"), and *jiga* (自我), another term relevant to the concept of self, can be translated as the perceived sense of self. *Jinkaku* (人格) is yet another word relevant to the concept of self, referring to the concept of one's personality. According to many psychological theories (e.g., Messer and Gurman 2011), it is *jinkaku* (personality) that is said to determine who a person "is"; that is, what one does or says and how one behaves. Finally, *ningensei* (人間性), which can be roughly translated as humanity and human beingness (Lebra 1976), is particularly relevant to the concept of self in Japanese culture. *Ningensei* is considered an esteemed quality of character valued by many Japanese people. Typically, it includes empathic interaction, reciprocity, commitment to the betterment of common goal, and emotional expression aligned with these three characteristics (Goldman 1994; Lebra 1976).

Whereas traditional values and practices (e.g., religion, culture) have historically played a significant role in forming and shaping individual character, we now are in an era in which traditional social processes and practices are increasingly devalued as formative determinants of individual character. Consider that in the past, identifying individuals as having "good" personal characteristics was made simple by linking them with the socially agreed-upon characteristics associated with their particular sociocultural groups. These characteristics were often informed by religious practices or cultural myths, and behaviors reflecting these characteristics were maintained and transmitted through generations (Skinner 1974). However, it is

Translated and Edited by Akihiko Masuda and Kayla Sargent, University of Hawaii at Manoa.

H.S. Okajima (✉)
Aichigakuin University, Aichi, Japan
e-mail: okajimah@dpc.agu.ac.jp

A. Masuda (✉) · K. Sargent
University of Hawaii at Manoa, Honolulu, USA
e-mail: amasuda4@hawaii.edu

K. Sargent
e-mail: kaylansargent@gmail.com

A. Masuda and W.T. O'Donohue (eds.), *Handbook of Zen, Mindfulness, and Behavioral Health*, Mindfulness in Behavioral Health, DOI 10.1007/978-3-319-54595-0_10

increasingly difficult to accurately identify such personal characteristics today, which is likely the result of globalization. This begs the question of whether or not such characteristics even exist anymore. Whereas we have achieved freedom and equality unthinkable to our ancestors, we are at ground zero for identifying and establishing who we are in character. It is as if we must start from the beginning again with a clean slate.

Although disparities in the distribution of wealth are pervasive issues in many parts of the world, most contemporary societies have achieved material wealth greater than ever before. In developed countries across the globe, multiple options are often available for aspects of living that were once quite limited in terms of personal choices (e.g., things to eat for dinner and places to live). Whether this change in circumstance is beneficial or not, we now live in an era of materialism, utilitarianism, and individualism where basic human rights are more or less protected in developed countries.

Also important are the associations among personal characteristics, ideal personal characteristics (e.g., humanity), and culture (e.g., historical and situational context). Personal characteristics are said to be developed through the will, values, and preferences shared by the members of the sociocultural group where one belongs. Thus, it is plausible that the development of personal characteristics functions as an interaction between the two (i.e., the interaction of ones' will and his or her sociocultural context). As such, we must consider the extent to which these two factors contribute to the development of personal characteristics.

The Place Where the Self Abides

Kodo Sawaki (沢木 興道; 1889–1965), a prominent Japanese Sōtō Zen teacher of the twentieth century, stated that Zen is "the self selfing the self" (Uchiyama and Okumura 2014). According to Sawaki, the self selfing the self is to seek the self wholeheartedly, and it is often called *kojikyume* (己事究明) in Japanese Zen.

The practice of *kojikyume* includes the various Japanese senses of self mentioned above (i.e., *jiko*, the self; *jinkaku*, personal characteristics; and *ningensei*, humanity). Furthermore, in the search for true self, Zen emphasizes the significance of *action* that one persistently takes (Dogen and Tanahashi 2010). Through the process of seeking the true self, one becomes aware of his or her own preconceptions as well as beliefs derived from a narrowly defined sense of self, thereby learning to let go without attachment. According to Zen, we cannot grasp the true self until we first let go of the conventional sense of self as a unique and perpetual being. Just as Jesus of Nazareth explained to John the Baptist's disciples in the Book of Matthew, new wine cannot be put into old wineskins; similarly, one cannot absorb new teachings fully if he or she maintains outdated perspectives or preconceptions of self.

In Buddhist practice and training, letting go of the self is an essential process for embodying the Buddha Way (Uchiyama et al. 2004). Through a continuous, often lifelong Zen practice, a student of Zen learns to let go of preconceptions, including that of self. Zen practice in this context includes, but is not limited to, *henzan* (遍参; trainings under different Zen teachers over years) and *haju* (把住; an intense training from a Zen teacher for break through one's preconceptions).

Dogen Zenji (道元禅師; 1200–1253), the founder of the Sōtō school of Zen in Japan, described the process of letting go of the self in the chapter of *Shoji* (Birth and Death) in *Shobogenzo* (Treasury of the True Dharma Eye) as follows:

> This life-and-death is the life of a buddha. If you try to exclude it, you will lose the life of a buddha. If you cling to it, trying to remain in it, you will also lose the life of a buddha, and what remains will be the mere form of a buddha. Only when you don't avoid birth-and-death or long for it do you enter a buddha's mind.
>
> However, do not analyze or speak about it. Just set aside your body and mind, forget about them, and throw them into the house of the buddha; then all is done by the buddha. When you follow this, you are free from birth and death and become a buddha

> without effort or scheme. Who, then remains in the mind? (see Dogen and Tanahashi 2010, p. 885)

The part of the quote above "… set aside your body and mind, forget about them, and throw them into the house of the buddha" is particularly relevant to the present chapter. It is equivalent to "let go of the self." According to Dogen et al. (2011), once we let go of the preconception of self, we become fully open to the teachings of Buddha Way without defense. As compassion and earnest endeavoring for the benefit of mankind and all myriad beings (the Buddha Way) reside within the Buddha Way, letting go of the self itself is naturally transformed to the dedication to humanity.

In practice, the students of Buddha Way continue to ask themselves who they are and what their heart (e.g., mind) is. There is an interesting *koan* (e.g., a paradoxical anecdote or riddle used in Zen Buddhism for learning the Buddha Way), *niso anjin* (二祖安心; Pacifying the Mind of the Second Patriarch), which reflects this questioning:

> Huike, the Second Patriarch, said to Bodhidharma, "My mind is not yet at rest. Master, I implore you, set my mind to rest."
> The Master (Bodhidharma) replied, "Bring your mind here, and I'll set it rest for you."
> Huike said, "I've searched for my mind, but am unable to find it."
> "There," said the master, "I've set your mind to rest" (see Kirchner 2013, p. 33)

In this *koan*, Huike (487–493; 慧可; Eka in Japanese), the Second Patriarch of Chinese Chán (Zen), asked his master Bodhidharma (菩提達磨), the original transmitter of Chan Buddhism to China, to ease his mind. However, as the *koan* goes, it is unclear where the mind resides and what the mind actually is; our mind may not be what we think it is. We often perceive our mind to be a concrete entity residing inside our body, but what if understanding the mind as an organ-like feature of our bodies is incomplete? Rather, it could be like a word with nothing solid, distinct, or concrete about it.

The body is emphasized in Zen training. Dogen stated that the whole universe is the Buddha Body and that through embodying the true body, a person becomes one with the universe. In the chapter *Shinjingakudo* (身心学道; Body-and-Mind Study of the Way) in *Shobogenzo*, Dogen wrote the following passage for the students of Buddha Way:

> … the moment the dharma wheel is turned, the true human body covers the whole universe and extends throughout all time. It is not that the true human body is unlimited; true human body is just true human body. At this moment, it is you, at this moment, it is I, that is the true human body, the entire world of the ten directions. Study the way without missing this point (see Dogen and Tanahashi 2010, p. 428).

Once again, embodying the true body is the commitment to letting go of the self. This standpoint is also consistent with what William James referred to as self-surrender. In the Varieties of Religious Experience, William James (1902) argued that an individual cannot make a radical change (*eshin*; 回心, conversion) unless he or she lets go of himself or herself (i.e., self-surrender); once the person is able to let go of the old self, the new self or new universe naturally unfolds and the self and the world become one.

The Significance of Others in Seeking the True Self

Although Zen is often associated with the importance of self-discipline, others in Zen training, such as teachers and fellow students, play crucial roles in studying the Buddha Way. For example, Baizhang Huaihai (720–814; 百丈懐海; Hyakujō Ekai in Japanese) emphasized the influence of our teachers by saying "my father and my mother gave birth to me, and that my fellows in training have made me who I am." Dogen and Tanahashi (2010) in his teaching stated that it is extremely important to meet the right teacher and fellow students in training.

In Zen training, teachers and fellow students often help an individual student to face the world from a new perspective that is free from his or her own biased assumptions. These biased assumptions include the complete cessation of personal suffering or becoming a superior being once embodying the true self. The following is a story of Qingyuan Xingsi (660–740; 青原行思; Seigen Gyōshi in Japanese) that captures the importance of others in studying the Buddha Way. Qingyuan was an eminent student of Hui-neng, the Sixth Patriarch of Chinese Chan (Zen), and he was known for many vivid episodes of his encounters with his students and other teachers. This brief story goes:

> A monk asked Qingyuan, "What is the great meaning of the Buddha dharma?"
> Qingyuan said, "What is the price of rice in Luling?" (see Ferguson 2011, p. 58)

In this dialog, the monk asked Qingyuann the above question while holding a particular view or assumption about the nature of the Buddha dharma. That is, there was something mystical about the Buddha Way, and the monk wanted to ask Qingyuan about the *secret* of Buddha dharma. Despite the monk's expectation that he would provide a profound or unprecedented answer, Qingyuan asked the monk a question instead. Furthermore, the question appeared to be irrelevant to the question the monk posed. From a perspective of conventional discourse, the exchange between Qingyuan and the monk was disorganized and illogical. However, from a Zen perspective, presenting an unexpected (and seemingly irrelevant) answer was quite significant. That is, Qingyuan's answer allowed the monk to experience a radical shift in perspective and helped him realize the preconceptions that the he had toward the Buddha Way. Through this narrative, that monk witnessed the depth of Qingyuan who embodied the universal self (i.e., the self who becomes one with the whole universe without boundaries). If the monk also experienced wholeness (e.g., enlightenment) in the interaction, true dialog is said to have been established.

The experience of wholeness can unfold in a relational context. The following is an example of enlightenment in an interaction with a Zen teacher, described in a koan known as Gutei's finger. Gutei Isshi (倶胝一指; Jinshua Juzhi in Chinese) was a ninth century Chinese Chan (Zen) master. The story of Gutei's finger goes:

> …
> Master Gutei, whenever he was questioned, just stuck up one finger. At one time he had a young attendant, whom a visitor asked, "What is the Zen your master is teaching?" The boy also stuck up one finger. Hearing of this, Gutei cut off the boy's finger with a knife. As the boy ran out screaming with pain, Gutei called to him. When the body turned his head, Gutei stuck up his finger. The boy was suddenly enlightened (Shibayama 2000, p. 42).

Generally speaking, a superficial conceptualization may not be encouraging. However, imitation may be useful and justifiable especially for dedicated beginning students, such as the boy in the story. Additionally, many of us who read this koan are disturbed by the boy's finger and the apparent cruelty inflicted upon the boy. Without justifying Gutei's actions, we can evaluate the important meaning within the narrative, particularly in its later portions. What would be Gutei's true intention in cutting off the boy's finger? One possibility was Gutei's greater compassion toward the boy, although his actions appeared extremely cruel. It was possible that for Gutei, the boy was a precious disciple, and that by cutting his finger, Gustei was willing to share the pain with the boy fully for the service of the boy learning the Buddha Way. In fact, the boy was said to be enlightened through the experience, as Gutei might have hoped.

The significance of others in Zen practice (e.g., the practice of true self) parallels that of others in the process of self-introspection for personal growth. When we do not find an answer ourselves, we seek others for their perspectives. We do so because we may find an answer (or a hint that helps us along in our search) through this process, thus giving us the ability to integrate the new wisdom from this process into our own. As such, introspection, which is usually considered an act of a single person, is also quite relational and interpersonal.

So far, I have discussed the significance of others in seeking the true self (i.e., the Buddha Way). Similarly, Dogen (Dogen et al. 2011; Okumura 2010) stated that one's entire surroundings (e.g., historical and situation environment) play crucial roles in studying the Buddha

Way. In *Genjokoan*, (現成公案), which is sometimes translated as Actualizing the Fundamental Point, Dogen stated the following:

> To practice and learn about the Buddha Way is to practice and learn about *jiko*. To practice and learn about *jiko* is to forget *jiko*. Forgetting about *jiko*, one is affirmed by all things, all phenomena (all dharmas). To be affirmed by all things means to be made to let go of all concepts and artificial divisions of one's body and mind, as well as the body and mind of others, by those very things that affirm us (see Uchiyama et al. 2004, p. xxiv).

Nishiari Bokusan (1821–1910), the father of the modern Sōtō Sect, described enlightenment in his commentary by relating to the above passage in Dogen's *Genjokoan* as follows:

> We normally talk about enlightenment this and enlightenment that, but what do we actually regard as enlightenment? I want you to fully understand this point (the immovable principle of enlightenment). To regard one person's one-time experience of realization, or an insight leading to a prediction of the future, as enlightenment is absolutely demonic. When we have a true enlightenment there is not even a speck of what you thought was enlightenment (see Dogen et al. 2011, p. 51 for Nishiari's comment).

He then states:

> … to be enlightened is no other than fully experiencing the self and fully experiencing myriad dharma. The self and myriad dharmas are originally one thusness. There is no self apart from myriad dharmas. There is no myriad dharmas apart from the self. Therefore, when dharma is actualized, the ten directions are comprehended. It is essential in the practice to "fully experience one dharma." In whichever practice, it is good to solidly master one dharma. When we fully experience the self, it is not betrayed by myriad dharmas. When we fully experience myriad dharmas, the self drops off spontaneously (Dogen et al. 2011, p. 55).

What Nishiari referred to as myriad dharmas above is what is meant by one's entire surrounding as well as what Suzuki (1996) referred to as Nature, "all that constitutes what is commonly known as Man's objective world" (p. 231). Fully experiencing the self and fully experiencing myriad dharma is to become one with what shows up as an experience as if the whole self is melted into the experience.

When we read books and communicate with others, we may catch ourselves wondering who we really are and where the self as a solid and actual entity exists. By facing the events (e.g., knowledge and books) and others, we may feel disappointed by the sense of self that feels fragile, ambiguous, or non-existing. Studying *koans* as well as studying Zen with teachers and fellow students elucidates the transient nature of self that is formless and interdependent without boundaries. Buddhism teaches us to let go of self. This necessitates that we must let go of ego, a narrowly perceived version of the self, as a unique and essential entity. In Zen, a *koan* practice serves as a mirror that reflects our extant sense of self and gives an opportunity to experience the one thusness (i.e., true self).

Features of Human Mind

No-self is one of the most challenging teachings of Zen Buddhism (Mathers et al. 2009). No-self can also be referred to as a state of no-mind. Suzuki (1996, 1997, 1998) sometimes described no-self as the act of taking a leap. It is to let go of all of the experiences and wisdom that one has already established. The *koan*, which is often called "The peak of great valor," is said to capture the experience of no-mind. Baizhang Huaihai (百丈懷海; Hyakujo Ekai in Japanese) was a Chinese Zen master of the eighth century. The *koan* goes:

> A monk asked Hyakujo, "What is a matter of extraordinary wonder?" Hyakujo said, "Sitting along on the Peak of Great Valor." The monk bowed, whereupon. Hyakujo hit him (see Cleary 2002, p. 80).

According to D.T. Suzuki, the exquisiteness and the crucial point of the story is found in the transition from the bow of the monk following Hyakujo's answer and Hyakujo subsequently hitting him. If the story ended with Hyakujo's answer (i.e., "Sitting along on the Peak of Great Valor"), the monk could only experience a fragment of the original wholeness. However, with the body being brought into the interaction (i.e., the act of hitting), the monk was able to see the contrast between the conceptualized world and the undivided world and experienced the latter fully.

Life is never free of contradictions, and the experience of no-mind resides in this contradicting world. We human beings put one foot into the divided world (i.e., divided and categorized experiences) and the other into the undivided (e.g., whole experiences). Similarly, our mind can be linked to both the conscious world and the unconscious world. Perhaps, this is the very nature of human existence. This perspective is similar to the concept of anamnesis in Plato's epistemological and psychological theory, which states that humans are constantly in a state of re-learning and discovering knowledge gained from previous lives.

The unconscious layer of human mind may be experienced as something ambiguous existing behind our consciousness. However, there is a deliberate effort to form a personality via grasping the interaction of consciousness and unconsciousness. For Zen Buddhism, it is the act of a whole person (*gyo*; 行) that is thought to integrate and adjust the two layers of human mind to form the true self. In other words, focusing on practice as the act of a whole person is the very attempt to integrate the unconsciousness into the development of spiritual and universal self.

Development of Personality and Act of a Whole Person

From a Zen perspective, Buddhism is a religion of action, and the action that one takes plays a crucial role in forming and developing her or his personality. For example, in the chapter of *Shoakumakusa* (Not Doing Wrongs) of *Shobogenzo*, Dogen stressed the importance of action in practice and morality (see Dogen et al. 1994, p. 81). More specifically, the chapter started with:

> The eternal Buddha says,
> Not to commit wrongs,
> To practice the many kinds of right,
> Naturally purifies the mind,
> This is the teaching of the buddhas

Following this passage, Dogen elaborated on the importance of refraining from wrong doings as part of the Seven Buddhas' Universal Precept. The Seven Buddhas here refer to the Original Buddha (Shakyamuni Buddha) and six legendary buddhas who preceded him. Dogen then suggests a shift in practice from refraining from doing wrongs as a rule-following endeavor to refraining from doing wrong as a product of having internalized the Way. More specifically, at the beginning of training, students of the Way refrain from doing wrong because they are told to do so. However, as the practice continues, the precept becomes one with the body-and-mind of students, and they simply let go of wrongs and engage in many kinds of rights instead.

From his own personal experience, Dogen also stated that practice is the Buddha Way itself: When one does zazen (i.e., zen mediation), washes the face, or engages in daily activities wholeheartedly, the students of the Way become one with the Buddha Way. Furthermore, the action itself is critical because it also connects the disciples of the Way with their teachers, fellow practitioners, and ancient buddhas.

Zen and Indiscriminating Mind

In many religions, a person is well-regarded if the person devotes himself or herself to one religion or one true teaching. On the other hand, Eastern religions, especially Zen, seem to be open to the existence of diverse ideas and practices, including different religions. Zen even values a stance of acknowledging the perspectives of others openly and allowing them to be what they are, without being pushed around by them. In Zen, this stance is often called *Samadhi*. The chapter of Bodhidharma in China in the Records of Transmission of the Lamp exemplifies this point:

> After nine years the master already wished to return to the Western Land of India, so he said to his disciples, "The time has come, so why should not each of you show what you have understood?" At this time, there was a disciple called Daofu who said, "According to my understanding, it is neither

> to hold on to words nor abandon words; this is the Way's functioning."
> The master replied, "You get my skin."
> The nun Zongchi said, "What I understand now is that it's like Ananda seeing the Realm of Akshobhya Buddha—once seen, never seen again."
> The master said, "You get my flesh."
> A certain Daoyu said, "The four great elements are originally empty, the five aggregates without existence and according to my understanding there is not a single Dharma which can be obtained."
> The master said, "You get my bones."
> Finally Hike bowed reverently, and then remained standing.
> The master said to Huike, "You inherit my marrow," and turning to him he addressed him thus, "In days gone by the Tathagata transmitted the eye of the True Dharma to the Great Master Mahakasyapa and from him it was repeatedly passed down until it reached me. I now hand it over to you. You should guard and nurture it. Furthermore, I give you the Robe as the faith in the Dharma. Each has a significance which it is proper to know of." (Daoyuan and Whitfield 2015, pp. 151–152)

A general interpretation of this story is that Huike received the marrow, the center of the body, because of his answer superior to other three. However, according to Dogen, Bodhidharma did not discriminate these four answers and valued them equally. His open attitudes toward different answers from the four disciples demonstrated his indiscriminating mind for diversity.

Individuality in Personality

Zen encourages personality that is free from egocentric views and preconceptions. As noted elsewhere (Uchiyama et al. 2004), this does not mean that Zen pursues the complete elimination of egocentric views and preconceptions. Rather, being free from egocentric views means *not being affected by them*. According to Buddhism, egocentric views and preconceptions are closely linked to one's preferences, which determine the event to which desire is directed. In Buddhism, the egocentric views and preconceptions are often considered the source of sufferings that are unique to humans. The Original Buddha sought freedom of all myriad beings from these egocentric perspectives.

Similarly, in practice, the students of the Buddha Way are taught to let go of their conventional ideas of self. Once again, this is the perceived sense of self as a unique, independent, and autonomous being (Markus and Kitayama 1991, 2010), and this self is said to be an entangled self, which is restrained by traditional or status-quo cultural practices. Just as Jesus of Nazareth taught that new wine must be put into fresh wineskins, one cannot become open to new teachings and new perspectives unless he or she opens the hand of the old preconceptions.

Nevertheless, many of us think that our personality consists primarily of elements that make us unique and autonomous beings (e.g., ego). For many of us, it appears that if our egos are removed from our personalities, nothing is left in us. However, Zen states that rich personality and individuality remain after egos become less dominant. This rich personality, according to Zen, is the true self as a transient and interdependent being without boundaries.

The heart of the teacher–student relationship in Zen is the mutual wholehearted understanding and transmission. For a student, the transmission is to find her or his original path (rather than replication of the teacher's path) and to surpass the teacher. Whereas the student and teacher share the fundamental wholeness (Dogen et al. 2011), the student must learn to express and embody the original self that is free from their teacher. Surpassing the teacher and receiving the transmission means that the student awakens to this individuality. An old koan attributed to Linji exemplifies this point:

> Followers of the Way (of Chan), if you want to get the kind of understanding that accords with the Dharma, never be misled by others. Whether you're facing inward or facing outward, whatever you meet up with, just kill it! If you meet a buddha, kill the buddha. If you meet a patriarch, kill the patriarch. If you meet an arhat, kill the arhat. If you meet your parents, kill your parents. If you meet your kinfolk, kill your kinfolk. Then for the first time you will gain emancipation, will not be entangled with things, will pass freely anywhere you wish to go (see Watson 1999, p. 52).

It is important to clarify that we should not take this koan literally. The Buddha, parents, and others in the koan are symbolic, pointing to various preconceptions, including that of Buddha Way. What Linji said in the koan is that, to study the Buddha Way, one must become free from preconceptions and teachings, including those of Buddha or enlightenment. It is crucially important for the student of the Way to become settled in the here-and-now fully. If the student desires enlightenment, he or she is not in the moment of here-and-now. Reflecting this koan by Linji, Shunryu Suzuki (1970) highlighted the importance of being in the present moment, the manifestation of true individuality. He said:

> When you try to attain something, your mind starts to wander about somewhere else. When you do not try to attain anything, you have your own body and mind right here. A Zen master would say, "Kill the Buddha!" Kill the Buddha if the Buddha exists somewhere else. Kill the Buddha, because you should resume your own Buddha nature (pp. 26–27).

Another point to be clarified is the role of others in honing the individuality in Zen practice. In the Koan, Linji did not say that students of Buddha Way should isolate themselves from others. As mentioned above, the student of the Buddha Way learns the Buddha Way through the relationship her or she has with teachers and fellow students. Linji and Suzuki simply stated that one must be present fully and that being present wholeheartedly is itself the embodiment of Buddha nature.

Compassion and Humanity: A Conclusion

For Buddhism, the most important individual characteristics include humanity, benevolence, and compassion. The act of humanity, benevolence, and compassion as core values has been transmitted to the Mahayana tradition, and from the Mahayana tradition to Zen Buddhism. As mentioned above, Zen, like other sects in Mahayana Buddhism, seeks complete enlightenment for the benefit of all sentient beings, and these core values are reflected within everyday activities of Zen practitioners (Dogen et al. 1995). In this final section, worth noting are three sets of behaviors that reflect humanity. These are *fuse* (布施; giving), *rigyo* (利行; beneficial action or helpful conduct), and *doji* (同事; identity-action, sharing the same aim). *Fuse* is to give. *Rigyo* is an act for the wellness of others without expecting return. Finally, *doji* is to identify oneself with others without seeking benefit or rewards for doing so. Dogen in the chapter of *Bodaisattashishobo* (菩提薩埵四摂法; the Bodhisattva's Four Methods of Guidance) of *Shobogenzo* explains *fuse*, *rigyo, and doji* as follows:

> "Giving" means nongreed. Nongreed means not to covet. Not to covet means not to curry favor. Even if you govern the Four Continents, you should always convey the authentic path with nongreed. It is like giving away unneeded belonging to someone you don't know, offering flowers blooming on a distant mountain to the Tathagata, or, again, offering treasures you had in your former life to sentient beings…
>
> "Beneficial action" is skillfully to benefit all classes of sentient beings; that is, to care about their distant and near future, and to help them by using skillful means. In ancient times, someone helped a caged tortoise; another took care of a sick sparrow. They did not expect a reward; they were moved to do so only for the sake of beneficial action.
> Foolish people think that if they help others first, their own benefit will be lost, but this is not so. Beneficial action is an act of openness, benefiting self and others together.
>
> … Thus, benefit friends and enemy equally. Benefit self and others alike. If you have this heart, even beneficial action for the sake of grass, trees, wind, and water is spontaneous and unremitting. This being so, make a wholehearted effort to help the ignorant.
>
> "Identity action" means nondifference. It is nondifference from self, nondifference from others…" "Action" means right form, dignity, correct manner. This means that you cause yourself to be in identity with others after causing others to be in identity with you. However, the relationship of self and others varies limitlessly according to the circumstance (Dogen and Tanahashi 2010, pp. 473–476).

These are at the heart of Buddha Way, and even to this date, benefiting others and compassion are included in the standards of conduct in various Zen communities (e.g., Dogen et al. 1995). Furthermore, benevolence, compassion, and humanity as core values are not limited to Zen or Buddhism. These seem to be the universal values shared by many sociocultural groups, including other religions.

References

Cleary, T. (2002). *Secrets of the Blue Criff Record: Zen comments by Hakuin and Tenkei*. Boston, MA: Shambhala.

Daoyuan, S., & Whitfield, R. S. (2015). *Records of the Transmission of the Lamp: Volume I The Buddhas and Indian Patriarchs*. New York: Books on Demand.

Dogen, E., Leighton, T. D., & Okumura, S. (1995). *Dogen's pure standards for the Zen community: A translation of Eihei Shingi*. Albany, New York: State University of New York Press.

Dogen, E., Nishiari, B., Okumura, S., Suzuki, S., & Weisman, S. M. (2011). *Dogen's genjo koan: Three commentaries*. Barkeley, CA: Counterpoint.

Dogen, E., Nishijima, G. W., & Chodo, C. (1994). *Master Dogen's Shobogenzo: Book 1*. Los Angeles, CA: Dogen Sangha.

Dogen, E., & Tanahashi, K. (2010). *Tresury of the true Dharma eye: Zen Master Dogen's Shobo Genzo*. Boston, MA: Shambhala.

Ferguson, A. (2011). *Zen's Chinese heritage: The masters and their teachings*. Somerville, MA: Wisdom Publications.

Goldman, A. (1994). The centrality of 'ningensei' to Japanese negotiating and interpersonal relationships: Implications for U.S.-Japanese communication. *International Journal of Intercultural Relations, 18*(1), 29–54. doi:10.1016/0147-1767(94)90003-5

Kirchner, T. Y. (2013). *Entangling Vines: A classic collection of Zen koans*. Somerville, MA: Wisdom Publications.

Lebra, T. (1976). *Japanese patterns of behavior*. Retrieved from Honolulu, HI, US.

Markus, H. R., & Kitayama, S. (1991). Culture and the self: Implications for cognition, emotion, and motivation. *Psychological Review, 98*(2), 224–253.

Markus, H. R., & Kitayama, S. (2010). Cultures and selves: A cycle of mutual constitution. *Perspectives on Psychological Science, 5*(4), 420–430. doi:10.1177/1745691610375557

Mathers, D., Miller, M. E., & Ando, O. (2009). *Self and no-self: Continuing the dialogue between Buddhism and psychotherapy*. New York, NY: Routledge/Taylor & Francis Group.

Messer, S. B., & Gurman, A. S. (2011). *Essential psychotherapies: Theory and practice* (3rd ed.). New York, NY: Guilford Press.

Okumura, S. (2010). *Realizing Genjokoan: The key to Dogen's Shobogenzo*. Boston, MA: Wisdom Publications.

Shibayama, Z. (2000). *The gateless barrier: Zen comments on the mumonkan*. New York, NY: Shambhala Publications.

Skinner, B. F. (1974). *About behaviorism*. Oxford, England: Alfred A. Knopf.

Suzuki, D. T. (1996). *Zen Buddhism: Selected writings of D. T. Suzuki*. New York, USA: An Image Book.

Suzuki, D. T. (1997). *Eastern perspective [Toyoteki na mikata]*. Tokyo, Japan: Iwanami Shoten.

Suzuki, D. T. (1998). The Zen doctrine of no-mind. In A. Molino (Ed.), *The couch and the tree: Dialogues in psychoanalysis and Buddhism* (pp. 26–36). New York, NY: North Point Press.

Suzuki, S. (1970). *Zen Mind, Beginner's Mind: Informal talks on Zen meditation and practice*. Boston, MA: Weatherhill.

Uchiyama, K., & Okumura, S. (2014). *The Zen teaching of homeless Kodo*. Somerville, MA: Tuttle Publications.

Uchiyama, K., Wright, T., Warner, J., & Okumura, S. (2004). *Opening the hand of thought: Foundations of Zen Buddhism practice*. Somerville, MA: Wisdom Publications.

Watson, B. (1999). *The Zen teachings of Master Lin-chi*. New York, USA: Columbia University Press.

Every Day is a Fine Day

A Zen Take on Problems

Mike K. Sayama

Keywords
Zen · Attachment · Behavioral health · Desire

"Every day is a fine day." Omori Sogen, a leading Zen master, *Kendo* (fencing) teacher, and calligrapher of modern Japan, used this saying to describe how someone, matured through long and hard training in Zen, experiences life. After Japan's defeat in World War II, Omori *Roshi* (title for Zen Master, literally old teacher) and his family, like many others, were impoverished and had little to eat. In his words, "We were sometimes so poor that even if we looked all over the house, we could not find one penny. That is how poor a life I caused my wife to have. At the longest we went five days to one week without food, but we did not starve. If we drank only water, we could live" (Hosokawa 1999, 61–62). His three-year-old daughter got sick with tuberculin meningitis and might have been cured with penicillin, but the cost was beyond reach. Omori *Roshi* recounted, "In the end, the only thing that we could do was to watch our own child suffer and die before our eyes. After that child died, my wife cried by herself every night for three years. For a parent, there is no sadder thing than to have your own child die before you" (Hosokawa 1999, 67). In the face of such sadness, what could Omori *Roshi* mean that every day is a fine day? What could he mean in the face of the tragedy and terror so routinely seen on the evening news, which at the time of this writing were the Syrian refugees and the massacre in Paris?

"Every day is a fine day" is not a Pollyannaish perspective that denies all this suffering. "Existence is suffering" is often portrayed as Buddha's First Noble Truth. "Every day is a fine day" must mean that the human spirit can transcend existence as suffering. To Omori *Roshi,* a person who has realized the True Self through long and hard training in Zen will be able to express the brightness of the original nature even in the midst of suffering. For such a person, every day is a fine day.

Fudoshin: The Immovable Mind

If you took "Everyday is a fine day" as a *koan* (a problem impenetrable to rational solution, such as "What is the sound of one hand clapping? Or what is the meaning of life?"), you could ask yourself every night, "Was today a fine day?" To answer, you might consider wasted moments,

M.K. Sayama (✉)
Chozen-ji, International Zen Dojo, Honolulu, HI, USA
e-mail: msayama@communityfirst.co

A. Masuda and W.T. O'Donohue (eds.), *Handbook of Zen, Mindfulness, and Behavioral Health*, Mindfulness in Behavioral Health, DOI 10.1007/978-3-319-54595-0_11

moments of pride and regret, moments of joy and sadness, moments of anxiety and ease, moments of loss and gain, and so on and on. From the Zen perspective, if it was not a fine day, your mind must have stopped; your flow of consciousness must have gotten stuck on an attachment; and your thoughts became delusions that caused you to suffer. During the day, you must have abided in what Takuan Soho (1573–1645) called "the dwelling place of ignorance and its affective disturbance." To experience everyday as a fine day is to experience the mind that does not move because it does not stop moment by moment with whatever it encounters, not even pain. More to the point, if today is not a fine day, at this very moment your mind is stopped.

Takuan was teacher to the Shogun Tokugawa Iemitsu, the ruler of Japan from 1623 to 1651, and to the great swordsman Yagyu Tajima Munenori (1568–1646). He wrote letters to Yagyu instructing him on the Immovable Mind in the context of sword fighting. These letters were compiled into a collection called *Fudochi Shimmyo-roku* (The Records of the Wondrous Mind of Immovable Wisdom), which is studied as a fundamental text at Chozen-ji, a Rinzai Zen temple founded by Omori *Roshi* and his student Tanouye Tenshin (1938–2003) in Hawaii. Tanouye *Roshi* was a genius in the martial way, expert in arts such as *Kendo*, *Judo*, *Karate*, *Iaido* (the art of drawing the sword), and *Jojitsu* (the art of the staff). Tanouye *Roshi* was also an advisor to many of the political, business, and community leaders in Hawaii. The interpretation of Zen in this chapter is based mainly on his teachings.

If we take sword fighting as a metaphor for living, Takuan's instructions on the Immovable Mind tell us to encounter the problems in our lives without stopping to make every day a fine day. The central teaching follows:

> Not to move means not to stop with an object that is encountered. Not to move means not to stop with an object that is seen. Because if the mind stops on any object, the mind will be disturbed with thoughts and emotions. This will lead to movement in the heart and mind. The stopping inevitably leads to the moving that is disturbance; therefore, there will be no freedom of movement. For example, suppose ten men are opposing you, each in succession ready to strike you down with a sword. *Ukenagasu* (deflect, parry, but literally, receive and let flow away) the first one without your mind stopping. Forget that man and encounter the next and in this way, although there are ten men, all will be dealt with successively and successfully (Tanouye 1989, 10).

> In the case of your swordsmanship, for instance, when the opponent tries to strike you and your eyes at once catch the movement of his sword and you may strive to follow it, but as soon as this takes place your mind stops on the opponent's sword. Your movements will lose their freedom, and you will be killed by your opponent. This is what I mean by stopping (Tanouye 1989, 6).

> In Buddhism, this "stopping" mind is called *mayoi* (delusion); hence, "the dwelling place of ignorance and its affective disturbance" (Tanouye 1989, 7).

When the mind stops, deluded thoughts are created, and emotions are agitated. From the Zen perspective, this mind stopping is the problem, not anything external to yourself. The mind stops because of attachments. The samurai's problem was to free himself from even the instinctual attachment to life, so that his mind would not stop in a fight to the death. If he were attached to life and feared death, his mind would be moved and stopped on the opponent's sword. In the critical moment, when swords are crossed, he will freeze and be killed.

In life, not moving means not stopping with whatever problems come your way. The problems in life differ from sword fighting in two critical ways, however. The natural action that flows from the mind not stopping may in fact require thinking, in the sense of rational problem-solving and may not require dramatic physical movement. The "thinking" that is deplored in Zen is empty speculation, regretting the past, and worrying about the future not rationality. This thinking results in "the anguish of thoughts feeding on thoughts." Rational problem-solving is a technique necessary to modern life, but when a person limits cognition to this technique, he can only understand reality dualistically and reduces the True Self to an ego. The actions of his life will not be wondrous, and he will not be able to transcend the existential problems of life. Wondrous does not necessarily mean miraculous. Ordinary behavior and rational thought happening naturally without the mind stopping are wondrous.

To offer a mundane example of the difference between rational problem-solving and mind stopping, let us take doing taxes. Doing taxes with the mind not stopping means not procrastinating, being focused and rational when sorting out income and expenses, and accepting the civic obligation and legal requirement without emotional disturbance. If the mind stops while doing taxes, there is avoidance of the task, unproductive speculation about paying too much or too little, and anxiety about an outcome that you cannot change. Doing taxes will be an inefficient and unnecessarily stressful process. If a swordsman fought like that, he would be killed.

Attachments as Fixations

If your mind stops and you get stuck in a situation, it means you have an attachment that you must let go. Attachments may be considered fixations, the freezing of the sentient energy that is the essence of consciousness. We can imagine three different levels of attachments: emotional, psychological, and karmic.

At the emotional level, they lead us to cling to people, things, ideologies, situations, abilities, and so on; these are all "objects" that can cause the mind to stop when there is an attachment. This stopping leads to delusive thoughts or ignorance. Delusions and ignorance leads to affective disturbance or suffering. When attachments are threatened, the mind stops, and we experience anxiety or at the extreme, fear and panic. We become defensive and psychologically regress to less mature coping mechanisms. Physiologically the fight/flight reflex is triggered, and we suffer the negative effects of being aroused to take dramatic physical action when none is appropriate. Emotional attachments untainted by unconscious fixations are rational or "normal." These are the attachments we must resolve as we pass through the stages of life given our society and times.

At the psychological level, an attachment is an unconscious complex, a fixation of consciousness in a pattern of behavior, feeling, and thought assimilated as a child or adopted as a once necessary attempt to cope with trauma or overwhelming stressors but which is eventually self-defeating. These fixations draw a person into situations, relationships, and so on that are associated with the unconscious complex. Out of the many possibilities we have, we create the reality which forces us to address our repressed trauma and other issues. If we succeed, we free consciousness and energy for growth. If we fail, we face another round of suffering.

At a karmic level, an attachment is *vasana*, habit-energy, a pattern in the universal mind reflecting the course of individual consciousness from time immemorial. It is a memory in the storehouse unconscious. Daisetz Suzuki explains as follows:

> Psychologically *vasana* is a memory, for it is something left after a deed is done, mental or physical, and it is retained and stored up in the storehouse unconscious as a sort of latent energy ready to be set in motion. This memory or habit-energy, or habitual perfuming is not necessarily individual; the storehouse unconscious being super-individual holds in it not only individual memory but all that has been experienced by sentient beings. When the Sutra [Lankavatara Sutra] says that in the storehouse unconscious is found all that has been going on since beginningless time systematically stored up as a kind of seed, this does not refer to individual experiences, but to something general, beyond the individual, making up in a way the background on which all individual psychic activities are reflected. (Suzuki 1975, 184)

> In the beginning there was the memory amassed in the storehouse unconscious since the beginningless past as a latent cause, in which the whole universe of individual objects lies with its eyes closed; here enters the ego with its discriminating intelligence, and subject is distinguished from object; the intellect reflects on the duality, and from it issues a whole train of judgments with their consequent prejudices and attachments, while the five other senses force them to become more and more complicated not only intellectually, but affectively and conatively? All the results of these activities in turn perfume the storehouse unconscious, stimulating the old memory to wake while the new one finds its affinities among the old. (Suzuki 1975, 191–192)

To summarize: The immovable mind is the mind that does not stop with whatever object it encounters. The mind stops because of attachments. Our emotional, psychological, and karmic attachments lead us to create our reality and our problems, but these problems are essentially opportunities for personal growth. Tanouye *Roshi* used to say, "If you don't have problems, you better go buy some."

The Marvelously Illuminating Dynamic Function of the Buddha Mind and the Screen of Many Possibilities

We are born with our karma, our metaphysical/psychological genetics from beginningless time. Our karma includes not only our DNA, but the *vasana*, the latent habit-energy or "memories" embedded in the line of consciousness that has become a human being in you. You are the culmination of a line of consciousness originating in the depths of the storehouse unconscious. In Buddhist metapsychology, the storehouse unconscious is a level of mind deeper than Jung's collective unconscious, containing within it not only the archetypes of the human species but the habit-energy, the memories of all sentient beings. Given our karma and the circumstances of our birth, our karma plays out as we move through the stages of life.

In psychoanalysis in the process of free association, the patient projects thoughts and feelings associated with repressed memories onto the blank screen of the analytic situation. These projections come from unconscious, emotionally charged memories seeking expression. Through analysis, the repressed trauma is made conscious, and behavior is freed from the neurotic complex. In life, we are presented with a screen of many possibilities from which we "choose" depending on our karma. Imagine life flowing toward us, the possibilities continually shifting according to choices we make as well as conditions beyond our control. Whether by choice or destiny, we find ourselves in situations where we have something to learn, an attachment to let go. If not for our attachments, we would not get stuck in suffering. We would move along in our lives like a round ball in a swiftly flowing stream, turning and turning as it slips past rocks. Existence is impermanent and ever changing. When things stay the same, we are clinging to something that prevents it from changing. We are suffering from delusions arising from the stopping of the mind.

Bankei Yotaku (1622–1693) was an iconoclastic Zen master whose teaching was to abide in the Unborn Buddha Mind. Tanouye *Roshi* was surprised at how much the spirit and energy of Bankei's calligraphy matched his own. Below Bankei explains how we create our delusions by attaching to the traces of our karma.

> All delusions, without exception, are created as a result of self-centeredness. When you're free from self-centeredness, delusions won't be produced. For example, suppose your neighbors are having a quarrel: if you're not personally involved, you just hear what's going on and don't get angry. Not only do you not get angry, but you can plainly tell the rights and wrongs of the case—it's clear to you as you listen who's right and wrong. But let it be something that concerns you personally, and you find yourself getting involved with what the other party [says or does], attaching to it and obscuring the marvelously illuminating [function of the Buddha Mind]. Before, you could clearly tell wrong from right; but now, led by self-centeredness, you insist that your own idea of what's right is right, whether it is or not. Becoming angry, you thoughtlessly switch your Buddha Mind for a fighting demon, and everyone takes to arguing bitterly with each other.
>
> Because the Buddha Mind is marvelously illuminating, the traces of everything you've done are [spontaneously] reflected. It's when you *attach* to these reflected traces that you produce delusion. Thoughts don't actually exist in the place where the traces are reflected, and then arise. We retain the things we saw and heard in the past, and when these things come up, they appear as traces and are reflected. Originally, thoughts have no real substance. So if they're reflected, just let them be reflected; if they arise, just let them arise; if they stop, just let them stop. As long as you're not *attaching* to these reflected traces, delusions won't be produced. So long as you're not attaching to them, you won't be deluded, and then, no matter how many traces are reflected, it will be just as they weren't reflected at all. (Haskel 1984, 24–25)

> Because the Buddha Mind is marvelously illuminating, mental impressions from the past are reflected, and you make the mistake of labeling as 'delusions' things that aren't delusions at all. Delusions mean the anguish of thought feeding on thought. What foolishness it is to create the anguish of delusion by changing the precious Buddha Mind, pondering over this and that, mulling over things of no worth! If there were anyone who actually succeeded at something by pondering it all the way through, it might be all right to do things that way; but *I've* never heard of anyone who, in the end, was able to accomplish anything like this! (Haskel 1984, 68–69)

Bankei's "marvelously illuminating dynamic function of the Buddha Mind" spontaneously reflects the traces of everything we have done. We cannot escape everything being revealed to us, and where there is unfinished business, we attach to these reflected traces. The mind stops on them, and we produce thoughts upon thoughts regretting the past and worrying about the future. We create a self-centered reality and suffer "the anguish of thought feeding on thought." To use psychoanalytic terms, we project our emotionally charged, self-centered karmic and repressed memories onto the screen of the many possibilities of our lives to create the reality we need to become enlightened of our attachments.

The Immovable Body

Although Takuan's teaching of the Immovable Mind and Bankei's teaching of the Unborn Buddha Mind are pointing at an actual state of being which must be directly experienced, we are likely to try to grasp them conceptually. A Zen saying warns this is like washing blood with blood. A more accessible, practical approach is entering Zen through the body. Takuan says *Fudoshin*, the Immovable Mind must also be *Fudotai*, the Immovable Body (Tanouye 1989, p. 10). This is the approach emphasized at Chozen-ji. Omori *Roshi* goes so far as to say in the canon of Chozen-ji, "Zen is a mind, body, and spiritual discipline to transcend life and death (all dualism) and to thoroughly (truly) realize that the entire universe is the "True Human Body."

Omori *Roshi* details the mechanics of breath, posture, and energy in his instructions for zazen in *An Introduction to Zen Buddhism* (Omori 1996, 35–63). Generally the practice is to breathe from the *hara* which is the lower abdomen, hips, and buttocks functioning as a unit with the center at the *tanden*. The *tanden*, an area two inches below the navel, is considered the psychophysical center of the human being and body. By breathing from the hara, energy radiates throughout the body. When exhaling, it feels that the tension in the body sinks into the lower abdomen as the breath is directed to the *tanden*. As the tension sinks down, the top of the head goes up, and the body stands taller. In the beginning of training a long, slow conscious exhalation is emphasized. We approximate this naturally when we sigh, drop the tension in our neck and shoulders, and clear our minds. When we sigh, however, there may be a tendency to collapse the body into an expression of despair rather than to expand the body into a feeling of spaciousness.

When inhaling, the lower abdomen is relaxed, like releasing the head of an eye dropper, allowing air to fill the vacuum in the lungs created by deep exhalation. Exhalation is more conscious exertion while inhalation is a controlled letting go. In both exhalation and inhalation, the breath is directed to the *tanden*, and the tension in the body set in the *hara*. Needless to say actual practice and face-to-face instruction would be far more effective than these words on paper, and even still, in the end refinement of our breathing can only occur by becoming increasingly sensitive to our own bodies.

When the body is centered at the *tanden*, it is immovable. The body is immovable because it is centered, balanced, and thus capable of movement in any direction. In the school of Aikido founded by Koichi Tohei, "the unliftable body" is practiced and demonstrated by a student first tightening his body up. In this state, he is easily lifted by two students standing at either side. When he centers himself, it is much more difficult to lift him. Paradoxically, this state of being centered and harder to move leads to the ability to move in any direction. From martial arts, both agility of action and power to throw or strike depend on movement from the *hara*. The immovable body is the immovable mind.

Entering Zen through the body does not mean only the use of its musculature. One can enter through the senses as described below by Tanouye *Roshi* in a talk given to students training at a *sesshin* (literally meaning to collect the mind and referring to a week-long retreat of intensive training) in Chicago in October of 1984.

> The mind would be helped with the eyes if you can look at things 180 degrees, always 180 degrees. Look forward as though looking at a distant mountain. Look as though you are not looking. Take a panoramic view. With the same panoramic view, just drop your eyes. As you sit here with this view, a funny phenomenon may happen. Your vision may become round as though there is only one eye. That is what they call the Third Eye. Instead of two eyes, there is just one big eye looking. Do not get attached to that. That is just a part of the *samadhi* (state of consciousness developed in training, a state of relaxed concentration in which the mind is fully present without thought). So look 180 degrees and lower your eyes. If you try to close your eyes halfway, like the books tell you, your focal awareness comes to your eyes which is not good. Some people stare, but staring is not looking 180 degrees which is a relaxed state where you can see more. Hold your two fingers out like this (arms extended to sides), see both fingers.
>
> The best is this: Listen to all the sounds that you hear. Let the total sound come to you. I'm talking to you, but you all can hear a buzzing. You can hear that buzzing because that's part of *samadhi*. You can hear everything. So you do zazen, hear all the sounds but don't identify any. Let all the sounds come to you and you'll hear a ringing in your ears. It's a high pitched ringing.
>
> Another way to do this, the book *Mumonkan* (The Gateless Barrier) says let the 84,000 pores in your body breathe. Feel your body totally. Imagine there's 84,000 hairs on your body. Feel every hair on your arms, legs, and on your body. You'll go into *samadhi*.
>
> Smell every smell in this room. Smell, try to smell every smell. You just have to let your body go. Gradually doing these things will put you into *samadhi*.
>
> So the very senses that cause delusions, you can turn it around and use them as a means to enter *samadhi*.

The direction to see 180° also means to hear, feel, and smell everything as well. It means to come back to your senses and be fully present.

Ukenagasu: To Receive and Let Flow Away

Returning to sword fighting as a metaphor for living, imagine problems in life as opponents we must face to realize our True Self. These opponents may be as trivial as cold water or distasteful food. If you think, "I do not want to wash my face, or I do not want to eat it," your mind has stopped, and the water and the food has taken a point on you in Kendo terms. Or the challenges may be as major as milestones in self-development as we go through the stages of life from being a baby, to an adolescent, to an adult, to a mature adult, and ultimately to realize the True Self. In Buddhist metapsychology, each of these stages can be associated with the emergence of specific structures of mind and related cognitive and motivational functions. I attempted to sketch such a developmental theory based on the metapsychology found in the *Lankavatara Sutra* (Sayama 1986, 91–98). Whether trivial or major, Takuan's teaching of the Immovable Mind instructs us to *ukenagasu* the opponent, to receive and to let flow away.

Let us imagine the flow of life. You are in the present, the past is behind you, and the future is coming. Each day brings challenges, opponents ranging from the mundane to the existential. How can you *ukenagasu* whatever problem you encounter so that even in a day filled with problems each is successively and successfully dealt with? What does it mean "to receive and let flow away"? To receive means to experience fully, not flinching, not turning away, and not repressing. It means facing your problems with your belly button forward and letting all the feelings and ramifications related to the problem come to you while you see 180°.

To let flow away means to cut your thoughts, let go of your attachments, and let things take care of themselves. In swordsmanship, it means to proceed just as you are when facing the opponent. Takuan explains as follows:

> Although you see the sword about to strike you, do not let your mind stop there. Do not intend to strike him by according his rhythm. Cherish no calculating thought whatsoever. You perceive the opponent's move, but do not let your mind to stop with it. You move on *sonomama* (just as you are), entering, and upon reaching the enemy's sword, wrench it away. Then the enemy's sword meant to strike you will instead become the sword which will strike the enemy. (Tanouye 1989, 6)

It must be remembered, however, that Takuan was instructing a master swordsman who has trained to the point of being able to throw away technique. Similarly, letting things take care of themselves is only good instruction for a mature person who is skilled in the technique of the ego. In this context, the ego is a technique for living in a civilized manner to be able to delay gratification, to learn forms, and to dualistically and rationally understand reality. A mature person in the modern world has mastered the ego and must throw it away to follow what Takuan advises and move on *sonomama*, just as you are.

In a sermon titled, "Letting things take care of themselves," Bankei said to a visiting monk:

> Your wanting to realize Buddhahood as quickly as you can is useless to begin with. Since the Buddha Mind you have from your parents is unborn and marvelously illuminating, before even a single thought is produced, all things are recognized and distinguished without resorting to any cleverness. Without attaching to [notions of] 'enlightened' or 'deluded,' just remain in the state where all things are recognized and distinguished. Let things take care of themselves, and whatever comes along will be smoothly managed—whether you like it or not! That's the [working of the] Buddha Mind and its marvelously illuminating dynamic function. Like a mirror that's been perfectly polished, without producing a single thought, with no awareness on your part, without even realizing it, each and everything is smoothly dealt with as it comes from outside. (Haskel 1984, 86)

Let me use myself as a bad example. I am in my early 60s facing my mortality and the diminution of possibilities and physical capabilities. My left knee is creaky; my right shoulder has limited mobility and often pain; yardwork which I could do in a day now takes four. I wonder about retirement, but I have twins just starting college. I live in Honolulu on a ridge overlooking Diamond Head in a small, old house for 20 years, but it has a tea room in which my wife passionately pursues her Way of Tea. The backyard borders the woods of a conservation area. We have a beagle which is an escape artist and can do all kinds of tricks. I really have nothing to complain about.

This year was one of transitions for our family with my twin sons going off to New York and Shanghai for college and my wife going to Kyoto to train in the Way of Tea for a year. It is just me and the dog holding the fort. My friends joke that I am a bachelor. That would not be bad, but I am a bachelor with a house, yard and plants, bonsai which are older than me, and a dog to take care of. I feel I am always busy with something to do. I meditate at least once a day for 30 min, often twice. Most mornings I start with zazen, set my mind, and try to face the day in *samadhi.*

A week ago my son came home from New York where he is studying dance. He has had a stressful but in the end exhilarating first semester struggling with roommates and a dance program which was not what he expected. After serious discussions over the phone and getting our approval to take a leave of absence from college, he changed roommates and talked to his teachers who helped him find new meaning in his classes. He really wanted to come home during the winter break.

For the first night back home his happiness sincerely showed through, but then he broke up with his high school girlfriend and failed the test for his driver's license. We had to adapt to living at home, just the two of us. My routine, busy as it was, and the clean, clear space I had created for myself was disrupted. Life was a lot more stressful having to drive him around, having him leave his stuff around, having to let him practice driving for his road test again and again, and having to endure teenage attitude. He was stopping my mind, but in a moment of irritation I realized I was acting like my father when the two of us lived together some 30 years ago. With that insight life with my son became more amusing and less irritating, not that there are not still moments.

Several days ago, I had to take the family van in for repairs. The hope was my son would have his license and he could drive the van. Since he failed, I asked a neighborhood friend to pick me up from the service station. Since the service station was close to our houses, my friend told me to call him after I checked the car in. The service station was short-staffed, and the owner who has been servicing my cars for 20 years was running around keeping things going. It took him some time to get to me, and when he did, he told me that one of the mechanics had called in sick and the valve cover gasket replacement I needed was a big job so we would have to reschedule. He assured me we could drive the car without problems, so based on my son's next driving test in several days, we settled on the next week. I called my friend to tell him he did not have to pick me up, but there was no answer. I called again a little later, but still no answer. I drove home, and when I got home, my son told me my friend just called and was looking for me at the service station. We did not have his cell, so I called the service station and had to explain the situation to an attendant. This took several attempts. I was on hold. Meanwhile, my friend called, so I told him what happened. He said he saw my car was gone so came down despite our agreement.

Next, as my son and I were about to leave for his dance studio, a college student, rooming at my house, walked out to catch the bus. I offered her a ride, and since my son told me it would not matter if we were a little late, I decided to drop her off first. I had forgotten that we also had to pick up his friend which meant backtracking and being later. My son was practicing driving and almost made a left turn into oncoming traffic at a somewhat complicated intersection. His cell phone rang. I answered and told his friend that we were on the way. His friend thought I was my son and said that he was just wondering if I was awake. Next a text came in. My son picked the phone up, but I told him just drive. He protested saying that it was a text from his friends waiting at the studio. He then ran a yellow light turning red after I told him to stop. I ordered him to pull over and took over driving. We are both pissed. I dropped him and his friend off and went to work out at the gym. The fire alarm went off at the gym, but happily I am almost finished, so I went to the car to leave. The parking structure is narrow with weird angles. As I turned to go down the ramp, a fire engine pulled up at the bottom with sirens going. My mind stopped on that, and I made the turn onto the ramp too sharply and scraped the right rear of the van. The side of the building had hit me on the head. The next day, my son was backing out of the garage. I told him watch out for the left front of the van, but he continued and hit the wall. The good thing was that it was hard to get mad since I put a bigger dent in the car the previous day.

Clearly in one morning, despite 40 years of Zen practice, my mind stopped several times on trivial matters. It is often one thing after another, the eternal recurrence of the small that gets us because with each small thing part of our mind gets stuck and we end up being out of touch with the present reality.

A more serious matter which stops my mind is the cost of college education for my children. Both are going to private universities, one in New York and one in Shanghai. I am financing it with a home equity line of credit. I make a good living but nothing that can handle the cost of their tuitions. I am on a project with only a year to go with the audacious goal of making structural changes in the healthcare system, focusing on payment reform, information integration, care coordination, and community engagement. The goal is a sustainable healthcare system in East Hawaii on the Island of Hawaii. It feels like climbing Mt. Everest. Our team of four has made great progress, but the summit does not look closer. When I dwell on the future, my mind stops on the financial uncertainty because I still have an attachment to die in my house.

It is embarrassing to admit the things my mind stops on given the major problems we have in America and the world. I take some consolation in knowing that Omori *Roshi*, when he was in his seventies, once told his attendant that he would die a happy man if he could have the right concentration for one day. Endless refinement is possible. As a matter of practice, we should strive to prevent mind stopping from turning into anxiety. Though the mind may stop when an attachment is threatened, with mind/body training, we can short circuit the fight/flight reflex that triggers anxiety and instead center ourselves through breathing from the *hara* and opening our senses to the present moment. Then in *samadhi*, we move on just as we are, illuminating the sit uation with the Buddha mind and let things take care of themselves.

If we can *ukenagasu* the existential problem of death, the small problems fall away. Life is the blink of an eye. Our time is short. What should we do with it? What is meaningful? What gives joy? What is worth caring about? Is caring the same as attaching, once again giving reality to reflected traces of unfinished business? Although these questions can only be answered by going deeply within, once we truly realize the imminence of our death, our perspective becomes existential. The petty problems drop away. When I was the vice president of customer relations at an insurance company, I once told Gladys, a supervisor of customer relations representatives who was bent out of shape by all the problems of the day, "Gladys, I know the secret about how not to get stressed. Do you want to know?" Of course, she said, "Yes." And I told her, "Gladys, you're going to die." Her eyes rolled, and she cracked up.

Let me share the story of Paul Nishimura who died in 2001 as an example of someone whose mind did not stop in the face of death. Paul was a big man who owned an auto body shop and who was a high ranking teacher of Aikido. He was the first president of Chozen-ji. He was diagnosed with cancer in July of 1999 and refused treatment, choosing to live fully as long as he could. He told me, "I'm not clinging to life. Life is clinging to me." In May of 2000 he wrote, "CT Scan-Liver almost half gone. Into left hip bone. Maybe a year left." In fact Paul had 13 months, and they were not easy for him or Junko, his wife of 29 years. Some nights when Paul could not sleep because of the pain, he would express his regret about hurting people's feelings with his manner and strong words. Junko said he limited his use of painkillers so he would not do that again. Paul considered his pain "*bachi*" (punishment) for hurting so many people.

In his last year, Paul found talking to Tanouye *Roshi* especially meaningful. He told me "Tanouye's showing me all kinds of things." and taking a stance with a bamboo sword, he said, "This is the Unborn Mind." Tanouye *Roshi* would tell him to ask questions, but Paul said, "I do not have any more questions. I answered them all by myself already. Next time I hope I train harder so I can ask questions I can not answer by myself." On one occasion, Paul and Tanouye *Roshi* were sitting on the lanai at the temple, and Tanouye *Roshi* was feeding birds. One dove landed on the lanai, cocked its head back and forth, hopped into Paul's lap, and stayed there for several minutes. Paul said, "Now I can make the Kannon (the Goddess of Compassion.)

The time came, however, when Paul felt he was only existing. Although he had Bankei's book on the Unborn Mind on his bed stand, he could not read because his eyes could not focus well enough. He had to fight through the stupor of pain medication to be alert and laid in bed most of the time. He found some comfort in incense and Japanese and classical music. Around the end of May, Paul decided it was time to go and stopped eating and drinking, figuring it would take 7–10 days to die. But he was afraid he might die on Junko's birthday on June 1, so he resolved to strengthen himself to celebrate her birthday. He told me, "I never knew a papaya could taste so good."

On Monday June 4 Paul walked into the hospice at the hospital on his own using his bamboo sword as a cane. He predicted he would die on the 10th. He had figured out his insurance policies would cover hospice expenses completely for one week. When I saw him the next day, he asked me to get cards and addresses for the people who had visited him. From memory, he dictated at list of these people. He wanted to write thank you notes and "clear the decks." I asked him when he was planning to do this, and he said "Within the next 12 hours."

He was still bright and playful when visitors came. Once he was describing how his mouth felt stuck together with super glue and that this was his punishment for talking so much before. When a visitor said that he was looking good, he responded, "You must be kidding. I look like a ghost. I scare myself when I look in the mirror." Another visitor encouraged him to at least drink juice because he had loss so much weight. Paul responded, "I'm trying to be like Mahatma Gandhi." On Friday Junko said Paul laughingly told her this would be his last day. He said, "I did one thing right in my life. I married you. *Arigato* (Thank you.)"

Paul expended his remaining strength to go to the bathroom that night. He climbed from his bed to a chair, rested, climbed from the chair to the bed closest to the bathroom, rested, and then entered the bathroom. After using the bathroom, he finally opened the door and collapsed. His sons carried him back to bed. From then through Saturday, it seemed that his consciousness had left and we were simply waiting for his body to follow. But around 2:15 in the afternoon, he gave a distinct order, "Pull me up." I pulled him up, and he tried to sit on his own but collapsed. We raised the hospital bed, so he was in a sitting position. He would gradually slip down and would reach for the guardrail on the bed, so we helped him straighten up. At 4:30 he died quietly. The periods between breaths became longer and longer till finally he just never took another breath. Paul died sitting up, one day ahead of schedule. Particularly toward the end of his life, despite his physical weakness, his energy was clear and bright, and being around him made my anxieties and pettiness disappear.

Facing fearlessly whatever happens from the eternal recurrence of the small to life and death issues, fully present moment by moment with the immovable mind, receiving and letting flow away everything enables one to say, "Every day is a fine day." Tanouye *Roshi* when asked about how to live, once said, "Row, row, row your boat gently down the stream. Merrily, merrily, merrily, life is but a dream."

References

Haskel, P. (1984). *Bankei Zen, Translations from the Record of Bankei*. New York: Grove Press.

Hosokawa, D. (1999). *Omori Sogen, the art of a Zen master*. London: Kegan Paul International.

Omori, S. (1996). *An introduction to Zen Buddhism*. London: Kegan Paul International.

Sayama, M. (1986). *Samadhi, self-development in Zen, swordsmanship, and psychotherapy*. Albany: State University of New York Press.

Suzuki, D. T. (1975). *Studies in the Lankavatara Sutra*. London: Routledge and Kegan Paul.

Tanouye, T., tr. (1989) Takuan Soho's, *Fudochi Shimmyo Roku* Honolulu: Daihonzan Chozen-ji/ International Zen Dojo.

Zen and Forgiveness

Shoryu Bradley

Keywords
Zen practice · Zazen · Buddhism · Forgiveness · Eihei Dogen · Three Minds · Angulimala

I am grateful to have this opportunity to share some thoughts on the topic of Zen and forgiveness. First, however, I will share a bit about my past and current Zen practice. I began practicing in the Soto Zen tradition in the late 1990s, and I was ordained as a Zen monk in 2002. During the course of my Zen training, I have lived at various Zen centers and monasteries. It was at my teacher's temple, Sanshinji, in Bloomington, Indiana, where I inherited the style of practice I currently follow at my monastery, *Gyobutsuji*, located in the Ozark Mountains of Northwest Arkansas. Zazen, or zen meditation practice, is the primary activity of the monastic day at *Gyobutsuji*, but we engage in study, chanting, and work practice as well. We also do a monthly sesshin, or meditation retreat, every month, and during these retreats, we focus almost solely on zazen practice for either five or seven days.

Forgiveness realized through Zen practice has had a powerful effect on my life, and I have seen its healing power working in the lives of others. I hope this essay will in some small way helps those who read it to deepen their connection with forgiveness's restorative influence.

Most of us likely do not normally associate the word *forgiveness* with Zen practice, but I do think they are genuinely linked. Seeing this link, I believe, is mostly dependent upon having a clear understanding of what forgiveness actually is, and we must also keep in mind certain points that allow Zen practice to be genuine.

I believe there are two aspects involved in realizing the healing power of forgiveness: the forgiveness we offer individually to one another and to ourselves, and the absolute forgiveness we receive or realize as the reality of our lives beyond individuality. In my understanding, Zen teaching shows us that these two types of forgiveness are actually inseparable. One type cannot be complete without the other; they are, in fact, one and the same.

Forgiveness of Others and Ourselves

To begin, let's examine conventional forgiveness, the forgiveness we offer to others and to ourselves. Are there differences in this form of

S. Bradley (✉)
Gyobutsuji Zen Monastery, Kingston, USA
e-mail: shoryu@gyobutsuji.org

A. Masuda and W.T. O'Donohue (eds.), *Handbook of Zen, Mindfulness, and Behavioral Health*,
Mindfulness in Behavioral Health, DOI 10.1007/978-3-319-54595-0_12

forgiveness as it is encountered in our general culture and in the way it is presented in Zen teachings? I actually believe we encounter genuine forgiveness quite rarely because its true meaning is not well understood, or at least it is not understood on its deepest level. To illustrate what in my view this misunderstanding is, I would like to offer two entries for the word *forgive* as they appear in two different dictionaries. First, here is an entry from Collins English Dictionary:

1. to cease to blame or hold resentment against (someone or something)
2. to grant pardon for (a mistake, wrongdoing, etc.)
3. *(transitive)* to free or pardon (someone) from penalty
4. (*transitive*) to free from the obligation of (a debt, payment, etc.)[1]

Next follows an entry from Webster's New World College Dictionary:

1. to give up resentment against or the desire to punish; stop being angry with; pardon
2. to give up all claim to punish or exact penalty for (an offense); overlook
3. to cancel or remit (a debt)[2]

Both entries include all the basic definitions of forgiveness we usually associate with the word, yet notice there is a subtle but important difference between the two listings. The first entry offers four clear, distinct definitions, while in the second, there are only three. Webster's New World College Dictionary combines meanings of the word that appear as separate meanings in the Collins Dictionary.[3] To my mind, this combination presents a confused understanding of the meaning of forgiveness, and it gives us a hint as to why the deepest levels of forgiveness's healing power are not commonly encountered.

Definition 1 of Webster's New World Dictionary implies that our emotional attitude toward someone we believe has wronged us is inseparably linked to our ability to pardon or forgive them. In our society, it is the norm to feel one who has been wronged is "owed" an apology before a pardon or forgiveness can be given to the perpetrator. One cannot stop being angry with someone unless the person we are angry with shows remorse and apologizes, and we cannot forgive or pardon until our anger is assuaged. Yet what can we do with our anger if we receive no apology, if the person we are angry with, for example, feels neither remorse nor a need to apologize? What becomes of our anger if the person who has harmed us remains unknown to us, as in the case of an unsolved crime against us? Further, what if the object of our anger is not a person at all? We might find ourselves becoming resentful due to some misfortune caused by a natural disaster, for instance. Many of us probably know people who have seemingly become angry and resentful with life itself, having found no way to reconcile with some great pain or loss.

The definition also seems to subtly equate our emotional attitude toward someone with our *right* to *pardon* them. This is problematic because to pardon someone one must in some way hold legal or moral power over that person. As a recipient of some wrongdoing, we might consciously or unconsciously feel as if the principle of justice itself elevates us to a higher moral or ethical status than the person who hurt us. If we are not careful, this kind of judgment can become confused–even to the point of thinking the mere fact we are angry or annoyed with someone gives us moral or ethical superiority over them. In such a case, our emotions alone seem to make us "right," "justified," "innocent," etc., while the other person becomes "wrong,"

[1]"Forgive." Collins English Dictionary, n.d. Web. 25 September 2015. http://www.collinsdictionary.com/dictionary/english/forgive.

[2]"Forgive." YourDictionary, n.d. Web. 25 September 2015. http://www.yourdictionary.com/forgive.

[3]This is the dictionary's entry for British English. Interestingly, the American English entry for the Collin's Dictionary was the same as the Webster's New World College Dictionary. This leads me to believe the slight difference in definitions is cultural.

"unethical," "blameworthy," etc. It is as if that person is unworthy of forgiveness until they adopt our own point of view.

The primary problem is, of course, we cannot always trust the accuracy of our thoughts and feelings concerning people and things. According to Zen, our observations are always colored by the particular circumstances of our individual lives. Most all of us have "emotional baggage," for example, that triggers emotions in certain circumstances that would not arise in most other people. Yet we tend to truly believe in what we think and feel as "truth" itself. And even if we do doubt some of our emotions and thoughts, it is nonetheless very difficult for most of us to loosen the influence they have on our behaviors and general attitudes.

Realizing there is no separate, unchanging, fundamental "truth" underlying our own thoughts and emotions is a key practice and teaching of Zen. Since all aspects of our experience are always changing and are influenced by other things, we cannot grasp our experience as "the truth" in an ultimate sense. Applied on a practical level, we can say this simply means we can be pretty certain there is another perspective from which to view most any situation we encounter. When we first hear this teaching, it can seem absurd, frightening, or even nihilistic. But this teaching is actually the foundation for freedom, growth, and joy in our lives. It is the key to practicing with a flexible mind and an open heart. In other words, it is the key to forgiveness.

Taking Responsibility

Embracing this magnanimity of the flexible mind and open heart is a primary teaching and practice in Buddhism. Shakyamuni, the founder of Buddhism, taught that clinging to our own particular views and investing in beliefs based on comparisons between ourselves and others is a fundamental source of suffering. When we feel we have been wronged, we might also feel we are entitled to judge the moral character of the offender, and we are often quite sure and unwavering in such judgments. Yet if we stop and think about this for a moment, we can see that such certainty about the moral status of others and our right to judge them is actually dangerous to everyone involved. It is just this sort of certainty, in fact, adopted on a broad scale, that underlies many of our world's most serious problems, including prejudice, discrimination, and war.

Shakyamuni, however, advised us to give up interpersonal comparisons altogether, seeing ourselves as neither superior, inferior, nor equal to others.[4] Consider these words of the founder of Buddhism:

> Focus, not on the rudeness of others,
> not on what they've done
> or left undone,
> but on what on what you
> have and haven't done
> yourself.[5]

Here the Buddha tells us coming to terms with the perceived offenses of others is *our* responsibility. When it comes down to it, we cannot really change the behavior or thoughts of others; we can only genuinely, on a deep level, affect our own minds and actions. So the responsibility for forgiveness is ours.

This teaching might strike us as quite sensible, even obvious. Yet in all probably many, if not most of us, feel receiving some indication that our "offender" is remorseful is a prerequisite for forgiving that person. Yet, as I mentioned above, this prerequisite is not always met. What then? If we make our forgiveness dependent upon certain conditions, we limit it severely. Sooner or later, lack of forgiveness or partial forgiveness gives rise to lingering anger and resentment, two poisons that can gradually darken our hearts and minds and drain our life energy.

I feel the need to note here that with this teaching the Buddha in no way intended to morally or ethically absolve wrongdoing or

---

[4]See, for example, H. Sasshatissa, trans., *The Sutta-Nipata* (Richmond Surry 1994, p. 94).

[5]Thanissaro Bhikkhu, trans., "The Dhammapada: A Translation," *Access to Insight (Legacy Edition)*, 30 November 2013, http://www.accesstoinsight.org/tipitaka/kn/dhp/dhp.intro.than.html, p. 36.

release criminal offenders from social responsibility. Shakyamuni taught that cause and effect is also a fundamental aspect of human life, so all of us, both those of us who have been wronged and those who have behaved wrongly, must accept responsibility for our actions.

In the case of a woman who is married to an abusive husband, for example, does forgiveness demand that she repeatedly "forgive and forget" and stay in the relationship, even if the abuse continues?[6] Here, it becomes important to remember that we are discussing what I feel is the deepest, most genuine type of forgiveness, and this forgiveness is not synonymous with granting a pardon. As I stated above, I believe if we forgive only when we are able (or seemingly able) to pardon those who have wronged us, we limit our capacity to express and receive the genuine healing and compassionate power of forgiveness.

For this reason, the practice of forgiveness would not necessitate a woman pardoning her abuser and releasing him from responsibility. In fact, true forgiveness, I believe, would help give this woman the clarity and strength to more wisely deal with the abusive situation, seek suitable help, and even leave her marriage if needed. From what I understand, complex and contradictory emotions can make it very difficult for a woman to leave an abusive relationship. She might intellectually realize that she should extricate herself from a harmful situation, but difficult emotions such as fear, anger, shame, anxiety, despair, and helplessness can seem paralyzing to anyone suffering from abuse. As I will further discuss below, forgiveness on a deep level means letting go of our clinging to our mental and emotional experience. It neither rejects nor negates this experience, but on the contrary, it holds all experience magnanimously and without bias. It is this lack of clinging and bias that can allow one in a difficult emotional situation, such as an abusive relationship, to make decisions with more clarity and to seek help. This deep forgiveness does not pardon unwholesome behavior, rather it sees more clearly how to deal with it wisely and compassionately, and it impels us to act accordingly.

Forgiveness Is a Practice

But of course truly taking responsibility for forgiving others and holding our experience magnanimously and unbiasedly is all too often easier said than done. Sometimes we just cannot seem to find an opening in our hearts to begin letting in forgiveness, even in situations far less provocative than abusive relationships. In such cases, what can be done? I remember one such time in my life. It happened many years ago, not long after I first began practicing Buddhism. I felt that I had been wronged by a close friend, and the incident affected me in a very deep emotional way. The pain was so intense and blinding that it was quite some time before I even *wanted* to forgive. The events precipitating my pain could not be undone, and I had not received the sincere, remorseful apology I felt I deserved.

Eventually I realized I had to give up the pain and resentment. At that point they had been plaguing me for quite some time, and it became apparent that they were a hindrance to my practice and well-being. I realized they had been serving me in a way, giving me a sort of ground to stand on, a way to deal with what I perceived as the humiliation and injustice of the situation. In my mind I had been standing on morally and ethically higher ground than my friend, since I was a "victim" and my friend was a "perpetrator." It felt rather good to cling to this subtle sense of superiority. It allowed me a defense against my feelings of inferiority and a means to be "in the right." But eventually I began to realize this ground I stood on was becoming sodden with judgment and self-righteousness. It seemed that it would soon become a deep quagmire, eventually engulfing my entire being. At that point I finally found the true desire to let go of the judgments and anger that I feared might continue to pull me down ever deeper into resentment.

[6] I would like to thank Dr. Masuda and Dr. O'Donohue for suggesting to me that I discuss this hypothetical example.

So I tried to let go of the "victim and perpetrator" narrative. I reasoned with myself and told myself how I "should" feel, and I told myself that the narrative was wrong. Sometimes the narrative did abate for short periods, but sooner or later it returned. I wanted to be magnanimous and understanding, and I tried to cultivate these qualities. I thought if all else failed, at least the "time heals all wounds" principle would eventually take care of the situation. But it just did not seem to be happening. Would I end up a bitter old man in later life?

Eventually, I began to think I was approaching the situation from a misguided direction. I had been emphasizing how I *felt* about the situation rather than how I *practiced* with it. In Soto Zen (the type of Zen I practice), *expressing* awakening is emphasized as opposed to *having the feeling or knowledge* one has awakened. Perhaps the important point was to *express* magnanimity, regardless of whether I *felt* magnanimous or not.

At some point I decided to try practicing with my resentment by doing prostrations. In Buddhism bowing practice is seen as an expression of veneration and humility, two qualities I definitely wanted to express in my life. For me, the practice of bowing to a Buddha statue, for instance, is a way to honor practice itself. The statue is not an idol of worship, but rather an expression carved in wood or cast in metal, plaster, etc., of awakening in practice. Practice has produced the statue, and we continue that practice by honoring the stature. Bows are offered regardless of our mental or emotional attitude, and we are not asking for anything when we bow. When it is time to bow, we just bow.

So, somewhat out of desperation at first, I began a bowing practice. Each morning I offered incense to a Buddha image and bowed. While I did so, I offered wishes of well-being to my friend. I tried to *offer* these wishes rather than make them a *request*. I felt that was important. At first this practice was almost painful; I noticed a lot of resistance coming up. But within a short period I began to enjoy the practice. This was one of the few times during my day I could let go of my difficult feelings, but the practice also became joyful in itself. It was as if the act of bowing allowed a mind of magnanimity and joy to arise.

Eventually, I felt the grip of anger and resentment easing in my heart and mind. Later I hardly felt the pain at all. That is not to say angry or resentful thoughts of the painful situation never arose, but rather when they came up, they could naturally fade away without my believing them or taking them too seriously. The change seemed almost miraculous, and it was such a relief!

Absolute Forgiveness: Letting Go

At this point I would like to begin speaking more explicitly about the second type of forgiveness that I previously mentioned: the absolute forgiveness we can receive or realize. But what does bowing have to do with that? Well, after my bowing practice experience I got to wondering how simply doing prostrations could be so powerful, and I came to the conclusion that it could be considered a form of zazen, or Zen meditation.

Strictly speaking, it would not be appropriate to call bowing practice a type of zazen since that Japanese word means "*sitting* meditation". And even the word *meditation* itself can be considered a misnomer when taken in the context of the teachings of Eihei Dogen (1200–1252), the founder of Japanese Soto Zen. Dogen wrote in his *Shōbōgenzō-Zazengi*:

> *Zazen is not learning [step-by-step] meditation. Rather zazen itself is the Dharma-gate of great peace and joy (nirvana). It is undefiled practice-enlightenment.*[7]

"Dharma gate" is a teaching of the Buddha that allows us to express nirvana, which in Dogen's teaching refers to awakening/practice, i.e., reality or "truth" itself. The important point here is that genuine Zen meditation in Dogen's tradition is not actually meditation in the way we

[7]Shohaku Okumura, trans., *The Heart of Zen: Practice Without Gaining-mind* (Tokyo, Sotoshu Shumucho, 2006), p. 76.

normally think of it. Commonly, meditation is considered a practice of cultivation or self-improvement. One might do it to gain spiritual insight, calm the mind, or relieve stress, for example, and of course all of these things are fine and good. Yet Dogen's zazen holds none of these things, or anything else, as its goal. We practice zazen just for the sake of zazen.

When we first encounter this teaching, it may seem strange or even absurd. Why would we want to do anything that has no goal or benefit? One way we could answer this question is to say that such an attitude is a necessary aspect of the absolute forgiveness we receive in practice.

To really understand this, we need to understand how to do zazen, and then actually do it. In zazen, one simply sits upright in the zazen posture, allowing the body, mind, and breath to naturally harmonize. When thoughts, sensations, feelings, emotions, etc., enter the mind, the zazen practitioner neither entertains nor rejects them. In explaining this aspect of the practice, Zen Master Shunryu Suzuki Roshi (1904–1971) said in zazen you should "leave your front door [of the mind] and back door open. Let thoughts come and go. Just don't serve them tea."[8]

Kosho Uchiyama Roshi called this "opening the hand of thought." The original Japanese word he used, *omoi*, here translated as "thought," actually includes all ideas, thoughts, emotions, and feelings.[9] Usually we grasp and cling to our sensations, emotions, thoughts, and ideas as real and belonging to "me." We invest ourselves in them completely. But Uchiyama Roshi said that in zazen we loosen our "grip" on all of our experience and let thoughts, feelings, sensations, etc., simply arise, change, and fade away as they will. We do not grasp them as real or unreal; we just let them be. But why would we want to do such a thing?

Shakyamuni Buddha taught that we create suffering for ourselves and others when we cling to our views as fixed truths. We usually identify deeply with our views of who we and others seem to be. Yet any person's view is limited; none of us is omniscient. Still, all too often we feel our perspective is "the truth." When I thought about my friend, for example, I defined that person in terms of one event; I saw that person only as a person who harmed me. In doing so, I disregarded all of the times I experienced my friend as kind, sincere and loving. The mind likes to latch onto one aspect of its experience and label it as the truth. Yet reality does not fit so neatly into categories. This is an extremely important point, I believe.

And even when we do intellectually understand that a view we hold is limited or mistaken, if the emotions we experience in association with that view are very deep, intellectual understanding alone will not be enough to truly change or broaden the view. Eventually I came to see intellectually, for example, that my judgmental views of my friend were useful to no one. Yet even though I wanted to let go of these judgments, I just could not do it solely with my willpower and intellectual reasoning.

Of course it is necessary for us to think, feel, conceptualize and judge in this life in order to live as human beings. Yet we create problems when our thoughts and feelings become our "idols," when we live in service of them. In that case, they drag us here and there in an aimless cycle of suffering. However, when we encounter our sensations, feelings, thoughts and concepts with wisdom, letting go of our clinging and holding them with care, they become of great service to us and allow us to express a wholesome way of life.

When we allow our zazen practice to be our life foundation, our ever-changing thoughts and emotions can begin to fall into perspective since we "step back" from them. This is a primary reason zazen practice is foundational for the practitioner of Dogen's style of Zen. It is the only time during our busy lives when we can completely let go of all views, judgments, sensations, feelings, concepts etc. We sit in the zazen posture and allow all of the various aspects of our experience to simply arise and subside, without

[8]David Chadwick, *Crooked Cucumber: The Life and Zen Teachings of Shunryu Suzuki* (New York, Broadway Books, 1999), p. 301.

[9]See *Opening the Hand of Thought* by Kosho Uchiyama (Somerville, Wisdom Publications, 2004), p. 179, n. 22.

"having tea with them." We completely let go of our grip on views and emotions. Of course we will eventually notice that we *are* having tea with some thought or emotion. Perhaps we suddenly notice we are planning our vacation or refining the details of tomorrow's presentation at work. That is OK. There's no need for judging or fretting. When we notice our engagement in thoughts, we simply return to the here and now of the zazen posture, letting go again of our little "tea party." We do this over and over again in zazen.

Zazen can be considered absolute forgiveness because in it we truly forgive every person, place, thing, event, situation, etc., of our lives; we completely let go of the views and emotions we usually associate with them. This is an unconditional forgiveness void of stipulations or demands. It is in this act of forgiveness that we are forgiven. We are forgiven of all things that define and limit us, regardless of whether we usually judge these things as positive or negative. In zazen we let go of memories of the past and concerns for the future, settling down into the here and now. So in a way we are "born again" in the freshness of the present. We are forgiven in an ultimate sense.[10]

In today's complex and competitive world, most of us expend a tremendous amount of energy trying to live up to some societal or personal expectation. But in zazen, we can settle down into the simplicity of the here and now, in the refuge of the body and mind simply being rather than striving. When we come to truly realize and embrace this force of forgiveness in our lives, our minds become more flexible and our hearts begin to open.

When we allow this zazen practice to be our refuge and our life guide, our grip on views and emotions in our daily lives beyond the meditation cushion can become less tight. We can begin to see things from a broader perspective, and we begin to take our fluctuating emotions less seriously. Then we have the opportunity to let go of the judgments of people and situations we encounter, as well as judgments of ourselves. Receiving the healing, absolute forgiveness of practice allows us to practice forgiveness toward others.

Yet at this point I feel the need to add a caveat. It is important that we do not sit zazen for the sake of broadening our views or becoming more emotionally healthy. Why is that? If we do so, we are doing zazen under the subtle influence of our views or desires, so we are not truly letting go of everything. This is why we are told over and over again by Zen teachers to sit zazen only for zazen's sake. It seems like a contradiction, but it is actually the only way we can let down the heaviest burdens of our lives. It is the only time in our waking lives neither we nor our performance is subject to anyone's judgment. We just sit. What a relief!

In terms of my bowing, I think it was important that I made an effort to avoid approaching it as a means of easing my mental state. I realized that if I was focused on myself when making that offering, it was not really an offering. I remember my attitude at the outset was actually closer to one of exasperation, to tell you the truth. It was as if I had become so tired of fighting myself that I essentially just gave up and began bowing; I could not think of anything else to do. Later when I realized some joy and lightness was actually arising during my practice, I discovered quickly that if I held on to any thought of doing something "good" or "noble" while bowing, the real joy of the practice disappeared. It was as if it became tainted, in a manner of speaking, with self-centeredness.

In order to practice sincerely, we must let go of acquisitive thoughts and emotions when they arise and simply return to our practice. It is essential to practice for the sake of practice, rather than for the sake of our own agendas. That is the only way we can release our grip on views that limit us and bind us to our suffering. When acquisitive thoughts come up while sitting zazen,

[10]One might ask just who is offering this forgiveness in zazen, since Buddhism, unlike most other religious traditions, recognizes no supreme creator/deity as an object of worship and bestower of forgiveness. But I think the point is that letting go of such concerns (and all others) is how forgiveness is realized in zazen. In accordance with the Zen Master's exclamation of "zazen does zazen!," we might just say "forgiveness forgives."

we just return to sitting, and when they come up while bowing, we just return to bowing. We simply keep doing this over and over again.

Absolute Forgiveness Beyond the Meditation Cushion: Dogen's Three Minds

Yet the refuge and guidance that zazen offers us is not limited to meditation and bowing practice. If we wish to live a life guided by the compassion and forgiveness of zazen, we must endeavor to express zazen in all of our activities. In fact, Dogen wrote of how we can actively allow zazen to guide our lives in our daily routines. In his *Instructions For The Cook* (*Tenzokyokun*)[11], he used the practice of cooking in a Zen monastery to illustrate how we can adopt the sincere attitudes that allow our activities beyond the meditation cushion to be expressions of zazen, of true practice. There Dogen said embracing the Three Minds (*Sanshin* in Japanese), Joyful Mind, Nurturing Mind, and Magnanimous Mind, are essential to this endeavor. Since the Japanese word *shin* (心) carries meanings associated with the English word "heart" as well as "mind," we might say Dogen's teaching of the Three Minds describes both mental and emotional attitudes one can embrace in order to sincerely and actively express the wisdom of practice. The first of these, Magnanimous Mind, is the mind that welcomes all experience with neither clinging nor aversion. In his commentary on the *Tenzokyokun*, Uchiyama Roshi said this is the mind that recognizes "everything I encounter is my life." Nurturing Mind, the mind that impels us to actively care for ourselves and others, arises in conjunction with Magnanimous Mind, according to Uchiyama Roshi, as well as Joyful Mind, the mind that finds joy and gratitude for the opportunity to support others. So in my view, these Three Minds are inseparable and can actually be seen simply as different perspectives from which we can invite sincere practice into our daily lives.

Although Dogen does not explicitly mention forgiveness in *Tenzokyokun*, I believe that we can see a deep connection between the Three Minds and the mind of forgiveness. I first began to realize this as I considered the powerful effect of my bowing practice. I came to the conclusion bowing practice can be an activity that invites the expression of the Three Minds. Actually, I believe any wholesome activity can be such an expression, and like the relationship between zazen and our sitting posture, we cannot really separate the Three Minds from the activity that invites them. We cannot just think to ourselves "now I will adopt the Three Minds" and then expect they will appear in our lives. We need a way to express zazen, or forgiveness, just as a musician needs an instrument in order to make music.[12]

According to Dogen, Magnanimous Mind is the mind like a mountain or a great ocean, void of bias or contention. Because it is as vast and unshaken as a mountain, the mind of forgiveness tolerates whatever it encounters, just as our zazen practice tolerates any thought, sensation, or emotion. It is the mind of just here and just now. To express Magnanimous Mind when we cook, we just focus our entire being on cooking. When bowing, we focus on just bowing. This mind is not biased or judgmental because it clings neither to past experiences nor future expectations.

Resentment is an emotion that toys with the past, but it cannot take hold of us when we focus on an activity in the present moment. My bowing practice did not erase my feelings of anger and resentment, but when they came up, I just kept returning to my bows. Then, the negative feelings could simply run their course. No feeling or emotion lasts forever, and they linger even less if we do not grasp them. Even if thoughts and emotions rage torrentially like a flooding river, Magnanimous Mind, the mind of forgiveness, can absorb them like a great calm ocean. It is vast and powerful, yet fluid and accepting.

[11]For a translation and excellent commentary on this text see *How to Cook Your Life: From the Zen Kitchen to Enlightenment* by Kosho Uchiyama (Boston, Shambala Publications, 2005).

[12]Of course the instrument can be the human body itself, as in the case of singing.

Nurturing Mind is the mind that cares for and nurtures all it encounters in the way parents care for and nurture their children. It is also like a mountain or ocean since it supports all life it meets, yet we might consider Nurturing Mind as the active aspect of genuine practice. It is the mind of offering.

A resentful and wounded mind is focused on itself. Its world is restricted, dark and self-absorbed. Nurturing Mind asks what it can do to help, and it takes into consideration the perspectives of others. When we feel we are wronged, do we consider the position of those who wronged us? Do we ask ourselves what part we might have played in creating the harmful action? It is very difficult to do these things unless we have a practice that helps to loosen our grip on our own pain and judgment. When we give sincerely, we offer ourselves up, so to speak, to the act of giving in the here and now. In this way our world can shift from a prison of self-absorption to a boundless mountain or ocean of offering.

When I consider Nurturing Mind in relation to my bowing practice, I see that the acts of bowing and offering good wishes for my friend helped direct my attention away from my own self-absorption and brooding. Shifting our focus from our own emotions to the well-being of others can end up being a powerful balm for our own suffering.

I saw this especially clearly on one occasion quite a few years ago when I was practicing at Tassajara Zen Monastery, the oldest Japanese Buddhist Soto Zen monastery in the USA, founded in 1966. There the practice schedule is divided into three distinct kinds of periods: two traditional, formal 90-day practice periods, two multi–week work periods, and a summer guest season. The practice environment at the monastery shifts quite dramatically during the transition from the focused quiet of practice period to the productivity-oriented work period. Some students who had enjoyed the six months of the cloistered, contemplative environment of practice period found it a challenge to deal with all the new guests and the relatively boisterous activity of the work period. This was the case for me during my first year at Tassajara.

At the end of one long day during a work period, I found myself tired and irritable as I walked toward the meditation hall to participate in evening zazen. I had worked very hard that day and was really not so excited, to tell the truth, about sitting zazen. I would have much preferred going to my bed. The tiredness seemed to fill my entire world and grumpiness colored all my thoughts and perceptions. At that time I saw there was a long line of people waiting to enter the meditation hall as the person in charge assigned seats. All resident students at Tassajara received longer-term seat assignments, usually for the entire work period, but sometimes the seat would be given away by mistake, especially if the zendo was very full. At that time I was quite attached to my particular seat because it was home to a special set of cushions I could arrange in a way that helped me sit in a comfortable and stable meditation posture. I remember grumbling to myself, "I sure hope my seat hasn't been given away this evening, I don't want to deal with a flat, spongy cushion and aching legs tonight!" As I came closer to the meditation hall door, I could see that indeed my seat had been given to someone else. I felt my mind sink and my heart shrivel as I walked through the doors to get my seat assignment. My bleak little world was definitely limited to my own suffering in that moment.

When I met the meditation hall manager, she looked at me with a hint of distress in her eye and said, "Can you help?" In that moment, my view of my entire world changed. I looked around. A second before I had seen a room full of people who were crowding our meditation hall and preventing me from sitting on my special cushions. Now I saw with wonder that close to 90 people (in a room build to accommodate around 60) were there to engage in the way of practice; what a wonderful and joyful occasion to have the fortune to encounter! In one instant my world changed from a dark sky of self-focused suffering to the clear joyful sky of offering. I got busy setting out cushions on the floor and showing visitors where they could sit.

This occasion also illustrates to me how Joyful Mind, another of the Three Minds, can influence our lives. Dogen said this is the mind that recognizes the good fortune of having the opportunity to make an offering, to practice. It is the mind of gratitude. Forgiveness comes easily when we recognize we are fortunate, as does joy. How foolish I was to be so upset at being deprived for one meditation period of my special cushions, when I actually had so much support in so many ways during that time! I had the rare opportunity to focus full-time on Zen practice with a large community of like-minded people. I was instructed, cooked for, advised, befriended, and sustained in innumerable ways by those around me and by those who had practiced there before me. I was indeed fortunate, and it was a privilege to encounter the opportunity to in some small way support the 90 people who had come to sit zazen that evening; it was a chance to return at least a tiny portion of the immense support I had received at Tassajara and beyond.

If we settle down and reflect in most any situation, we can see through the eyes of Joyful Mind and allow forgiveness to enter our lives. We are always being supported in innumerable ways, and we can almost always, I believe, with sincere practice, find the mind of gratitude. This Joyful Mind prompts us to offer ourselves in service, and an act of offering in turn promotes even more deeply the mind of offering.

It is important to stress that the forgiveness arising in zazen and in practicing with the Three Minds is not only forgiveness of "others." It is also fundamentally forgiveness of the self, and it therefore leads us to absolute forgiveness. When we let go of our grudges, biases, and discontents by focusing totally on bowing, cooking, sweeping, or any wholesome activity in the here and now, we can be released from the burdens of our hearts and minds. In the immediate here and now, we can be freed from our own expectations, definitions, and judgments of ourselves. Dogen wrote "to study the self is to forget the self,"[13] and perhaps, we can also say, "to study the self is to forgive the self." We might even say forgiving the self on a deep level is simultaneously forgiving others. According to Zen teaching, there is no fundamental, unchanging difference between ourselves and others since we are all interconnected, sharing, essentially, the same life. True forgiveness of self and forgiveness of others are one and the same on this deep level.

Angulimala as a Story of Forgiveness

To end my discussion of forgiveness, I would like to present an ancient story found in the early texts of Buddhism. It is the story of Angulimala, the ferocious murderer who is redeemed by the power of practice and the compassionate insight of Shakyamuni Buddha. For centuries it has been used to illustrate that the healing power of forgiveness is open to anyone, regardless of social status or past actions. In conclusion, I will present a few comments on the story that I hope will help illustrate a few more points on the relationship between forgiveness and Zen.

But before proceeding, I would like to say a few words about the seemingly "supernatural" events that take place in the story. I believe it is important to understand these events were not necessarily recorded with the intent that they be taken literally. In fact, I think we often find the deepest "truths" of ancient stories embedded within events of those stories that most likely did not actually occur.[14] These events were often added over time to historical incidents and were passed down from generation to generation not as records of historical happenings but rather as parables or metaphors intended to transmit some type of spiritual understanding or wisdom. I think this is the case with the story of Angulimala. Many if not most of the events occurring in the story may indeed have actually taken place,

[13] Shohaku Okumura, *Realizing Genjokoan: The Key to Dogen's Shobogenzo* (Somerville: Wisdom Publications, 2010), p. 2.

[14] The first of the "Rules of Zen Studies" of the late Buddhist Scholar John Macrae is "It's not true, and therefore it's more important." Dr. Macrae specialized in the study of Chinese and Japanese Buddhism, but I imagine his rule may apply to ancient religious stories in general. See John R. Macrae, *Seeing Through Zen* (Berkley and Los Angeles: University of California Press, 2003).

but I believe we find the key teachings of the story are emphasized and summed up by two metaphorical events: the calmly walking Buddha's remaining beyond the reach of the running Angulimala, and the transformed Angulimala's blessing helping a suffering woman. Of course many modern people would have difficulty believing these events actually happened, yet I do believe they bring to light some very important points of the Angulimala story.

What follows is an edited version of the story of Angulimala as it appears in the *Majhima Nikaya*, an early Buddhist scripture[15]:

> I have heard that on one occasion the Blessed One was staying near Savatthi at Jeta's Grove, Anathapindika's monastery. And at that time in King Pasenadi's realm there was a bandit named Angulimala: brutal, bloody-handed, devoted to killing and slaying, showing no mercy to living beings. He turned villages into non-villages, towns into non-towns, settled countryside into unsettled countryside. Having repeatedly killed human beings, he wore a garland (mala) made of fingers (anguli).
>
> Then the Blessed One, early in the morning, having put on his robes and carrying his outer robe & bowl, went into Savatthi for alms. Having wandered for alms in Savatthi and returning from his alms round after his meal, he set his lodging in order. Carrying his robes & bowl, he went along the road to where Angulimala was staying. Cowherds, shepherds, and farmers saw him going along the road to where Angulimala was staying, and on seeing him said to him, "Don't go along that road, contemplative, for on that road is Angulimala: brutal, bloody-handed, devoted to killing and slaying, showing no mercy to living beings. He has turned villages into non-villages, towns into non-towns, settled countryside into unsettled countryside. Having repeatedly killed human beings, he wears a garland made of fingers. Groups of ten, twenty, thirty, and forty men have gone along that road, and even they have fallen into Angulimala's hands." When this was said, the Blessed One kept going in silence.
>
> A second time... A third time, cowherds, shepherds, and farmers said to the Blessed One, "Don't go along that road, contemplative...." When this was said, the Blessed One kept going in silence.
>
> Then Angulimala saw the Blessed One coming from afar and on seeing him, this thought occurred to him: "Isn't it amazing! Isn't it astounding! Groups of ten, twenty, thirty, and forty men have gone along this road, and even they have fallen into my hands, and yet now this contemplative comes attacking, as it were, alone and without a companion. Why don't I kill him?" So Angulimala, taking up his sword and shield, buckling on his bow and quiver, followed right behind the Blessed One.
>
> Then the Blessed One willed a feat of psychic power such that Angulimala, though running with all his might, could not catch up with the Blessed One walking at normal pace. Then the thought occurred to Angulimala: "Isn't it amazing! Isn't it astounding! In the past I've chased and seized even a swift-running elephant, a swift-running horse, a swift-running chariot, a swift-running deer. But now, even though I'm running with all my might, I can't catch up with this contemplative walking at normal pace." So he stopped and called out to the Blessed One, "Stop, contemplative! Stop!"
> "I have stopped, Angulimala. You stop."
>
> Then the thought occurred to Angulimala, "These Sakyan[16] contemplatives are speakers of the truth, asserters of the truths, and yet this contemplative, even while walking, says, 'I have stopped, Angulimala. You stop.' Why don't I question him?"
>
> So Angulimala the bandit addressed this verse to the Blessed One:
> "While walking, contemplative, you say, 'I have stopped.'
> But when I have stopped you say I haven't.
> I ask you the meaning of this: How have you stopped?
> How haven't I?"
>
> [The Buddha:] "I have stopped, Angulimala, once & for all, having cast off violence toward all living beings. You, though, are unrestrained toward beings. That's how I've stopped and you haven't."
>
> [Angulimala:] "At long last a greatly revered great seer for my sake has come to the great forest. Having heard your verse in line with the

[15]Thanissaro Bhikkhu, trans., "Angulimala Sutta: About Angulimala" (MN 86). Access to Insight (Legacy Edition), 30 November 2013, http://www.accesstoinsight.org/tipitaka/mn/mn.086.than.html. I have condensed the story quite a bit in the interest of space. Brackets appear in the original translation; double brackets indicate my own editing.

[16]A person of the Sakya clan, the Buddha's clan.

> Dhamma,[17] I will go about having abandoned evil." So saying, the bandit hurled his sword & weapons over a cliff into a chasm, a pit.
>
> Then the bandit paid homage to the feet of the One Well-gone, and right there requested the Going-forth.[18]
>
> The Awakened One, the compassionate great seer, the teacher of the world, along with its devas,[19] said to him then:
>
> "Come, bhikkhu.[20]" That in itself was bhikkhuhood for him.

At this point, the story relates how Angulimala, having accompanied the Buddha as his attendant to Anathapindika's monastery, receives a reprieve from King Pasenadi. The king, having come in search of the bandit with an army and the aim to "stamp him out," is so impressed that Angulimala has become a monk under the Buddha's guidance that he offers Angulimala material support.

Next, we hear how Angulimala, while on his alms rounds, encounters a woman suffering a breech birth. He is very moved, saying to himself, "How tormented are living beings!" After his meal, he returns to the Buddha and reports with distress what he saw. Their conversation follows:

> "In that case, Angulimala, go to that woman and on arrival say to her, 'Sister, since I was born I do not recall intentionally killing a living being. Through this truth may there be wellbeing for you, wellbeing for your fetus.'"
> "But, lord, wouldn't that be a lie for me? For I have intentionally killed many living beings."
> "Then in that case, Angulimala, go to that woman and on arrival say to her, 'Sister, since I was born in the noble birth, I do not recall intentionally killing a living being. Through this truth may there be wellbeing for you, wellbeing for your fetus.'"[21]
> Responding, "As you say, lord," to the Blessed One, Angulimala went to that woman and on arrival said to her, "Sister, since I was born in the noble birth, I do not recall intentionally killing a living being. Through this may there be wellbeing for you, wellbeing for your fetus." And there was wellbeing for the woman, wellbeing for her fetus.

The story next relates how the monk Angulimala, dwelling alone in resolution, attains complete spiritual liberation. Later we find him having gone into town to gather alms:

> Now at that time a clod thrown by one person hit Ven. Angulimala on the body, a stone thrown by another person hit him on the body, and a potsherd thrown by still another person hit him on the body. So Ven. Angulimala — his head broken open and dripping with blood, his bowl broken, and his outer robe ripped to shreds — went to the Blessed One. The Blessed One saw him coming from afar and on seeing him said to him: "Bear with it, brahman! Bear with it! The fruit of the kamma[22] that would have burned you in hell for many years, many hundreds of years, many thousands of years, you are now experiencing in the here-&-now!" [[...]]

Some Teachings of the Angulimala Story

In my view, we encounter the most important point of this story with the initial meeting of the Buddha and Angulimala. Here the horrible slayer of hundreds of men and indiscriminate leveler of towns and villages meets his match in the form of a quiet contemplative. Although Angulimala, who was said to have outrun deer, elephants, and horses, runs with all his might, he is unable to overtake the Buddha peacefully walking at a normal pace. Up to this point, Angulimala had been able through brute strength to destroy any being or village he encountered. Though it once seemed the world cowered at his feel, he is thwarted by a single quiet, mendicant teacher, finally facing a being he cannot overcome. In keeping with a point I mentioned above, I believe the fact that we modern readers might doubt the historical veracity of this particular event is actually an indication its teachings are very

[17]The word "Damma" has multiple meanings; in this case it means the teachings that lead to the end of suffering; i.e. the teachings of Buddhism.

[18]Becoming a Buddhist Monk or nun.

[19]A being dwelling in a heavenly realm.

[20]A Buddhist mendicant monk.

[21]Translator's note: This blessing is often chanted at house blessings in Theravada countries.

[22]Action. Kamma produces either wholesome or unwholesome effects.

important, so I'll speak a bit more about Angulimala's "running."

To me it is very interesting that in some versions of the story, Angulimala's running has a more complex and even more sinister motivation beneath it. He intends to take the life *and the finger* of the Buddha in order to fulfill a specific goal. He has been sent on a quest by his spiritual teacher to gather the fingers of 1000 victims. When he finishes his collection, he has been told, he will obtain the ultimate spiritual fulfillment. The plot is a ruse concocted by his misguidedly jealous teacher to get Angulimala out of the way, but it turns out that Angulimala is so powerful and committed that he almost achieves his gruesome goal.

Unfortunately, Angulimala's approach to life in that version of the story is all too common in our society, and if we are honest with ourselves, we might reluctantly have to admit we can identify with Angulimala's motivation. No doubt all of us have found ourselves deeply desiring that very special something (it may actually have been a desire for the *removal* of something) we think will finally make us happy or content, yet we just cannot get the thing we think we need.

Today more than ever, it seems human beings generally believe that life fulfillment comes through some form of acquisition; if one obtains enough of something one desires, or perhaps even just one very special thing, one will find fulfillment. So we set out to get what it is we think we need, pursuing or "running after" that thing at all costs. We might be running after material wealth, status, romance, fame, power, or whatever, and the capture of our object of desire becomes all important.

Consciously or unconsciously, we become like Angulimala. Even when we do find success in our pursuits, sooner or later we find the success is not quite enough to completely fulfill us after all. So, we continue to run. Of course we don't murder and pillage, yet we do adopt forms of domination and manipulation much more subtle than brute strength in our efforts to get what we want. We might use wealth, intelligence, artistic expression, wit, technological savvy, or sexuality, to name just a few examples, as tools to get what we think we need, usually at the expense of others. "Looking out for number one" becomes consciously or unconsciously "the bottom line" in our lives.

The point is that we are always competing with others and with ourselves, and we are always running to stay ahead of the game, whether we realize it or not. It is true that a few of us do seem to find success in most all of our endeavors, seemingly conquering all obstacles, as Angulimala did. Yet sooner or later everyone encounters some person, event, or situation that cannot be overcome, just as Angulimala could not overcome the Buddha. Whether it be a bitter divorce, the death of a loved one, or a serious illness, sooner or later we all meet our match in this life.

The Buddha taught that the relentless pursuit of our desires only worsens our situation in the long-run. Due to the principle of causality, the more we blindly seek fulfillment in ego-centric pursuits, the more suffering we create for ourselves and others since our desires can never be completely fulfilled. The wisdom to live well eludes us since we are always moving. When we run away from the truth of our lives unfolding in the present, our activities create increasingly unwholesome effects.

It's important to note that if we, like Angulimala, approach our spiritual practice as a quest for attainments or some ultimate goal, our practice is no different than the "running" we have undertaken in other aspects of our lives. We are simply "gathering fingers" if we fail to settle down in the here and now of sincere practice.

When we do stop running away from the past and rushing toward the future, we can receive the forgiveness of the present moment. We stop the indiscriminate harm we cause ourselves and others when we no longer allow the fulfillment of our self-centered desires to be our ultimate motivation.

The Buddha taught there is no fixed, unchanging nature that ultimately defines a human being. One becomes reborn in a sense in every moment, since we and everything we encounter are always changing. Fixed definitions of who we are exist only as concepts in our minds, so when we truly let go of clinging to those concepts, we become free of their limiting boundaries. That is why in one instant Angulimala was able to change from a horrible murderer to a humble monk.

When we see the simple reality of impermanence before us, we no longer have to dwell in the past or run away from the past because we realize on a deep level only the reality of now is genuine; we can only come to terms with the past by taking responsibility in the here and now. We no longer need to run toward the future because we realize it, too, is not our reality. The future never comes, essentially, since life unfolds only as the present. We can care for the future and make amends for the past only in the here and now. This is the reality that our zazen practice shows us. It is the reality of absolute forgiveness and redemption in the present.

In the story, it took some time for Angulimala to truly come to terms with his past. His meeting with the suffering woman shows he was likely feeling remorse for all the suffering he had created. With this meeting, it seems his heart opened, perhaps enabling him to feel compassion for the suffering he encountered in the present, while at the same making the suffering he had created in the past more palpable. His offering of a "blessing" to aid the healing of the woman shows us perhaps that he was taking responsibility for with his past by making an offering to aid the suffering he encountered in the present.

Again, I believe the fact that this part of the story involves a supernatural element (the woman's receiving well-being as a result of Angulimala's "blessing") indicates it contains a key teaching. This event represents and underscores, I think, Angulimala's transformation: The former indiscriminate *creator* of suffering here has become the compassionate and sensitive *healer* of suffering.[23] And perhaps the woman's recovery represents the healing power of compassion and forgiveness in the here and now.

This part of the story also illustrates how the process of forgiveness unfolds in our lives. We cannot forgive ourselves until we have the courage and strength to truly see and accept ourselves; we must acknowledge and accept who we are and who we have been. We must accept that we have caused suffering for ourselves and for others, and we cannot let go of our suffering until we truly accept our suffering. Yet this acceptance gives us the freedom to forgive ourselves, because it allows us to see there is no unchanging essence to who we are. And forgiveness of ourselves, in turn, naturally promotes a forgiveness and concern for others.

In our zazen practice, we accept everything we encounter. We may encounter thoughts and emotions that are angry, remorseful, childish, vengeful, happy, ecstatic, or morbid. They may be brilliant, foolish, insightful or dull, and everything in between. Yet we accept all of them and let all of them go. We accept ourselves completely in this way, and yet we are released from ourselves completely at the same time. This is the way zazen becomes the foundation for our understanding of absolute forgiveness.

The Buddha understood that Angulimala had been "cleansed" of his past actions in the power of the present. That is why the Buddha suggested to Angulimala he tell the suffering woman, as a blessing, that he had no recollection of ever harming beings. We can interpret this blessing, I believe, as a way to symbolically offer the woman the healing power inherent in the "purity" of the present. Yet it seems Angulimala was still in the process of accepting his past since he was only able to see his blamelessness at this point in terms of his becoming a monk. Eventually, he does come to complete awakening in the story. Perhaps we can infer that an element of his awakening involved his complete understanding of the nature of his life and his ability to completely accept it.

Angulimala's concern for the woman illustrates another important point: receiving absolute forgiveness prompts us to offer ourselves to others in service. We want to give because we realize we have received so much from our forgiveness and from our lives in general. Our eyes begin to open to the gift of life that is all around

[23]The symbolism of Angulimala's interaction with the suffering woman was brought to my attention by the Reverend Zuiko Redding. I appreciate her help and insight.

us. Our perspective broadens and we are more able to understand the perspectives and sufferings of others.

Yet, absolute forgiveness does not absolve us of responsibility for our actions. Being cleansed in the present does not erase the functioning of cause and effect in our lives. On one hand, Angulimala essentially "repented" of his crimes by returning to the reality of the present. In that reality, he was moved to adopt a wholesome way of life and became a monk, and that act of sincerity had a beneficial effect on his social standing. As a result of his "going forth," the King absolved him of legal responsibility for his crimes. On the other hand, Angulimala still had to suffer the effects of his past unwholesome actions, at least to some degree. His robes became torn, his alms bowl was broken, and his body became bloodied when people threw objects at him. No doubt they were seeking some level of justice for his past crimes. One can easily see, in fact, how a person in Angulimala's situation could have had his own life taken in vengeance for his past actions.

Taking responsibility in our practice is a very important point. It is critical that we do not misinterpret the Zen teachings of absolute forgiveness. The fact that we are "born again" in every moment does not give us license to act irresponsibly, and it does not erase the effects of our past behaviors. When we are truly in accord with the freedom of the present, we deeply understand the importance of the Buddha's teachings of causality. And when awake, we are not duped by an arising impulse to act irresponsibly.

In conclusion, I would like to express my appreciation for the opportunity to share some thoughts concerning this important topic. It is my great wish that the practice of forgiveness may begin to more deeply influence the lives of all of us inhabiting this troubled world. May the healing power of forgiveness increasingly awaken, cleanse, and guide us and our descendants.

Zen and Science: Zen as an Ethical Guideline for Scientists' Conducts

Rosan Yoshida

Keywords
Ethics · Science · Zen Buddhism · Zen · Humanity

Since it was first introduced to the West in early 1900s, many scholars and practitioners have discussed Zen along with sciences in various foci. The most topic of discussions focuses on characterizing Zen and delineating whether Zen is or is not a form of science (Muramoto 2002; Rosemont 1970). Whereas fitting Zen into categories may not be wholly adequate (Wallace 2003), Buddhism in general and Zen in particular are generally viewed as more empirical, scientific, and philosophical than other world religions and spiritual traditions. Although it tends to reject other spiritual traditions, the realm of science seems to have a favorable attitude toward Zen as a distant relative.

Another common theme is the identification of similarities and differences between science and Zen. For example, the Dharma of Dependent Co-origination is considered to be a shared concept between Zen and science (Iino 1962; Kurak 2003; Mikulas 2008). For Zen, this wisdom emphasizes the interrelatedness where multiple conditions may serve as causal factors of a particular event in a reciprocal fashion (Iino 1962): For a seed to germinate and grow, there must be sufficient water, nutrition, light, and other things. Unlike theistic religions, which may advocate creationism, providence, and original sin, the Dependent Co-origination in Buddhism is derived from direct observation and empirical verification (Gergen 1983). As the Buddha stated, the Awakened Way (Buddhism), especially Zen (*jhāna*), is the practice of "come and see" (*ehi-passika*).

Third, regarding the intersection between science and Zen, various fields of natural and social sciences investigate Zen and its effects on an individual and the society. Exemplars are psychology, physiology, and neuroscience, to name a few, that investigate the nature and health benefits of Zen and Zen meditation though various methods, such as behavioral health outcomes, the electroencephalogram (EEG), computed tomography (CT) scan, computerized axial tomography (CAT) scan, magnetic resonance imaging (MRI), and other behavioral measures such as personality (Chiesa 2009). To date, a growing body of empirical evidence is said to uncover and confirm the salutary benefits of Zen meditation; at the same time, many Zen scholars and practitioners argue that scientific

R. Yoshida (✉)
Missouri Zen Center, Webster Groves, MO, USA
e-mail: rdaido@gmail.com

A. Masuda and W.T. O'Donohue (eds.), *Handbook of Zen, Mindfulness, and Behavioral Health*,
Mindfulness in Behavioral Health, DOI 10.1007/978-3-319-54595-0_13

investigations may not fully grasp the heart of Zen as well as the supra-mundane realm of Zen practitioners (Suzuki 2010).

What has not been fully discussed, however, is the potential role of Zen as an overarching ethical guideline for the behavior of scientists as well as the consumers of science. According to Zen (Dogen et al. 2011), the fundamental problem of all living beings is the *karma* problem, which has arisen from the ongoing evolutionary process, especially from the birth of the human beings. The term *karmic conditions* in this chapter refers to our tendency to prioritize the narrowly identified ego (i.e., me-ism/selfishness/sinfulness) over others. This tendency can be called utilitarianism, materialism, militarism, and the money-ism (Suzuki 1996). Unlike our image of sciences as being value-free and bias-free, sciences are in fact forms of human enterprise vulnerable to these karmas like any other human activities.

The original Buddha foresaw the destruction of the world in the collections of karmas, called the triple poisons (see, for example, in Sammaditthi Sutta in Nanamoli and Bodhi 2005). The triple poisons include desire (e.g., craving, greed, thirst), divisiveness (e.g., hatred, anger), and delusion (of an independent eternal ego). The original Buddha also provided the solution for issues arising from the triple poisons. These include Zen, the embodiment of Dharma of Dependent Co-origination. This experience of wholeness is said to collectively transform our fundamental inclination from greed, anger, and delusion into generosity, compassion, and wisdom.

Once again, I do not argue that all scientific activities are toxic or that all scientists should practice Zen. Rather, my intention is to postulate that all human activities, including science, need ethics to follow and that Zen teachings can serve as an overarching guideline for scientists and consumers of science in order to promote humanities and the welfare of global ecosystems. The Dharma of Dependent Co-origination stipulates that any activity affects the whole system: all people, all organisms, and all environments. The claim that science is "value-free" is untenable because it is inherently connected to its surroundings, but in this chapter, I will discuss the harms of achieving a truly "value-free" science. Instead, the enterprise of science might engage in more beneficial activities by embracing globally common values.

Sciences

The word "science" is derived from the Proto-Indo-European root *skei* (split), as is the Latin *scientia* (knowledge) from *sciens*. The definitions and goals of science vary across individuals and disciplines. However, generally speaking, science is viewed as an organized human enterprise with the goal to *acquire* knowledge about the phenomena of the natural world or universal truths beyond time, space, and social conventions. Employing systematic verification strategies (e.g., experiments), modern sciences often claim to be value-free, especially from scientists' own preconceptions as well as biases from traditions, religious assumptions, faiths, and dogmas. Similarly, the public tends to follow in that science is one of the greatest authorities in decision-making and defining the "Truth." As Gergen (1983) noted that:

> It has been often ventured that the form of scientific understanding represents the highest level of understanding to be achieved by human beings. It is said to be more precise, more reliable, more flexible, less burdened by emotional baggage, and more functional in the real world, than common marketplace understanding (Gergen 1983, p. 135).

There is no doubt that sciences have advanced our understanding of the world, contributing to the welfare of human life and shifting our worldviews. Historically, scientists such as Kepler, Galileo, and Copernicus replaced religious dogmas with revolutionary worldviews through rigorous empirical verifications. Copernicus made the ground-breaking shift from the Earth-centered Ptolemaic model of the heavens to a heliocentric one. Einstein, with his theory of relativity, transformed the Newtonian mechanics of physics and astronomy, ushering in the nuclear age. To date, scientists have continued to advance our knowledge and technologies.

However, science as a human enterprise is a double-edged sword. While flourishing our lives, it has also threatened global life systems including that of human beings. Unfortunately, despite a conventional image of sciences as being value-free and bias-free, they are also human enterprises that are influenced by personal, social, and political contingencies (Kuhn 1996; Skinner 1974). As such, like any other human activities, sciences can be extremely vulnerable to ego-centered desires of individuals who are involved in these activities, creating materialistic, militaristic, and economical and political conflicts, including climate change and nuclear threats.

Recapitulating my points, we, as a whole, must constantly monitor the practice of sciences and evaluate whether and how the products of science affect human lives and global life systems at multiple levels. The intention of this chapter is not to blame sciences for all of the problems that we have faced today. Rather, it is important to continue the discussion of our own humanity as scientists, to remember that scientists are also humans, that sciences are not impervious to bias, and that the behavior of scientists as well as those of the consumers of science must be carefully reviewed to avoid errors in judgment and interpretation that harm the wholly wholesome life systems.

When findings and technologies derived from science are used to benefit only limited groups of individuals (e.g., the most wealthy or most educated), outcomes are often extremely destructive. We have already witnessed numerous times that sciences without clear ethical and aesthetic guidelines have contributed to the global problematique (i.e., intertwined global problems) including wars, nuclear weapons, nuclear power disasters, global warming, and mass extinction. Without the synthesis of ethics and scientific conduct, the world is simply a set of resources to be consumed. According to Zen teachings, the reality is the Dharma of Dependent Co-origination (縁起 in Japanese); all things arise in dependence upon other things. Those who are involved in scientific enterprises are living beings dependent on others. A scientific determinist would agree. Dogen, the founder of Soto Zen in Japan, states that we must strive to embody the true self, the interdependent being, the one with the whole. Prospering limited groups of individuals through science is not congruent with the stance of the true self. Science, then, must be the collective efforts of greater beings (true self) with ethics and aesthetics.

Zen as an Ethnical Guideline for Scientific Conducts

The goal of Soto Zen Buddhism is to awaken in nirvana and live an awakened life through the constant practice of *Zazen*, the solid still sitting called *shikan-taza* (只管打坐), literally meaning *devotion in total sitting*. *Shikan-taza*, the devoted total sitting stressed in Soto Zen, is the essence of Soto Zen in the unity of cultivation and verification. Solid sitting is itself the manifestation of awakening, according to Dogen et al. (1997). Soto Zen does not take the practice of sitting as the means to the end of enlightenment. This steadfast (*a-cala*, lit. un-moved, by anything) *shikan-taza*, the essential core of *Zazen*, is the witnessing of nirvana (no-wind of karma), permeating into meditation in awakening and awakened prognosis, the wakeful practice of mindful actions in daily activities. Dogen also called this “the Buddha Dharma of One Color (*Isshiki-no Buppō*),” life and practice in the Buddha Dharma. Life in the Buddha Dharma here and now, inclusive of all in time and space, is ongoing, absolute, and complete.

Practicing Zen is to live with proper perspective, priority, prognosis, and peace in and from nirvana and awakening. This is the realm of no discrimination by karma-conditioning, in which conceptualization, emotion, volition, and perception are quieted as the stages of Zen practice proceed.

As noted elsewhere in this book, our karmas (i.e., our physical, verbal, and mental actions and habits) discriminate between the self and others, here and there, and now and then. However, in a karma-less state, an individual stays with all, wholly, in a wholesome state, finding oneself being harmonious with the whole. Zen Buddhism is the holiness, a wholly wholesome way and world. The Buddha stated that one cannot reach the end of the world by walking. By this, he did not mean that it is too far to reach but that one must still one's karmas in still sitting to go beyond the conventional karmic world. As such, the transcendent and interconnected quality of the here-and-now experience as a whole person is a crucial to embody the true self, avoiding the fundamental delusion of the self as a separate substance from all in space and time, which leads to divisiveness and desire.

As the story goes, the original Buddha enjoyed nirvana/awakening for many weeks and was at first reluctant to go out into the world to share it with other people. This was because he saw that people were deeply immersed in the long and deep storage of karma. The story, which was told by him, that Brahma, the Supreme Being, besought him to go out into the world to share his aspiration to save the world.

The Buddha's epithet *Tathāgata* is usually translated as Thus-come (*Nyo-rai*: 如来: *Tathā-āgata*) and refers to the Returning Aspect (還相) of him as a Bodhi-sattva, Awakening Being. The term suggests that he was originally aspiring for awakening and later became a being aspiring for others' salvation, or saving others first and himself last, from his having become *Tathāgata*, Thus-gone (*Nyo-ko*:如去:*Tathā-gata*). When he visited the five practitioners who had once practiced with him in order to share the Dharma to which he had just awakened, he requested that they call him *Tathāgata*, rather than Gotama, the form of address associated with his past identification before becoming *Buddha.* His intention, given his aspirations and actions, seems to mean Thus-being or Being-in-Thusness (Truth) as in the compound *hasta-gata-āmra* (mango being in the hand, lit. hand-being mango, *gata* meaning "being in"). This obviates the elements of "go" (往相, Going Aspect) and "come," as there is no more going or coming, birth or death, oneness or diversity, interruption or eternity in the karma-less, selfless realm of nirvana, nor within the Eight Negations by Nagarjuna. The Great Vehicle Buddhists (Mahayana, usually identified as the Northern, but not space-specific), especially Zen practitioners, follow the Buddha's Path to live as Bodhisattvas who take vows to save all beings first and themselves last because of their clear understanding of the intertwined world, including all karmic delusions of the independent individual or separated self.

Scientists' activities are bonded to their individual karmas as well as karma dictated by the politics and culture at large. Some scientists may engage in science to fulfill ego-centered desires, such as the achievement of personal fame and success as defined by the karmic world they are in. On occasion, scientists have deeply regretted their scientific discovery. Responding to the dropping of the atomic bombs on Hiroshima and Nagasaki in 1945, Albert Einstein shared his dilemma of scientific discovery in relation to peace and concluded that his own situation mirrored Nobel's. In December 1945, Einstein stated:

> Alfred Nobel invented an explosive more powerful than any then known—an exceedingly effective means of destruction. To atone for this "accomplishment" and to relieve his conscience, he instituted his award for the promotion of peace. Today, the physicists who participated in producing the most formidable weapon of all time are harassed by a similar feeling of responsibility, not to say guilt. As scientists, we must never cease to warn against the danger created by these weapons; we dare not slacken in our efforts to make the peoples of the world, and especially their governments, aware of the unspeakable disaster they are certain to provoke unless they change their attitude toward one another and recognize their responsibility in shaping a safe future… The war is won, but the peace is not. The great powers, united in war, have become divided over the peace settlements. The peoples of the world were promised freedom from fear; but the fact is that fear among nations has increased enormously since the end of war. The world was promised freedom from want; but vast areas of the world face starvation, while elsewhere people live in abundance. The nations of the world were promised "liberation" firing on peoples who demand political independence and social equality, and supporting by the force of arms, those individuals and political parties which they consider best suited to represent their own vested interests. Territorial conflicts and power politics, obsolete as these purposes of national

> policy may be, still prevail over the essential requirement of human welfare and justice (Easlea 1980, p. 118).

Zen practitioners practice the Awakened Way of Holiness, the Wholly Wholesome Way, for the benefit of all beings to enjoy holy truth, goodness, and beauty in harmony, health, and happiness. Zen practice accepts all scientific truths, if such truths are wholly wholesome, ethical, aesthetic as well as viewed and valued from the embodiment of nirvana and awakening, Zen practitioners are advised to accept, adapt, and advance these truths for the benefit of all to enjoy holy truth, goodness, and beauty. In this sense, Zen practice is in harmony with scientific truths but also integrates religious goodness and nature's beauty (Uchiyama and Okumura 2014), unlike value-free sciences. It is important to note that "religion" in the context of Zen differs from the concept of religion often held in the West. Zen is a religion in the sense that it teaches an attitude and a way of life that embraces and embodies the true reality of the self. Thus, the point is in holiness, the wholly wholesome way world, as described in the Kalama Sutta (Thera 1981), rather than the achievement of a specific afterlife or adherence to routines prescribed by a certain God.

Anyone can witness calmness and clearness of mind and world after some duration of sitting in stillness and serenity with good posture and good breathing. Solid still sitting with the best balanced upright posture is conducive to achieve the best state of body, mouth, and mind, and it facilitates the best deep, long, and smooth breathing. Today, breathing is known to regulate our bodily functions, such as heart rate, blood pressure, blood circulation, body temperature, and immune system. This leads naturally to the holy wholesomeness of the whole system: the physical, mental, and environmental all in harmony, health, and happiness.

Breathing is crucial for facilitating life and life systems. Many Eastern traditions state that long breathing (i.e., *iki*) leads to long life (i.e., *iki* or *iki-ru*). In these cultural contexts, breath has been identified as life (cf. *Pāna*, *prāṇa*, *pneuma*, *humus*, etc.). The best posture (e.g., upright and tallest) facilitates the best breathing (e.g., long, smooth, and deep), leading to the wholly wholesome state of the whole system with free, full function in harmony, health, and happiness. The best posture happens within the inside of the torso (e.g., lungs and guts) as one mass makes the best breathing. I usually recommend that practitioners imagine the abdominal area as a plastic bag into which they pour in and push out water. Imagine filling it in from the bottom up and pushing out from the top with a smooth shift from exhalation to inhalation, making the shifting point from exhalation to inhalation smooth as if into a large circular motion from a small piston motion. Practitioners are encouraged to count breaths in and for concentration, going from one to ten, steadily repeating them. Through practice, the ordinary breathing of 15–16 times per minute can be cultivated to 4–5 per minute with ease. Breathing as the vital life function is said to be profoundly intertwined with the body, brain, mind, head, heart, and *hara* (i.e., guts).

Zen is for everyone. Dogen (2004) offers this unique message of the essence of the Awakened Way in its utmost aspiration in his *Fukanzazengi* (普勧坐禅儀; *Universal Recommendation for True Zazen*). Dogen stated that all may attain unconditioned peace and unsurpassed awakening, living in harmony with the entire world in pure bliss and peace. The unique difference of Buddhism, especially Zen Buddhism, from other human activities such as the sciences, religions, politics, or economics, lies within its ultimate truth in the awakened wisdom of nirvana, which goes beyond karmas. Buddhism works with karmas from the vantage point of perspective, priority, prognosis, and peace, while knowing the limitations of conventional sciences, ethics, and aesthetics. Further, Zen provides the skillful means to go beyond limited, selfish, tribal, nationalistic, and species-centered attitudes and actions.

Global Ethic

Ordinary, status quo worldly human activities are the very culprit of climate change and the sixth mass extinction. As such, sciences must shift their position from the so-called value-free to a paradigm of being value-friendly, embodying the true meaning of "free-dom" (Sanskrit: *priya-dhāman* Pali: *piya-dhāman*, meaning beloved-domain). In 1972, the Club of Rome, a global think tank dealing with a range of global and political issues, published *The Limits to Growth*, one of the best-selling books on environmentalism (Meadows et al. 1972). The book awakened and alarmed people in the world with the awareness that economic growth could not continue indefinitely; natural resources would be drained out sooner or later. The Intergovernmental Panel on Climate Change (IPCC), a leading international body for the assessment of climate change established by the United Nations Environment Programme (UNEP), has been warning of catastrophic disaster due to climate changes since its first report in 1990. However, even so, we have continued to be driven by our karma of self-centeredness. While some scientists have worked for industries that have contributed to the global crisis, other scientists and intellectuals work tirelessly to convince politicians, stakeholders, and businessmen of the dire consequences of climate change. Governments and private sectors in the world seem to be slow to react, however.

The importance of establishing and adhering to a global ethic applied to diverse human activities has been discussed at large across many countries. For example, in 1993, the second Parliament of the World's Religions issued the *Declaration toward a Global Ethic* (Kung and Kuschel 1993). Drawing on what is already common to the religions of the world, declared "what you do not wish done to yourself, do not do to others, or what you wish done to yourself, do to others," as the irrevocable, unconditional norm for all areas of life. It also highlights four guidelines that most of religions of the world affirm as the irrevocable directives. These include commitments to cultures of:

Non-violence and respect for life,
Solidarity and a just economic order,
Tolerance and a life of truthfulness,
And equal rights and partnership between men and women.

These four irrevocable directives are made from the first four precepts of the Buddhist Five/Ten Precepts (e.g., no killing, no stealing, no falsehood, and no sexual misconduct) related with the sixth and down of the Ten Commandments (e.g., no homicide). These concepts are uniquely universal and observable for anyone with or without religious beliefs anyone without faith in God or religion can agree in rational thinking. If everyone observed these four directives, there would be no war, pollution, global warming, or mass extinction. The global problematique comes from human karma or its triple poisons of desire, divisiveness, and delusion, which develop into killing, stealing, lying, and other social ills. *Zazen*, or sitting Zen, includes no killing, stealing, lying; *Zazen*, simple still sitting, can benefit all by returning to the original zero, *nirvana*.

At the Parliament of the World's Religions, the declaration was signed by over 200 leaders from more than 40 faith traditions with several thousand participants in attendance. In 1997, the InterAction Council, an independent international organization to mobilize the experience, energy, and international contacts of a group of statesmen who have held the highest office in their own countries took the tenet of the *Declaration toward a Global Ethic* and made it into the draft of the *Universal Declaration of Human Responsibilities*. The document was presented to the United Nations to commemorate the 50th anniversary of the *Universal Declaration of Human Rights* as the essential counterpart of this. Zen is uniquely able to provide guidance for the integration of all peoples because it precludes adherence to a specific religion, or belief in a specific God, from foundational elements of the practice. That is, it does not have a correlate to "Thou shalt have no other Gods" but includes overarching values that can be embraced by all.

Paradigm shifts are inevitable, not only in dominant instrumental ideas or concepts in sciences, as Kuhn (1996) suggested, but also in society at large. We are at the critical point that requires a shift from ego to eco, civilization to culture and cultivation, sinfulness to holiness, an artificial unidirectional individualistic pyramidal system to natural cyclical interdependent Indra-net system.

Barney (1999), in his book, *Threshold 2000: Critical Issues and Spiritual Values for a Global Age*, presented a way to a new dialogue among religions as well as those between religions and other guiding institutions regarding the future of the earth and humanity. He also identified and called five major agents in modern society (i.e., nation states, corporations, religions, media, and education institutions) arbitrary. These five institutions are all changing, usually without widespread environmental benefit, but in the service of benefitting the few instead. Corporations collapse, states sink, religions reform, media malfunction, and education evolves. There is neither self-sameness nor self-sovereignty; thus, there is no self-substance and the selfless nature of all things as Buddhism reveals is held captive. Our bodies and minds are further analyzed into the five components of physical forms. Masses of people, however, firmly believe in these misleading misplaced bodies as firm and fixed, especially their states and selves.

There exists a pattern of masses of separated people (*pṛthu-jana*/*pṛthag-jana*) living with "nescience," the non-witnessing egoless nature of all phenomena in the Dharma of Dependent Co-origination; this produces "craving," or thirst and "hatred" as the third poison. Our problems and sufferings persist and prevail as a result. If we truly want to stop them, we must witness the egoless nature of our life way and world by sitting still, stilling karmas, settling in nirvana, serving the Dharma, and saving all. We must work with a world that is afflicted and may be annihilated, along with other species in our spheres. For more than two millennia, Buddhas and Bodhisattvas have been striving to share the Buddha's unconditioned peace and unsurpassed awakening, but the human species has been slow to change.

For more than two decades, religious individuals and institutions have been striving to share the Buddha's five precepts as essential directives in the *Declaration toward a Global Ethic* (Kung and Kuschel 1993), but the world has been too slow to respond. The key that will open confining cells to the spacious sky is not intellectual, but existential, a witnessing of the work of egoless, limitless life, light, liberation, and love, like the ocean, by bubble bursting. This shift from sin (i.e., separation/selfishness) to holiness (i.e., wholly wholesomeness) is the essence of religion (from Latin *re-ligare*: reunion with holiness from sinfulness). This was the essence of religious founders in many religions, but religious institutions regressed into selfishness to protect their institutions. The Buddha "preached" that selflessness is the core of our being, regardless of national origin or religion. Jesus suggested we crucify our small selves every day. Muhammad said that killing a man is killing humanity. This is precisely why the global ethic is relevant across diverse and seemingly conflicting religious practices today. *Zazen*, sitting Zen, is stilling karma, seeing the Dharma, serving and saving all by witnessing or awakening in nirvana (no-wind of karma). This can be done by anyone regardless of age, gender, race, religion, etc. It is not acquiring anything, but eliminating acquired karma, reunifying or returning to the original zero (sunya, zifr, zero, emptiness of entity).

Our behaviors are conditioned by karmas in the intricately interdependent universe, globe, environments, ecologies, evolutions, events, climates, civilizations, cultures, societies, institutions, traditions, and habits. We must constantly witness the impacts of karmas and work with them to take our responsibilities to the wider world in a wholly wholesome way. The Buddha recommended that we practice the Fourfold Exertions (e.g., *padhāna*, *pradhāṇa*) of decreasing and stopping existing bad karmas, increasing existing good karmas, and starting new good karmas. We cultivate our worldly (e.g., sinful = separated, selfish) behaviors (*lokiya-vohāra*, *laukika-vyavahāra*: worldly-convention) in this way to verify holy behaviors (*ariya-vohāra*, *ārya-vyavahāra*, *ariya*/*ārya*:*hagia*: holy is mistranslated as noble in the Four Noble Truths, Eightfold Noble Way/Path but should be translated as the Four Holy Truths, Eightfold Holy Way/Path, as the wholly wholesome way and truth, wholesome truth/way of all and for all) and blisses (cf. the Five Blisses of awakening, freedom, equality, love, and peace).

We can learn solutions in concrete methods and practical methods for a *preventive and preservative way of the total system*. To actualize it, we must act for solutions in our concrete daily living. Table 1 is my proposal of how to act on and within the global system and global ethic, including a concrete method to approach material and information flows for easy memory and action. The points are essential for sciences, technologies, states, and civilizations to save our way and world from destruction and demise.

Zen and Science

Zen is scientific, but it is not science itself. Science is truthful, but not truth itself. Zen is true, good, and beautiful. Science may be truthful, but it is not necessarily good and beautiful. There are a number of harmful products of science: atomic, biological, chemical (ABC) weapons, pollutions, and sicknesses; weapons of mass destruction (WMD); robotic-cybernetic-chimera creations; nuclear holocaust; space, robotic, and drone wars; and gene manipulations. All of these and more are endangering the wholly wholesome life system constantly, creating catastrophe. Zen is value-oriented for wholly wholesome life and living. Science claims to be value-free, historically and most strongly in regard to religious dogma and domination.

The value-free position of the sciences can be the strongest virtue for human knowledge as well as the worst vice against human ethics and aesthetics. This is related to human karmas, our heredities, habits, and actions, especially since the time of the Civilization Revolution that began about five millennia ago. According to the Cosmic Calendar, which places the Big Bang at 0:00 a.m. on January 1 and the present moment at 24:00 p.m. on December 31, the Civilization Revolution began a mere 10 s ago. With it, however, came the Fivefold Calamities of delusion, bondage, discrimination, exploitation, and destruction. One can say that the Spiritual Revolution, especially the Religious Revolution, represents the countermeasure to this. Appearing about 2.5 millennia ago, five second ago in the Cosmic Calendar, it introduced the Fivefold Blisses of awakening, freedom, equality (i.e., all living beings are four billion years old, sharing the same genomic pattern), love, and peace.

Karmas created sciences and technologies for the human benefit of ever increasing matter and power, creating increasingly complex civilizations. Such urbanization (civilization means urbanization, deriving from Latin *civitas*, city), with its Fivefold Calamities or Damages of delusion of ego, desire, discrimination, domination, and destruction within a pyramidal system, has implemented that pyramidal power civilization with the global problematique: population explosion; mass production, consumption, and waste; depletion of resources; pollution of the environment; wars; nuclear Nemeses; loss of diversities and densities of species; and mass extinction. The words "tree" and "true" share the same etymological root of *deru* (durable, endure) or *dhṛ* (root of dharma: hold). Because they live in harmony with water, wind, the sun, stars, birds, and bees, giving all oxygen, shelter, flowers, and fruits, trees can survive many thousands of years, as in Japan and the USA, or even ten thousand years, as found in Africa.

The sciences and scientists are subject to their karma and its consequences. They are not really free from values, because they are also

Table 1 Global system and ethic: material and information flow

Global system: 5Ss	Global ethic: 5Ls	Material flow: 5Rs	Information flow: 5As
Systemic	Law = Dharma	Reduce	Access
Sustainable	Life	Reuse	Assess
Saving	Love	Recycle	Agree
Safe	Liberation	Rearrange	Act
Simple	Lielessness	Restore	Advise

karma-heirs, karma-owners, and karma-machines living in the conventional karma world with their karma ways. Without Zen practice, they have cravings and nescience expressed in hatred, anger, and divisiveness. They share the same world with other karma-owners and karma-machines, individually and institutionally, and are compelled by and competing for fame and fortune. Thus, scientists and sciences are not karma-free or value-free. In truth, they should be called "dogma-free." The sole solution is the karma-free, supra-mundane perspective of priority, prognosis, peace, and persisting perfection in process while avoiding preconceptions, prejudices, and pyramidal power politics.

Nescience has been built into our life organisms and systems through billions of years of evolution, and it enforces its power with enhanced sciences and technologies, enticing us with new methods of global destruction and degradation. This beginningless nescience not only continues *samsara* suffering, but also it intensifies and expands it. The advances in science and technology within our modern civilization are bringing about global catastrophe and species demise, including the human species. It can, however, be countered by knowing the truth of it and actualizing ethics to stop it. Now, with past experiences of trial and error, it is only by constant witnessing (*vijjhā*, *vidyā*) and committed practice of the truth of life that we may stop our Life Wheel.

Nirvana is stilling karmas, seeing and serving the Dharma/dharmas, and saving all beings from individual and institutional karmas. It is to change our common conventional karmas or behaviors, our conventional common course of action, to holy dharmas and behaviors. Nirvana is the sole definitive way to change *nescience* to *true science*, a synthetic, value-provided prognosis with peace. The holy (wholly wholesome) truth, goodness, and beauty of life are in the beginningless holy, not sinful, separated, selfish, short-lived, short-sighted, short-circuited sciences. It should be good in the beginning, in the middle, and in the end, for all time and all places, as aimed at by Zen practice. Only practice makes perfect. Sitting still and stilling karma is the most important matter, as the Buddha said:

> Enmity is never appeased by enmity here, but by non-enmity. This is the truth forever. (The Dhammapada, pg. 5)
>
> Better than the one conquering thousands upon thousands in wars is the one conquering oneself. He is the greatest of war conquerors. (The Dhammapada, pg. 103)

Religions and sciences must mutually learn their best virtues and values. Religion is by definition "reunion" with the ideal "way to life" or "way to the holy (wholly wholesome)" from the actual "way of life" or "way of sins (separations, selfishness)" in truth (*Dharma*, *Dao*, *Deo*, *Deva*, etc.) and peace (nirvana, *śānti*, *šalōm*, *salām*, etc.) with the ideal figure (*Mitra*, *Mithra*, *Maitreya*, *Messiah*, etc. meaning "friend" from *mit*: with, future savior expressing human potential). In actuality, religious people as karma-machines remain in selfish sins and *samsara* suffering. Their institutions are, thus, also karma-machines with selfish sins and samsara suffering, and so they often choose traditions with dogmas rather than truth (science), goodness, and beauty. Traditional religions must interact with scientific knowledge. Sciences must accommodate religious values, especially ethics for wholesome perspectives, priority, prognosis, and peace in holy truth, goodness, and beauty.

References

Barney, G. O. (1999). *Threshold 2000: Critical issues and spiritual values for a global age*. Ada, Minnesota: CoNexus Press.

Chiesa, A. (2009). Zen meditation: An integration of current evidence. *Journal of Alternative and Complementary Medicine, 15*(5), 585–592. doi:10.1089/acm.2008.0416

Dogen, E. and (2004). *Beyond thinking: A guide to Zen meditation*. In Kazuaki Tanahashi (ed.). Boston, US: Shambhala Publications.

Dogen, E., Nishiari, B., Okumura, S., Suzuki, S., & Weisman, S. M. (2011). *Dogen's genjo koan: Three commentaries*. Barkeley, CA, US: Counterpoint.

Dogen, E., Uchiyama, K., Okumura, S., & Leighton, T. D. (1997). *The wholehearted way: A translation of Eihei Dogen's Bendowa with commentary by Kosho Uchiyama Roshi*. North Clarendon, VT, US: Tuttle Publications.

Easlea, B. (1980). Einstein's political struggle. In M. Goldsmith, A. Mackay, & J. Woudhuysen (Eds.), *Einstein: The first hundred years* (pp. 117–125). Pergamon.

Gergen, K. J. (1983). Zen Buddhism and psychological science. *Psychologia: An International Journal of Psychology in the Orient, 26*(3), 129–141.

Iino, N. (1962). Dogen's Zen view of interdependence. *Philosophy East and West, 12*(1), 51–57. doi:10.2307/1397245

Kuhn, T. S. (1996). *The structure of scientific revolutions* (3rd ed.). Chicago, IL, US: University of Chicago Press.

Kung, H., & Kuschel, K. J. (1993). *A global ethic: The declaration of the Parliament of the World's Religions*. New York, US: Continuum.

Kurak, M. (2003). The relevance of the Buddhist theory of dependent co-origination to cognitive science. *Brain & Mind, 4*(3), 341–351. doi:10.1023/B:BRAM.0000005468.95009.86

Meadows, D. H., Meadows, D. L., Randers, J., & Behrens, W. W. (1972). *The limits of growth: A report for the club of Rome's project on the predicament of mankind.*

Mikulas, W. L. (2008). Buddhist psychology: A Western interpretation. In K. R. Rao, A. C. Paranjpe, A. K. Dalal, K. R. Rao, A. C. Paranjpe, & A. K. Dalal (Eds.), *Handbook of Indian psychology* (pp. 142–162). New Delhi, India: Cambridge University Press India/Foundation Books.

Muramoto, S. (2002). Buddhism, religion and psychotherapy in the world today. In P. Young-Eisendrath, S. Muramoto, P. Young-Eisendrath, & S. Muramoto (Eds.), *Awakening and insight: Zen Buddhism and psychotherapy* (pp. 15–29). New York, NY, US: Brunner-Routledge.

Nanamoli, B., & Bodhi, B. (2005). *The middle length discourses of the Buddha: A translation of the Majjhima Nikaya.*

Rosemont, H. J. (1970). Is Zen Buddhism a philosophy? *Philosophy East & West, 20,* 63–72.

Skinner, B. F. (1974). *About behaviorism*. Oxford, England: Alfred A. Knopf.

Suzuki, D. T. (1996). *Zen Buddhism: Selected writings of D. T. Suzuki*. New York, US: An Image Book.

Suzuki, D. T. (2010). *The training of the Zen Buddhist Monk*. New York, US: Cosimo, Inc. (original work published in 1934).

Thera, S. (1981). *Kalama Sutta: The Buddha's charter of free inquiry Berkeley*. CA, US: Buddhist Publication Society.

Uchiyama, K., & Okumura, S. (2014). *The Zen teaching of homeless Kodo*. Somerville MA, US: Tuttle Publications.

Wallace, B. A. (2003). Introduction: Buddhism and science—Breaking down the barriers. In B. A. Wallace (Ed.), *Buddhism and science: Breaking new ground* (pp. 1–30).

Part III

Application of Zen to Behavioral Healthcare Issues

Zen and Behavioral Health: A Review of the Evidence

Kenneth P. Kushner

Keywords
Zen · Buddhism · Behavioral health · Science · Meditation

Introduction

Generally speaking, Zen in modern cullture has become associated with greater physical and mental wellness as well as health-related products. These claims originate from more than simple trends in marketing. For example, in 1984, a team of Japanese researchers (Ogata et al. 1984) published a study showing that Zen priests living in Japan had lower mortality rates than age-matched male counterparts living in the general Japanese population. During the years studied (1955–1978), 18% fewer priests died than would have been expected of Japanese men overall, regardless of the cause of death. This decreased mortality was statistically significant for multiple causes of death: heart disease, cerebral vascular disease, hypertension, liver cirrhosis, and some forms of cancer. These results reinforce the popular wisdom that Zen promotes good health. For example, a Google search of the term "Zen and Health" resulted in roughly 54,600 hits. The word "Zen" is now ubiquitous in marketing health-related items from shampoo, to wellness and beauty spas, to exercise programs, to better nutrition.

Given the widespread assumption that Zen is good for health, it is not surprising that Zen has found its way into the medical examination room and psychotherapy office, as interventions based upon Zen principles have been adapted to clinical settings. In this chapter, I will explore the current state of scientific research supporting the efficacy of those interventions. In so doing, I will define "behavioral health" broadly as it applies to both traditional psychotherapy and the application of psychological principles for prevention and treatment of medical illnesses, psychosomatic conditions, and lifestyle modification related to health.

Reviews abound on meditation in general and on specific types of meditation as applied to health and mental health (Canter 2003; Canter and Ernst 2004; Chan and Larson 2015; Chiesa and Serretti 2011; Dear et al. 2008; Fortney and Taylor 2010; Grant 2013; Hofmann et al. 2010; Krisanaprakornkit et al. 2010; Marchand 2013; Ospina et al. 2007; Sedlmeier et al. 2012; Weaver et al. 2008; Zgierska et al. 2009). While some of these reviews show a wide range of positive effects for a variety of forms of meditation, others cite poor design and

K.P. Kushner (✉)
Department of Family Medicine and Community Health, University of Wisconsin, Madison, Wi, USA
e-mail: Kenneth.Kushner@fammed.wisc.edu

A. Masuda and W.T. O'Donohue (eds.), *Handbook of Zen, Mindfulness, and Behavioral Health*, Mindfulness in Behavioral Health, DOI 10.1007/978-3-319-54595-0_14

methodological flaws as reasons for not drawing conclusions about the efficacy of meditation.

The only previous review of research specifically on Zen was conducted by Chiesa (2009), who reviewed the literature through 2008. Limiting himself to stringently controlled studies, he concluded that "…actual evidence on Zen meditation is scarce and does not allow us to reach definitive conclusions. There is some evidence that Zen meditation practice is related to EEG alpha activity and theta activity (especially in more expert practitioners); that long-term Zen meditation might protect against cognitive decline; and that Zen meditation could be useful for reducing stress and blood pressure" (p. 591). More attention to mechanisms of action with better-designed and larger studies was recommended for future examinations on the effectiveness of meditation.

The intent of this chapter is to update Chiesa's review by including literature on *zazen* (usually translated as "Zen meditation") published since 2009. We will also expand upon Chiesa's review by including meditation research that does not involve rigorously controlled methodology. This is, in part, because much of the foundational psychophysiological studies of *zazen* were un- or poorly controlled. Regardless, they provide important insight into the effects of Zen meditation. Further, as Caspi and Burleson (2007) suggest, randomly controlled trials—the gold standard of medical research—may not be practical in meditation research. However, before proceeding, I would like to discuss two major influences that informed this updated review of the literature.

The Traditions of Zen

In a review of methodological issues in meditation research, Caspi and Burleson stressed the point that "different forms of meditation may have different therapeutic effects" (2007, p. 37). The practice of *zazen* is not uniform across the world of Zen practitioners; in fact, two major sects of Japanese Zen, Soto and Rinzai, exist. There are other smaller traditions such as the Obaku sect and Sanbo Kyôdan; the latter combines both Soto and Rinzai practices. Each tradition gives somewhat different instructions for the practice of *zazen*, particularly regarding the role of breathing.

The Rinzai sect emphasizes a type of breathing that is referred to in Japanese as *hara* or *tanden* breathing. *Hara* is a Japanese word that refers to the lower abdomen; the term is replete with physical, psychological, and spiritual connotations in Japanese culture (Von Durckheim 1980). *Tanden* is the Japanese pronunciation of the Chinese word, *dantien*,[1] which refers to a point roughly two inches below the naval. It, too, has significant physical, psychological, and spiritual meanings in both Japanese and Chinese cultures. *Tanden* breathing is a form of deep abdominal breathing in which the lower abdomen is expanded throughout the respiratory cycle. Whereas *tanden* breathing is not absent from Soto and other sects' practices, it may not be stressed to the same degree as it is in the Rinzai tradition (Lehrer et al. 1999). Given that changing breathing patterns can affect both physiological and psychological arousal (Cappo and Holmes 1984), it is conceivable that different methods of breathing employed by various Zen traditions may have different effects on physiological factors impacting health.

I will have more to say about the differences between traditions of Zen in the next section.

Mindfulness and Zen

Anecdotally speaking, considerable confusion exists regarding the relationship between Zen and mindfulness. There appears to be a conflation of Eastern meditative disciplines in general and mindfulness-based disciplines in particular; it is frequently assumed that any Eastern meditative technique involves mindfulness (Wilson 2014). Several prominent researchers and reviewers have described *zazen* as being mindfulness-based (Chiesa 2009; Chiesa and Malinowski 2011; Ospina et al. 2007; Pagnoni et al. 2008).

[1]There are actually three *dantien* in Chinese thought. In common use *dantien* refers to the lowest of the three, the location of which is described above, as does the Japanese word *tanden*.

As I have contended before (Kushner 2012), the blanket assumption that all Zen is mindfulness-based is erroneous. One way of characterizing meditative disciplines is to make a distinction between those that are mindfulness-based and those that are concentration-based (Goleman 1988; Sedlmeier et al. 2012). The practice of mindfulness has been described as "allowing any thoughts, feelings, or sensations to arise while maintaining a specific attentional stance." The same authors described concentration-based meditation as "involving focusing on specific mental or sensory activity; a repeated sound, an imagined image, or specific bodily sensations such as the breath" (Cahn and Polich 2006, p. 180). However, it is generally acknowledged that these differences are not hard and fast dichotomies; rather, they describe a continuum of meditation experiences with varying emphases on mindfulness and concentration. Some traditions of Zen fall more clearly toward mindfulness. In particular, the Soto sect emphasizes a practice called *shikantaza* ("just sitting"), which is closer to mindfulness. Other traditions, notably those of the Rinzai sect, emphasize *samadhi.* Although this term does not have a good equivalent in English, it has been described as a state of "relaxed concentration" (Sayama 1986).

Another schema categorizes meditative disciplines by those that attempt to regulate conscious awareness and those that do not (Chiesa and Malinowski 2011). By this classification, mindfulness-based practices are non-regulatory in nature. On the other hand, some traditions of Zen regulate attention by regulating breathing and posture. The differences between the two can be observed in instructions for mindfulness meditation compared to *zazen* in the Rinzai tradition (which I practice and teach). Kabat-Zinn describes mindfulness as "…observ[ing] the breath as it flows in and out. We give full attention to the feeling of the breath as it comes in and as it goes out… And whenever we find that our attention has moved elsewhere, wherever that might be, we just note it and let it go and gently escort our attention back to the breath" (Kabat-Zinn 1990, p. 64). In contrast, writing from a Rinsai Zen perspective, Sekida writes "it is the correct manipulation of the lower abdomen, as we sit and breathe, that enables us to control the activity of our mind" (Sekida 1985, p. 33).

Thus, because not all Zen involves mindfulness and all mindfulness meditation is not Zen, whether one characterizes a given Zen tradition as mindfulness-based or concentration-based may have implications for the practice of *zazen* and for its physiological effects on a practitioner. It might also affect the amount of time that it takes for a practitioner to learn the techniques. For those reasons, it is unclear what bearing the many studies on mindfulness meditation may have on the question of the effects of *zazen*; therefore, reviews of studies in this chapter are limited to those that are clearly identified as involving Zen or *zazen*.

Methods

In order to search the literature for research studies on Zen, online queries were made in the following databases using "meditation" as a keyword: PubMed, Google Scholar, JSTOR, and Web of Science. This resulted 1655 references between 1995 and June 1, 2015. Given the large number of references, the databases were searched using "Zen" as a title and "meditation" as a keyword. Additional references were gleaned from the articles reviewed. Included for this review was any study that involved quantitative data collection and analysis, clearly involved *zazen* or other aspects of Zen training as a focus, had outcome measures that could pertain to behavioral health (broadly defined as physical or mental health), and was written in English. For reasons described above, studies of mindfulness-based meditation were excluded if they did not explicitly involve Zen or *zazen*. This review is organized by the following categories relevant to behavioral health: relaxation, stress reduction, and anxiety; attention; cardiovascular health; depression; pain; and the training and efficacy of health professionals. In some cases, assignment of a study to one of these categories was somewhat arbitrary. For example, studies involving brain waves may relate to both attention and relaxation. In such instances, they are reviewed here within the category that seemed the most relevant for each particular study. Where it was available, the specific traditions of Zen described in each study are noted.

The Studies

Relaxation, Stress Reduction, and Anxiety

Perhaps more than anything else in Western culture, Zen is associated with relaxation. Some of the earliest research on the psychophysiology of Zen related *zazen* to decreased physiological parameters associated with relaxation. Both Nagashima et al. (1977) and Hirai (1989) cited a 1964 study conducted by Sugi and Akutsu which found that the respiration rates of experienced Zen priests during *zazen* ranged from two to five breaths per minute, with an average of four breaths per minute. The typical adult breathes at a rate of 16–20 times per minute when resting (Barrett et al. 2010). The priests' oxygen consumption decreased markedly at the beginning of *zazen* and recovered immediately afterward. Oxygen consumption is a good measure of relaxation because relaxed muscles do not require as much oxygen as tensed muscles. Nagashima et al. (1977) observed that the oxygen consumption of an 83-year-old Zen master decreased from his baseline by 50% during meditation. Hirai also reported data indicating that oxygen consumption in two experienced priests decreased by 20–30% during *zazen* (1989).

Research on brain wave changes also pertains to the role of *zazen* in relaxation. Kasamatsu and Hirai (1966) and Hirai (1989) reported on a series of EEG studies, which included recordings of 48 Zen priests of both the Soto and Rinzai sects. They also made recordings of 98 Zen trainees of the same priests. A control sample, including 18 research fellows without prior *zazen* experience, was subjected to the same measurements during *zazen*. A summary of their most salient results, as presented by Hirai (1989), is as follows:

- Alpha wave activity appeared shortly after *zazen* started.
- Over the course of a *zazen* period, the participants showed increasing alpha wave amplitude and decreased alpha frequency.
- In some participants, rhythmical theta trains appeared.
- The more experience with *zazen* a priest had, the more likely he was to show decreased alpha wave frequency and the appearance of rhythmical theta trains.
- They did not find similar changes among control participants with no prior *zazen* experience.
- There were no differences between Rinzai and Soto priests.

Alpha activity is associated with relaxation (Austin 1998); both increased alpha amplitude and decreased alpha frequency are associated with relaxed states. Alpha biofeedback paradigms have traditionally been used to induce relaxation (Yates 1980). Theta activity has been related to relaxation and decreased anxiety (Kubota et al. 2001). From this standpoint, the results of these Japanese studies suggest a relationship between *zazen* and relaxation, also implying this relationship strengthens with increased *zazen* practice.

Subsequent studies generally have corroborated Hirai's findings regarding EEG changes. Hardt (1994) found that the more adept in Zen a student was rated by his or her teacher, the more likely he or she was to show increased alpha amplitude and decreased alpha frequency during *zazen*. Takahashi et al. (2005) trained adults with no meditation experience in *susoku*, a technique of *zazen* involving counting one's breath. They found increased fast theta and slow alpha activity, predominantly frontal, during meditation. Huang and Lo (2009) found increased alpha activity in experienced *zazen* practitioners, but not in controls. Murata et al. (1994) found that theta activity, particularly frontal, was found predominantly in more, as opposed to less, experienced Soto Zen priests.

Fumoto et al. (2004) trained meditation-naïve participants in voluntary abdominal breathing (VAB), a technique clearly derived from *tanden* breathing. As described earlier, *tanden* is deep abdominal breathing in which the lower abdomen remains expanded throughout the respiration cycle. Participants reported increased vigor activity and a tendency for reduced anxiety during VAB, compared to a resting period. These states were correlated with high-frequency alpha activity. Using a similar paradigm, Yu et al. (2011) taught novices without any prior meditation experience how to perform *tanden* breathing. In the subsequent 20-min meditation trial, they were asked to focus their awareness on their breathing. Compared to a resting period, the participants showed increase alpha activity and a decrease in theta.

Three studies investigated the effects of *zazen* on the anxiety levels in nonclinical samples; all three used psychological inventories as dependent measures. Goldman et al. (1979) taught college students *zazen*, which they then practiced daily for five days. They were compared to another group that taught “antimeditation” (e.g., numbers cancellation and symbol-digit tasks while tuning out background music) and a no-treatment control. All groups reported reduced anxiety, and there were no differences between the groups. Gillani and Smith (2001) compared experienced Zen meditators performing *zazen* for 70 min to a control group of college students who were asked to silently read magazines for 60 min. The *zazen* group reported decreased worry compared to the control group. Tloczynski (1994) also taught *zazen* to meditation-naïve college students. The *zazen* instructions involved “following the breath” as adapted from Shapiro and Giber (1978). They were compared to a group given instructions to “just relax” and to a no-treatment control. After six weeks of practice, both meditation and relaxation groups showed statistically significant reductions in anxiety, whereas the control group did not.

Lin et al. (2008) investigated the effects of *zazen* on performance anxiety and musical performance quality in participants recruited from conservatories. Participants were randomly assigned to either a meditation group or a wait list control group. Those in the meditation group were assigned to an 8-week meditation course of Soto-style Zen. There were no differences between the two groups in either self-reports of anxiety or quality of music performance as judged in a recital at the end of the program. However, evidence of a positive correlation between anxiety and musical quality was found in the meditation group alone.

Attention

Whether it is called mindfulness or *samadhi*, the development of concentration is central to Zen training. It is not surprising, therefore, that some of the earliest research on the psychophysiology of Zen pertained to attention. The EEG studies described above are relevant in that regard. The development of theta activity has been related to states of relaxed concentration (Kubota et al. 2001).

Another line of research, also going back to the early days of research on Zen, pertains to attention: alpha blocking. Typically, alpha activity is interrupted when a participant is initially exposed to a novel stimulus, such as a clicking noise. Over repeated presentations of the same stimulus in short sequence, the amount of alpha disruption is diminished (i.e., alpha blocking), as the participant habituates to the stimulus. This habituation can be seen as the participant’s ceasing to pay attention to the new stimulus.

Kasamatsu and Hirai (1966) compared three Zen masters performing *zazen* to three control participants, sitting with their eyes closed, in their degrees of alpha blocking subsequent to the presentation of the regular presentation of a clicking noise. They found that the control participants, who were research fellows with no Zen experience, showed steadily decreasing durations of alpha blocking over the course of stimuli presentation. On the other hand, the Zen masters’ duration of alpha blocking stayed the same throughout. In other words, the Zen masters remained keenly attentive to their environment, regardless of repetition; that is, their concentration did not tire. They remained in the "here and now" as they treated every repetition of the stimulus as a unique occurrence. This indicates increased ability to sustain attention on the part of the Zen masters.

Hirai (1989) later described a series of studies in which he found that control participants sitting with their eyes closed showed greater alpha blocking than Zen priests performing *zazen*. This was true regardless of the alpha-blocking stimulus (hand clapping, calling out names). He concluded that *zazen* "produces a condition that may be called relaxed awareness accompanied by steady responsiveness" (p. 74). One priest in the experiment described this state as "noticing every person on a street without looking back at them in emotional curiosity" (p. 63).

Becker and Shapiro (1981) were unable to replicate Kasamatsu and Hirai's (1984) and Hirai's (1989) earlier results. They found that 10 experienced Zen students recruited from an American Zen center did not show inhibition of alpha blocking after repeated exposure to clicks while performing *zazen*. Nor did they find trends indicating that those with more *zazen* experience show less habituation to the stimulus than those with less experience.

Kozasa et al. (2008) reported on a preliminary study in which one Zen nun and four "regular meditators" were tested before and after an eight-day *sesshin* (i.e., Zen retreat). In these tests, they were administered the Stroop Color Word Test, a test with high demand on attention, while undergoing functional magnetic resonance imagery (fMRI). The authors noted "enhanced activation" of the anterior cingulate, right dorsolateral prefrontal, insular, occipital, and parietal cortices after meditation practice. According to the literature, these areas represent functional activation related to attentional circuitry and reinforce the idea that meditation can further develop attentional abilities that have lasting effects (p. 366).

Pagnoni and Cekic (2007) studied the effects of *zazen* on gray matter volume and attention in aging participants. Typically, both gray matter volume and attention decline with increased age. The participants were 13 experienced Zen trainees. Control participants were matched for age, sex, and education level. Both groups were administered a continuous performance test (i.e., a measure of sustained attention) while undergoing fMRI. They found less age-related decline in the volume of the putamen, a cerebral structure strongly linked to attentional processing, in the meditators than in the controls. They also found that gray matter volume and performance on the attention task both correlated negatively for control participants; the meditators did not show a correlation between the two variables. Their findings suggest that regular meditation may reduce cognitive decline associated with normal aging due to relative preservation of gray matter volume.

Cardiovascular Health

In Ogata et al.'s (1984) study of mortality among Japanese priests, death by heart disease accounted for approximately half of the comparison cohort. The authors suggested that diet may have been a factor of the priests' greater longevity; in fact, Japanese Zen priests who ate a strict vegetarian diet were found to have more favorable lipid levels than matched meat-eating controls (Kita et al. 1988). Ogata et al. did mention, almost in passing, that the monks' practice of "self-control" might also have contributed to their longevity. Presumably, they were referring to the monks' meditative practice, and it is reasonable to suspect that intensive practice of *zazen* may have influenced their longevity.

Kim et al. (2005) studied the effect of Zen meditation on serum nitric oxide and on oxidative stress. Nitric oxide is known to improve vasodilation (i.e., widening of the blood vessels) and to decrease atherogenesis (i.e., plaque builds up in the arteries linked to heart disease). Oxidative stress has been implicated as a cause of atherogenesis and chronic heart disease; it was measured by serum malondialdehyde (MDA). Twenty experienced members of a Zen center in Korea were compared to age- and sex-matched control participants with no previous stress management or meditation training. Blood samples drawn before and after a 70-min meditation period showed that the meditators had significantly higher levels of nitric oxide and lower levels of MDA compared to the controls. Kormanovski et al. (2009) found unfavorable changes in serum lipid levels after six weeks of practice among Transcendental Meditation instructors who were taught *zazen*.

Heart rate variability (HRV) refers to variation in the intervals between heartbeats. A related phenomenon, respiratory sinus arrhythmia (RSA), occurs when HRV is synchronized with respiration (Yasuma and Hayano 2004), more specifically when heart rate increases during inhalation and decreases during exhalation. By reducing unnecessary heartbeats during exhalation, RSA provides rest for the heart. Thus, high cardiac variability is related to aerobic fitness and general physical activity. It declines with age, is a risk factor for hypertension, and predicts mortality among patients with cardiac disease. Cardiac variability is also related to vagus nerve tone (Thayer and Lane 2007) which is associated with positive cardiovascular health, and greater amplitude of RSA has been related to increased vagal tone (Lehrer 2001). Therefore, it is logical to deduce that practices that increase HRV and RSA, particularly the amplitude of respiratory and heart rate waves, may improve cardiovascular health.

Lehrer (2001) and Lehrer et al. (1999) studied cardiac variability in six Rinzai and five Soto Japanese priests over the course of a 20-min period of *tanden* breathing. They found that heart rate amplitudes increased during *zazen* in low-frequency wave ranges but decreased in the high-frequency range. Rinzai priests breathed slower and had high amplitudes of low-frequency heart rate waves than Soto priests. The authors concluded that "the elevations in HR low-frequency waves among Zen monks may explain the apparently salutary effects of Zen on heart disease" (p. 819).

Cysarz and Büssing (2005) studied nine participants; one had "long experience" with zazen, and one was "experienced" with Vipassana meditation, which is mindfulness-based. The remaining participants had no previous experience with any meditative discipline. Researchers found that the participants exhibited RSA during both *zazen* (i.e., concentrate on "just sitting" and "just breathing") and *kinhin* (i.e., walking meditation). They did not, however, compare those who were experienced in meditation to those who were meditation-naïve. Peressutti et al. (2010) found greater resonance between respiration and cardiac variability in more experienced Soto *zazen* practitioners compared to less experienced ones. Fiorentini et al. (2013) found that higher cardiac variability during a Zen retreat persisted into the next day.

Stone and DeLeo (1976) taught what they referred to as "psychologic-relaxation training" to mild-to-moderate hypertensive patients. This training, which was clearly modeled after *zazen*, involved sitting in a chair and counting breaths, as in *susoku*. The 19 patients were newly diagnosed, having previously had untreated hypertension, and were receiving care at a Veterans' Administration Hospital. Fifteen patients were arbitrarily assigned to the medication group on the basis of the researchers' perceptions of their abilities to understand the instructions, their motivation, and their willingness to participate in an experimental protocol. They were asked to practice the relaxation exercise for 10–15 min, twice daily, for six months. The remaining five patients were assigned to a control group and received only monthly blood pressure measurements. The blood pressure of the meditation group was significantly lower after six months of meditation, but there was no significant change of blood pressure in the control group. The average reduction in combined systolic and diastolic blood pressure in the former group was 12 mm Hg. Fifty-seven percent of the meditation group participants experienced at least a 14 mm Hg reduction with a range up to 30 mm Hg.

Pain Management

The traditional practice of Zen involves performing *zazen* in a seated cross-legged posture for long periods of time; moving is not permitted. This can become uncomfortable, if not painful, but Zen practitioners learn to cope with the pain through distraction, breathing, and relaxing tense muscles (Kushner 2000). It is conceivable, then, that the practice of *zazen* may have a role in pain management.

The analgesic effects of *zazen* have been studied in a series of reports by Grant and colleagues. Grant and Rainville (2009) compared 13 experienced Zen meditators, recruited from local centers, with matched controls. Participants in both groups were individually administered a painful thermal stimulus while they were in a supine position. The meditators required higher temperatures to elicit moderate pain. When instructed to attend to the pain "mindfully," the meditators reported decreased pain intensity, whereas the controls reported greater pain intensity when asked to concentrate on the pain. In the meditators, pain modulation was correlated with the slowing of respiration; no such association was found for the controls. The researchers concluded that Zen meditators have lower pain sensitivity and experience analgesic effects during mindful states. Using similar methodology, Grant's group (Grant et al. 2010) found that experienced *zazen* practitioners had greater cortical thickness (i.e., indicating more gray matter) than non-meditating controls in pain-related brain regions. Previous research (Teutsch et al. 2008) had shown that increased gray matter in pain-processing regions of the brain is associated with decreased pain sensitivity. Thus, the results of Grant et al. (2010) suggest that decreased pain sensitivity among Zen meditators may be related to morphological changes in the brain.

In yet another study, Grant et al. (2011) found that experienced Zen students, compared to non-meditating controls, had reduced activity in executive, evaluative, and emotional areas of the brain when exposed to a painful stimulus; additionally, the most experienced meditators showed the greatest reductions. They interpreted this to show that lower pain sensitivity in meditators was predictive of "a functional decoupling of the cognitive-evaluative component of pain, possibly allowing the practitioners to view painful stimuli more neutrally" (p. 151).

Depression

There are theoretical reasons why *zazen* may be beneficial for people with depression. The cognitive-behavioral model of psychotherapy for depression is predicated on the idea that fixation on dysfunctional automatic thoughts is implicated in the development and perpetuation of depression. Cognitive-behavioral therapists have developed techniques to "distance" patients from those negative cognitions (Teasdale et al. 1995). These techniques, in Beck's words, allow people to "examine thoughts as psychological phenomena rather than as identical to reality" (1976). I have previously written how the practice of *zazen* creates distance from unnecessary thought through the development of *samadhi* (Kushner 2012). By implication, *zazen* should enable an individual to create distance from negative automatic thoughts.

Yu et al. (2011) found that oxygenated hemoglobin (i.e., an index of activation of brain areas) in the anterior prefrontal cortex increased significantly during focused attention on *tanden* breathing in meditation-naïve participants. These changes were related to reductions in self-reported negative mood administered before and after the meditation task. Because previous research had implicated the anterior prefrontal cortex in emotion regulation, they hypothesized that the reduction in negative mood may have been mediated by activation of the anterior prefrontal cortex. Yu et al. and Fumoto et al. (2004) both found that serotonin (5-HT) levels increased during *tanden* breathing, compared to baseline measurements. Serotonin is a commonly known neurotransmitter implicated in the treatment of depression. Thus, on a theoretical level, zazen may improve mood through its actions on the serotonin system.

The Training and Effectiveness of Behavioral Health Practitioners

There are many theoretical reasons why the practice of *zazen* may enhance therapeutic effectiveness. In this section, we will focus our attention on the effects of behavioral health practitioners practicing *zazen*.

The development of empathy, intuition, and the ability to pay full and extended attention are key by-products of Zen training. This can result in enhanced therapeutic presence (Bruce and Davies 2005; Brenner 2009) or what my colleague, Gordon Greene Roshi (who authored Chapter "Zen, Pain, Suffering and Death" in this book) and I refer to as "Therapeutic Stance" (Kushner and Greene 2005). It has also been suggested that Zen training improves therapeutic intuition (Sayama 1986).

Lesh (1984) taught *zazen* to students enrolled in a master's degree program in counseling psychology. The specific *zazen* instructions included regulation of posture and counting one's breath while breathing diaphragmatically. The meditators were compared to two other groups: (1) master's degree students in other areas of study who were taking counseling psychology classes and volunteered to participate in the meditation program but who did not actually do so; and (2) another group of master's degree students in also other areas who were taking counseling psychology classes but who did not volunteer to participate in the meditation program. The *zazen* group practiced daily for 1 month. Lesh found that the meditation group improved on measures of empathy over the course of the study, whereas the others groups did not. However, level of concentration achieved in *zazen*, as determined by the ratings after each practice session, was not related to individual empathic abilities. They also found that participants who started out low in empathic ability were more likely to improve than participants high in this ability after 1 month of *zazen*.

Grepmair et al. (2006) compared the outcomes of patients who were in inpatient treatment with either psychotherapists in training who practiced Zen meditation before psychotherapy sessions or psychotherapists in training who did not practice Zen meditation. The setting was a "psychosomatic" hospital in Germany. The same psychotherapists participated in both nine-week phases of the study. In the first phase, no modifications were made to the therapists' training program. At the beginning of the second phase, the therapists all received instruction in *zazen* from a Zen master, who then led daily morning sittings for the group for the duration of the phase. Whereas the Zen master's tradition of Zen was not specified, his meditation technique involved focused attention on breathing while sitting on a cushion or chair. Data were collected on 196 patients throughout the study. The authors did not describe the diagnoses of the patients. Different patients were treated in each of the two phases of the study. Patients in both phases were blind as to whether their therapists were or were not engaging in *zazen*. The therapists and the Zen master were blind to the fact data had been collected on their patients. The results were that patients' symptom improvement was greater and ratings of their psychotherapy experiences were more favorable for the meditation phase than in the control phase.

Summary

What, then, have we learned from the studies reviewed above?

Relaxation, stress management, and anxiety. Early psychophysiological studies indicate that physiological parameters associated with relaxation (i.e., decreased respiration and decreased metabolism) are also associated with *zazen*, at least in experienced practitioners. The cumulative results of the various EEG studies described above strongly suggest that brain wave activity with relaxation (i.e., slow wave alpha and theta activity) is associated with *zazen*. The latter appears to be more prominent in more experienced Zen trainees; thus, it requires a considerable amount more experience and skill in the meditative discipline. It should be noted that the associations between *zazen* and increased alpha and theta activity has not been born out in all studies. Notably, Fumoto et al. (2004) found that *tanden* breathing was associated with high-frequency alpha. In a study using a similar methodology, Yu et al. (2011) found that *tanden* breathing was associated with decreased theta activity. However, both the studies used meditation-naïve participants who received minimal training in the breathing technique. This led Yu et al. to speculate that the increase of theta during zazen might be a function of experience with *zazen*. The literature to date on physiological parameters and *zazen* has focused almost exclusively on the changes during meditation or immediately after its termination. The lasting effects of *zazen* on brain waves have not been studied.

Despite the promise shown by the psychophysiological studies indicating that *zazen* induces relaxation, there is an almost total absence of studies that have examined the efficacy of *zazen* in stress management programs or clinically anxious populations. Lin et al.'s (2008) investigation of the effects of *zazen* on a self-identified anxious population of musicians is the exception. They demonstrated that *zazen* was beneficial to musicians with higher levels of performance anxiety.

Attention. There is physiological evidence that the practice of *zazen* may increase attention. In particular, theta activity, associated with *zazen*, at least in experienced meditators, promotes a state of relaxed alertness. Similarly, alpha-blocking studies provide evidence that experience with Zen training leads to sustained attention. The results of Kozasa et al. (2008) indicate that the benefits of *zazen* on attention may extend past periods of meditation. Results from Pagnoni and Cekic's (2007) work suggest that attentional improvements brought about by *zazen* may be due to morphological changes in the brain and that these changes may inhibit the decline in attention seen in the normal aging process. In spite of the psychophysiological evidence suggesting that *zazen* may improve attention, to date no studies have examined *zazen* as way of enhancing attention in nonclinical populations or as a treatment for Attention Deficit/Hyperactivity Disorder.

Cardiovascular health. There is evidence that HRV and RSA, which have been related to cardiac health, are strengthened with *zazen*. The results of Cysarz and Büssing (2005) indicate that this might be true for novice Zen practitioners, not just advanced practitioners. There is evidence that the practice of *zazen* may decrease oxidative stress and increase serum nitric oxide; both outcomes have been related to cardiovascular health. There is also evidence that *zazen* may reduce blood pressure among mild-to-moderate hypertensive patients.

Pain. There is evidence that experienced Zen practitioners may have lower pain sensitivity compared to non-meditators. To date, there have been no studies of the use of *zazen* as an analgesic measure in clinical populations.

Depression. There is evidence suggesting that *zazen* may increase positive mood, even in novice meditators, and that such improvement may be mediated by changes in blood serotonin levels. To date, there have been no studies of the use of *zazen* in the treatment of clinically depressed populations.

The Training and Effectiveness of Behavioral Health Practitioners. There is evidence that *zazen* may improve empathy of counselors in training. More impressive is evidence from a randomized double-blind study that the outcomes of psychotherapist trainees who participate in *zazen* are better than those of trainees who do not meditate.

Type of Zazen. There is little evidence of differences among the traditions of *zazen*. Whereas there are accounts of experienced Rinzai practitioners breathing more slowly than experienced Soto practitioners (Lehrer et al. 1999; Hirai 1989), these were based on observations of small samples and are almost anecdotal. Hirai (1989) found no differences in EEGs of experienced Soto and Rinzai practitioners. Similarly, there are no studies that have investigated whether modifications to *zazen* [e.g., performing it while supine (Grant et al. 2011) or sitting in chairs (Stone and DeLeo 1976)] affect its underlying physiological effects.

Experience with Zazen. The *zazen* training experience of the participants in the studies reviewed ranged from several hours to decades. The little data available on the effects of training are found in the EEG studies. These data suggest that slow alpha and theta activity increases with training. Few studies utilized internal measures to determine whether the participants had properly learned how to practice *zazen*. Lesh (1984) used logs of participants' subjective experiences with *zazen*. Both Fumoto et al. (2004) and Yu et al. reported that by using biofeedback, they were able to teach *tanden* breathing in one session to participants unfamiliar with meditation. This was confirmed by physiological monitoring of their breathing.

As noted above, both Fumoto et al. (2004) and Yu et al. (2011) obtained results that contradicted previous research on more experienced Zen practitioners (notably Hirai 1989). This prompted Yu et al. to suggest that their results may have reflected their use of novice practitioners. This raises the important but unanswered question of how long it takes to learn the techniques of *zazen* in order to experience health benefits. Based upon my experience as both a Zen student and Zen instructor, the learning curve for *zazen* can be steep. This can explain the somewhat surprising results of Kormanovski et al. (2009) who found that cholesterol levels changed in unfavorable directions after six weeks of *zazen*. Further, the fact that their participants were teachers of another meditative discipline (Transcendental Meditation) may not have predisposed them to attain proficiency in *zazen* more quickly than other people. One could argue that it might have taken them longer because they may have had difficulty abandoning their habitual way of meditating. On the other hand, other studies found positive benefits after minimal zazen training. Cysarz and Büssing (2005) found positive effects on HRV in their participants, most of whom had no prior *zazen* experience. Lin et al. (2008) found positive benefits on the music quality of performance-anxious musicians (albeit it only among the most anxious musicians) after eight weeks of *zazen* training. These studies suggest that it may be possible for people to experience health benefits after relatively little *zazen* training.

Discussion

In his 2009 review of research on Zen, Chiesa wrote, "In conclusion, actual evidence on Zen meditation is scarce and does not allow us to reach definitive conclusions" (2009, p. 591). The same can be said today. Chiesa did provide some evidence that zazen is related to increased (slow) alpha and theta activity, especially among more experienced practitioners, that it could be useful for reducing stress and high blood pressure, and that it might prevent age-associated cognitive decline. The current review provides additional evidence suggesting that *zazen* might have applicability in the promotion of cardiac health, to the treatment of anxiety, depression, and attention problems, and to the control of pain. There is also evidence that *zazen* might improve the therapeutic effectiveness of behavioral health practitioners, at least in trainees. Ultimately, there is an almost total absence of research on the effectiveness of *zazen* in clinical populations. In short, we are left more with a road map for future research than with a firm base of evidence supporting the clinical efficacy of *zazen*.

Of all the studies reviewed in this chapter, only two of them involved actual clinical samples: Stone and DeLeo's (1976) study of the treatment of mild-to-moderate hypertensive patients and Grepmair et al.'s study of the effects on patients of therapists in training practicing *zazen*. Both studies found *zazen* to be effective. In the case of Stone and DeLeo, patients who engaged in *zazen* experienced significant reductions in blood pressure. Grepmair et al. (2006) found that psychiatric inpatients in treatment with trainees who did *zazen* had greater symptom reduction and better evaluations of their therapy experiences. Both studies had design flaws. Stone et al. had a small sample size (19 in the treatment groups, 5 in the control group), and the selection and assignment of the participants were, in the words of the researchers, "arbitrary." Grepmair et al. had a fairly large sample size (119 patients), and they kept patients and therapists blind to their conditions, but the control participants were treated earlier in the year than the participants whose therapists were sitting *zazen*. Thus, the better outcomes of the patients in the second phase of the study may have been due to the fact their therapists were more skilled in general at that time. A third study, Lin et al. (2008), while failing to use an actual clinical sample, recruited musicians with self-described performance anxiety. They found that *zazen* was effective only for more anxious participants.

The American Psychological Association has established criteria for empirically supported treatments[2] (Task Force on Promotion and Dissemination of Psychological Procedures 1995). In them, a distinction is made between *well-established* and *probably efficacious* empirically supported treatments. Although these criteria have been controversial (Church et al. 2014; Norcross et al. 2006), and the designation "empirically supported" does not necessarily imply that it is more efficacious than others, the American Psychological Association criteria provide a good reference point of how many in the field evaluate the evidence base of treatments. On the basis of those criteria, *zazen* cannot be designated either a *well-established* or *probably efficacious* treatment for any specific behavioral or medical disorder.

Regardless, lack of evidence is not evidence of lack of effectiveness. The lack of empirical evidence of the efficacy of *zazen* is based largely on a paucity of empirical investigation of its utility and should not stifle innovation in the application of *zazen* in clinical contexts. Despite its prominence in the early days of meditation research, *zazen* has languished in a research backwater. This is unfortunate because *zazen* has much to offer, as should be evident from the other chapters of this book. Perhaps this chapter will serve as encouragement to include *zazen* in the research agenda of behavioral health researchers. Basic questions remain that should be addressed in the future:

- For what conditions is *zazen* appropriate as a treatment? The obvious first choices, based on the literature, are anxiety disorders, attention problems, depression, and hypertension.
- How can zazen be used in coordination with other treatments?
- How long does it take to attain adequate proficiency with *zazen* for a patient to receive benefit from it? Whereas the fact that an octogenarian Zen master can reduce his oxygen consumption by 50% may have scientific interest, it may not be relevant to the question of how quickly an anxious patient can expect to benefit from *zazen*.
- Are some techniques of *zazen* (e.g., following the breath versus regulating the breath, or *tanden* breathing) easier to learn or more efficacious than others? Which techniques are most effective for what problems?
- What modifications to *zazen* may be made for it to be more applicable in a behavioral health setting? Of particular concern is posture; many Westerners have difficulty with the traditional postures for *zazen*: the full and half lotus positions. Can the benefits of *zazen* be preserved if other postures are used?
- What is the role of zazen in the prevention of physical, psychological, or comorbid problems?

Limitations

This review has several limitations. First, it is not systematic in that I selected the articles; there was no independent vetting process. Second, I only reviewed publications written in English. Third, by limiting the search to publications specifically involving Zen *or zazen*, I did not

[2]**Criteria for Empirically Supported Treatments** (Paraphrased from Chamblis and Task Force on Promotion and Dissemination of Psychological Procedures 1995) *Well-established*: Manualized treatments researched by at least two different investigators, using well-specified client samples with either (A) two or more between-group studies showing superiority to placebo or another treatment, and/or equivalence to an established treatment in an adequately powered study or (B) a large series of well-designed single-case studies demonstrating efficacy compared to another intervention as in "A" above. *Probably Effective*: Two studies showing superiority to waiting-list control or one or more studies meeting criteria for A above but only one investigator or two or more positive studies but heterogeneous samples or a small series of well-designed single-case studies.

discuss contributions of research on other forms of meditation that may still relate to the efficacy of *zazen* in behavioral health.

Coda

Whenever a prospective Zen student contacts me, I first have a face-to-face meeting with them. I ask them why they want to study Zen. Almost without exception, they describe a utilitarian reason, such as wanting to feel less stressed, wanting to be more effective at work, or wanting to get over a breakup. Others hope to control long-standing depression or anxiety. One person told me he wanted to live longer. He believed that we are all born with an upper limit of the number of breaths we can take in a lifetime and he thought that he could extend his life by learning to slow down his breathing.

All of these motivations for starting Zen training are important and meaningful. They reflect a larger trend in our society as meditative disciplines become equated with health and mental health (Wilson 2014). However, it is misleading to view Zen or any Buddhist meditative tradition, if not any religion for that matter, solely in utilitarian terms.

In the foundational story of Buddhism, Shakyamuni Buddha left the comfort of his palace to find the answers to burning existential doubt. He did not leave to become less stressed or a more effective heir apparent to the throne of his kingdom. The religion that grew out of this experience was fundamentally designed to help people come to grips with basic questions of existence. States of relaxation or attention are perquisites for this; they are not ends in and of themselves. Benefits to health or mental health that arise from *zazen*, while certainly desirable, are essentially by-products of the search for one's true nature. To paraphrase my colleague, Stephen Kow Roshi, "the question of whether Zen training benefits your health is misguided. The question should be whether Zen can help you fearlessly face ill health and death."

In this review, I took a decidedly dualistic approach to Zen by focusing narrowly on scientifically based evidence for the applicability of *zazen* to behavioral health. But, from a different, hopefully less dualistic perspective, the research on Zen should have no effect on the practice or significance of Zen. It will remain a vital way for dedicated people to answer critical existential questions.

On the other hand, if aspects of Zen training can reduce the suffering of a larger group of people, this would be in keeping with a basic Buddhist tenet. Gordon Greene Roshi has articulated a distinction between training *in* Zen and training *by* Zen. Training in Zen refers to people who commit themselves to intensive Zen training. Training *by* Zen refers to the application of Zen principles to help people in their daily lives. The use of *zazen* in the context of behavioral health clearly fits into the rubric of training *by* Zen, and Zen has much to offer the world in that context.

References

Austin, J. H. (1998). *Zen and the brain*. Cambridge, MA: MIT Press.

Barrett, K., Barman, S., Boitano, S., & Brooks, H. (2010). *Ganong's review of medical physiology*. New Delhi: McGraw Hill.

Beck, A. T. (1976). *Cognitive therapy and the emotional disorders*. New York: International Universities Press.

Becker, D. E., & Shapiro, D. (1981). Physiological responses to clicks during Zen, Yoga, and TM meditation. *Psychophysiology, 18*(6), 694–699.

Brenner, M. J. (2009). Zen practice: A training method to enhance the skills of clinical social workers. *Social Work in Health Care, 48*(4), 462–470. doi:10.1080/00981380802589860

Bruce, A., & Davies, B. (2005). Mindfulness in hospice care: Practicing meditation-in-action. *Qualitative Health Research, 15*(10), 1329–1344. doi:10.1177/1049732305281657

Cahn, B. R., & Polich, J. (2006). Meditation states and traits: EEG, ERP, and neuroimaging studies. *Psychological Bulletin, 132*(2), 180–211. doi:10.1037/0033-2909.132.2.180

Canter, P. H. (2003). The therapeutic effects of meditation. *British Medical Journal, 326*(7398), 1049–1050.

Canter, P. H., & Ernst, E. (2004). Insufficient evidence to conclude whether or not transcendental meditation decreases blood pressure: Results of a systematic review of randomized clinical trials. *Journal of Hypertension.*

Cappo, B. M., & Holmes, D. S. (1984). The utility of prolonged respiratory exhalation for reducing physiological and psychological arousal in non-threatening and threatening situations. *Journal of Psychosomatic Research, 28*(4), 265–273.

Caspi, O., & Burleson, K. O. (2007). Methodological challenges in meditation research. *Advances in Mind-Body Medicine, 22*(3–4), 36–43.

Chan, R. R., & Larson, J. L. (2015). Meditation interventions for chronic disease populations: A systematic review. *Journal of Holistic Nursing: Official Journal of the American Holistic Nurses' Association*, 1–15. doi:10.1177/0898010115570363

Chiesa, A. (2009). Zen meditation: An integration of current evidence. *The Journal of Alternative and Complementary Medicine, 15*(5), 585–592. doi:10.1089/acm.2008.0416

Chiesa, A., & Malinowski, P. (2011). Mindfulness-based approaches: Are they all the same? *Journal of Clinical Psychology, 67*(4), 404–424. doi:10.1002/jclp.20776

Chiesa, A., & Serretti, A. (2011). Mindfulness-based interventions for chronic pain: A systematic review of the evidence. *The Journal of Alternative and Complementary Medicine, 17*(1), 83–93. doi:10.1089/acm.2009.0546

Church, D., Feinstein, D., Palmer-Hoffman, J., Stein, P. K., & Tranguch, A. (2014). Empirically supported psychological treatments: The challenge of evaluating clinical innovations. *The Journal of Nervous and Mental Disease, 202*(10), 699–709. doi:10.1097/NMD.0000000000000188

Cysarz, D., & Büssing, A. (2005). Cardiorespiratory synchronization during Zen meditation. *European Journal of Applied Physiology, 95*(1), 88–95. doi:10.1007/s00421-005-1379-3

Dear, J. W., Gough, K., & Webb, D. J. (2008). Transcendental meditation and hypertension. *Postgraduate Medical Journal, 84*(994), 417.

Fiorentini, A., Ora, J., & Tubani, L. (2013). Autonomic system modification in Zen practitioners. *Indian Journal of Medical Science, 67*(7), 161. doi:10.4103/0019-5359.125877

Fortney, L., & Taylor, M. (2010). Meditation in medical practice: A review of the evidence and practice. *Primary Care, 37*(1), 81–90. doi:10.1016/j.pop.2009.09.004

Fumoto, M., Sato-Suzuki, I., Seki, Y., Mohri, Y., & Arita, H. (2004). Appearance of high-frequency alpha band with disappearance of low-frequency alpha band in EEG is produced during voluntary abdominal breathing in an eyes-closed condition. *Neuroscience Research, 50*(3), 307–317. doi:10.1016/j.neures.2004.08.005

Gillani, N. B., & Smith, J. C. (2001). Zen meditation and ABC relaxation theory: An exploration of relaxation states, beliefs, dispositions, and motivations. *Journal of Clinical Psychology, 57*(6), 839–846.

Goldman, B. L., Domitor, P. J., & Murray, E. J. (1979). Effects of Zen meditation on anxiety reduction and perceptual functioning. *Journal of Consulting and Clinical Psychology, 47*(3), 551–556.

Goleman, D. (1988). *The meditative mind: The varieties of meditative experience*. New York: Putnam.

Grant, J. A. (2013). Meditative analgesia: The current state of the field. *Annals of the New York Academy of Science, 1307*(1), 55–63. doi:10.1111/nyas.12282

Grant, J. A., Courtemanche, J., Duerden, E. G., Duncan, G. H., & Rainville, P. (2010). Cortical thickness and pain sensitivity in Zen meditators. *Emotion, 10*(1), 43–53. doi:10.1037/a0018334

Grant, J. A., Courtemanche, J., & Rainville, P. (2011). A non-elaborative mental stance and decoupling of executive and pain-related cortices predicts low pain sensitivity in Zen meditators. *Pain, 152*(1), 150–156. doi:10.1016/j.pain.2010.10.006

Grant, J. A., & Rainville, P. (2009). Pain sensitivity and analgesic effects of mindful states in Zen meditators: A cross-sectional study. *Psychosomatic Medicine, 71* (1), 106–114. doi:10.1097/PSY.0b013e31818f52ee

Grepmair, L., Mitterlehner, F., Rother, W., & Nickel, M. (2006). Promotion of mindfulness in psychotherapists in training and treatment results of their patients. *Journal of Psychosomatic Research, 60*(6), 649–650. doi:10.1016/j.jpsychores.2006.04.003

Hardt, J. V. (1994). Proficiency in Zen meditation-correspondence with multichannel EEG coherence spectrum. *International Journal of Psychophysiology, 18*(2), 112–113.

Hirai, T. (1989). *Zen meditation and psychotherapy*. Tokyo; New York: Japan Publications.

Hofmann, S. G., Sawyer, A. T., Witt, A. A., & Oh, D. (2010). The effect of mindfulness-based therapy on anxiety and depression: A meta-analytic review. *Journal of Consulting and Clinical Psychology, 78* (2), 169–183. doi:10.1037/a0018555

Huang, H. Y., & Lo, P. C. (2009). EEG dynamics of experienced Zen meditation practitioners probed by complexity index and spectral measure. *Journal of Medical Engineering Technology, 33*(4), 314–321. doi:10.1080/03091900802602677

Kabat-Zinn, J. (1990). *Full catastrophe living: Using the wisdom of your body and mind to face stress, pain and illness*. New York, NY: Delta Publishing.

Kasamatsu, A., & Hirai, T. (1966). An electroencephalographic study on the Zen meditation (Zazen). *Psychiatry and Clinical Neurosciences, 20*(4), 315–336. doi:10.1111/j.1440-1819.1966.tb02646.x

Kasamatsu, A., & Hirai, T. (1984). An electroencephalographic study of the Zen meditation (Zazen). In *Meditation, classic and contemporary perspectives*. New York: Aldine Publishing Company.

Kim, D. H., Moon, Y. S., Kim, H. S., Jung, J. S., Park, H. M., Suh, H. W., et al. (2005). Effect of Zen meditation on serum nitric oxide activity and lipid peroxidation. *Progress in Neuro-Psychopharmacology and Biological Psychiatry, 29*(2), 327–331.

Kita, T., Yokode, M., Kume, N., Ishii, K., Nagano, Y., Mikami, A., et al. (1988). The concentration of serum lipids in Zen monks and control males in Japan. *Japanese Circulation Journal, 52*(2), 99–104.

Kormanovski, A., Padilla, E. L., Rodriguez, R. C., & Harasymowicz, J. (2009). Metabolic effects of a Zen meditation and qigong training program on sedentary people. *Archives of Budo, 5*, 15–19.

Kozasa, E. H., Radvany, J., Barreiros, M. A. M., Leite, J. R., & Amaro, E. (2008). Preliminary functional magnetic resonance imaging Stroop task results before and after a Zen meditation retreat. *Psychiatry and Clinical Neurosciences, 62*(3), 366. doi:10.1111/j.1440-1819.2008.01809.x

Krisanaprakornkit, T., Ngamjarus, C., Witoonchart, C., & Piyavhatkul, N. (2010). Meditation therapies for attention-deficit/hyperactivity disorder (ADHD). *Cochrane Database Systematic Reviews*, (6), CD006507. doi:10.1002/14651858.CD006507.pub2

Kubota, Y., Sato, W., Toichi, M., Murai, T., Okada, T., Hayashi, A., et al. (2001). Frontal midline theta rhythm is correlated with cardiac autonomic activities during the performance of an attention demanding meditation procedure. *Cognitive Brain Research, 11* (2), 281–287.

Kushner, K. (2000). *One arrow, one life: Zen, archery and enlightenment*. Boston: Tuttle.

Kushner, K. (2012). You cannot wash off blood with blood: Entering the mind through the body. *Explore (NY), 8*(4), 243–248. doi:10.1016/j.explore.2012.04.002

Kushner, K., & Greene, G. (2005). Seeing 180 degrees: A Zen perspective on the medical encounter. *Medical Encounter*, 3–5.

Lehrer, P. (2001). Biofeedback for respiratory sinus arrhythmia and tanden breathing among zen monks: Studies in cardiovascular resonance. In Y. Haruki, A. Umezawa, I. Homma, & Y. Masaoka (Eds.), *Respiration and emotion* (pp. 113–120). Tokyo: Respiration and Emotion. doi:10.1007/978-4-431-67901-1_11

Lehrer, P., Sasaki, Y., & Saito, Y. (1999). Zazen and cardiac variability. *Psychosomatic Medicine, 61*(6), 812–821.

Lesh, T. V. (1984). Zen meditation and the development of empathy in counselors. In *Meditation, classic and contemporary perspectives*. New York: Aldine Publishing Company.

Lin, P., Chang, J., Zemon, V., & Midlarsky, E. (2008). Silent illumination: A study on Chan (Zen) meditation, anxiety, and musical performance quality. *Psychology of Music, 36*(2), 139–155. doi:10.1177/0305735607080840

Marchand, W. R. (2013). Mindfulness meditation practices as adjunctive treatments for psychiatric disorders. *Psychiatric Clinics of North America, 36*(1), 141–152. doi:10.1016/j.psc.2013.01.002

Murata, T., Omori, M., Murata, I., Nishio, M., Koshino, Y., Sakamoto, K., et al. (1994). Quantitative EEG study on Zen meditation (Zazen). *Japanese Journal of Psychiatry and Neurology, 48*(4), 881–890.

Nagashima, C., Ikawa, Y., & Akishige, Y. (1977). Studies of "Josoku". In Y. Akishige (Ed.), *Psychology of Zen*. Tokyo: Komazawa University.

Norcross, J. C., Beutler, L. E., & Levant, R. F. (2006). *Evidence-based practices in mental health: Debate and dialogue on the fundamental questions*. Washington, DC: American Psychological Association.

Ogata, M., Ikeda, M., & Kuratsune, M. (1984). Mortality among Japanese Zen priests. *Journal of Epidemiology and Community Health, 38*(2), 161–166.

Ospina, M. B., Bond, K., Karkhaneh, M., Tjosvold, L., Vandermeer, B., Liang, Y., et al. (2007). Meditation practices for health: State of the research. *Evidence Report/Technology Assessment, 155*, 1–263.

Pagnoni, G., & Cekic, M. (2007). Age effects on gray matter volume and attentional performance in Zen meditation. *Neurobiology of Aging, 28*(10), 1623–1627. doi:10.1016/j.neurobiolaging.2007.06.008

Pagnoni, G., Cekic, M., & Guo, Y. (2008). "Thinking about not-thinking": Neural correlates of conceptual processing during Zen meditation. *PLoS One, 3*(9), e3083. doi:10.1371/journal.pone.0003083

Peressutti, C., Martín-González, J. M., García-Manso, J. M., & Mesa, D. (2010). Heart rate dynamics in different levels of Zen meditation. *International Journal of Cardiology, 145*(1), 142–146. doi:10.1016/j.ijcard.2009.06.058

Sayama, M. (1986). *Samadhi: Self development in Zen, swordsmanship, and psychotherapy*. Albany, New York: SUNY.

Sedlmeier, P., Eberth, J., Schwarz, M., Zimmermann, D., Haarig, F., Jaeger, S., et al. (2012). The psychological effects of meditation: A meta-analysis. *Psychological Bulletin, 138*(6), 1139–1171. doi:10.1037/a0028168

Sekida, K. (1985). *Zen training: Methods and philosophy*. New York: Weatherhill.

Shapiro, D. H. J., & Giber, D. (1978). Meditation and psychotherapeutic effects. Self-regulation strategy and altered state of consciousness. [Review] [132 refs]. *Archives of General Psychiatry, 35*(3), 294–302.

Stone, R. A., & DeLeo, J. (1976). Psychotherapeutic control of hypertension. *New England Journal of Medicine, 294*(2), 80–84. doi:10.1056/NEJM197601082940204

Takahashi, T., Murata, T., Hamada, T., Omori, M., Kosaka, H., Kikuchi, M., et al. (2005). Changes in EEG and autonomic nervous activity during meditation and their association with personality traits. *International Journal of Psychophysiology, 55*(2), 199–207. doi:10.1016/j.ijpsycho.2004.07.004

Task Force on Promotion and Dissemination of Psychological Procedures. (1995). Training in and dissemination of empirically-validated psychological treatments. *The Clinical Psychologist, 48*(1), 2–23. doi:10.1037/e554972011-003

Teasdale, J. D., Segal, Z., & Williams, J. M. (1995). How does cognitive therapy prevent depressive relapse and why should attentional control (mindfulness) training help?. [Review] [30 refs]. *Behaviour Research & Therapy, 33*(1), 25–39.

Teutsch, S., Herken, W., Bingel, U., Schoell, E., & May, A. (2008). Changes in brain gray matter due to repetitive painful stimulation. *Neuroimage, 42*(2), 845–849.

Thayer, J. F., & Lane, R. D. (2007). The role of vagal function in the risk for cardiovascular disease and mortality. *Biological Psychology, 74*(2), 224–242. doi:10.1016/j.biopsycho.2005.11.013

Tloczynski, J. (1994). A preliminary study of opening-up meTeutsch, S., Herken, W.,Bingel, U., Schoell, E. May, A. (2008). Changes in brain gray matter due to repetitive painful stimulation. Neuroimage, 42(2), 845-849.ditation college adjustment, and self-actualization. *Psychological Reports, 75*(1 Pt 2), 449–450.

Von Durckheim, K. G. (1980). *Hara: The vital centre of man*. London: Allen and Unwin.

Weaver, A. J., Vane, A., & Flannelly, K. J. (2008). A Review of Research on Buddhism and Health: 1980–2003. *Journal of Health Care Chaplaincy, 14* (2), 118–132. doi:10.1080/08854720802129075

Wilson, J. T. (2014). *Mindful America: The mutual transformation of Buddhist meditation and American culture*. New York, NY: Oxford University.

Yasuma, F., & Hayano, J.-I. (2004). Respiratory sinus arrhythmia: Why does the heartbeat synchronize with respiratory rhythm? *Chest, 125*(2), 683–690. doi:10.1378/chest.125.2.683

Yates, A. (1980). *Biofeedback and the modification of behavior*. New York, NY: Plenum.

Yu, X., Fumoto, M., Nakatani, Y., Sekiyama, T., Kikuchi, H., Seki, Y., et al. (2011). Activation of the anterior prefrontal cortex and serotonergic system is associated with improvements in mood and EEG changes induced by Zen meditation practice in novices. *International Journal of Psychophysiology, 80*(2), 103–111. doi:10.1016/j.ijpsycho.2011.02.004

Zgierska, A., Rabago, D., Chawla, N., Kushner, K., Koehler, R., & Marlatt, A. (2009). Mindfulness meditation for substance use disorders: A systematic review. *Substance Abuse, 30*(4), 266–294. doi:10.1080/08897070903250019

Zen and Psychotherapy

Peiwei Li and Daniel Rodriguez Ramirez

Keywords
Zen · Buddhism · Psychotherapy · Suffering · Self · No self · Emptiness · Liberation · Emancipation · Dialectics · Mindfulness

Your vision will become clear only when you can look into your own heart. Who looks outside, dreams; who looks inside, awakes.

Carl Jung, Memories, Dreams, Reflections

To study the Buddha Way is to study the self. To study the self is to forget the self. To forget the self is to be verified by all beings. To be verified by all things is to let the body and mind of the self and the body and mind of others drop off. There is a trace of realization that cannot be grasped. We endlessly express this ungraspable trace of realization.

Dōgen Zenji, Genjokoan

Introduction

In recent years, there has been an unprecedented influence of Buddhism in Western psychology and psychotherapy. Expressions such as "mindfulness," "meditation," and "Zen" have become buzzwords across the academic and the popular culture alike. This has been accompanied by the increased popularity of various mindfulness-informed therapeutic modalities, including acceptance and commitment therapy (ACT; Hayes 2004; Hayes et al. 1999; Hayes et al. 2006), dialectical behavioral therapy (DBT; Linehan 1987, 1995, 2013), mindfulness-based stress reduction (MBSR; Kabat-Zinn 1990, 1994; Kabat-Zinn and Hanh 2009), mindfulness-based cognitive therapy (MBCT; Teasdale and Segal 2007), and Zen therapy (Brazier 1997, 2001) (see more discussion below). Although these approaches do not always articulate an explicit connection to Buddhism as a religion, they all seem to draw insights from Buddhist teachings, at least through forms of secularized discourses such as mindfulness.

Meanwhile, the influence of Zen in psychotherapy seems to be cast against the backdrop of a surge of epidemics of mental health

P. Li (✉)
Springfield College, Springfield, USA
e-mail: pli@springfieldcollege.edu

D.R. Ramirez
University of California Santa Cruz, Santa Cruz, USA
e-mail: drodri37@ucsc.edu

A. Masuda and W.T. O'Donohue (eds.), *Handbook of Zen, Mindfulness, and Behavioral Health*, Mindfulness in Behavioral Health, DOI 10.1007/978-3-319-54595-0_15

conditions. World Health Organization reported that more than 350 million people suffer from depression globally (WHO 2012). In the USA alone, about 18.1% or 42 million people experience an anxiety disorder in any given year (Kessler et al. 2005). With these staggering statistics, we cannot help but ponder the meaning of this parallel: Why do we resort to Eastern ideas such as Buddhism now? What is the underlying impetus? Where do Buddhism, a 2500-year-old Eastern religion, and psychotherapy, a Western invention of psychological treatment, converge and diverge? Is Zen just an influence on psychotherapy, or is Zen psychotherapy a deliberate reaction to Western psychotherapy? These are the questions that we will be wrestling with throughout this chapter. It is worth noting that we will mainly focus on Zen Buddhism (hereafter "Zen") in our discussion although other forms of cross-fertilization between different sects of Buddhism (e.g., Tibetan Buddhism) and psychotherapy have flourished as well in recent decades.

Zen has been among the earliest influence of Buddhism in psychotherapy in the West. It was first brought to the USA by Chinese immigrants in the mid-nineteenth century[1] (Masis 2002) and became popular due to the teachings of Japanese Zen teachers and scholars such as D.T. Suzuki and Shunryu Suzuki, as well as the writings of psychoanalysts like Carl Jung, Karen Horney, and Eric Fromm (Ando 2009; Cooper 2010; Masis 2002). Interestingly, despite the existence of diverse sects of Buddhism, Zen has always been a primary focus of study for Western psychology (Muramoto 2003), likely due to the historical engagement between Western psychoanalysts and Japanese Zen Buddhists who opened the door for reciprocal learning and understanding.

To ground our discussion, we will first provide a brief historical sketch about the origin of the synergy between Zen and psychotherapy. We will then examine a few key underlying concepts that bind and distinguish the two traditions, followed by specific examples of how Zen and certain therapeutic orientations intersect, and a brief case discussion. With this foundation, we will critically reflect on the current trends and applications of Zen in psychotherapy. We will share our observations about potential problems that could hinder the full potential of their cross-fertilization toward emancipation and transformation.

The Encounter of Zen and Psychotherapy: A Brief Sketch

The increase of psychological interest in Buddhism coincided with the popularization of Buddhist practices in the West. When Buddhism became more mainstream in the 1960s in both Europe and America, it opened the door for communication and collaboration between Buddhist philosophers/practitioners and Western psychoanalysts. The encounter of Zen and psychotherapy has been documented by various scholars (Ando 2009; Kato 2005; Masis 2002; Maupin 1962). The impetus for dialogue between the two came from both the East and the West. On the one hand, a generation of Japanese scholars were interested in communicating to their Western counterparts about Zen, while others were studying Zen through psychological means (for a detailed account see Kato 2005). For example, the publication of "Psychology of Zen Sect" by Enryo Inoue in 1893 is considered the first academic publication regarding Zen and psychology. Similarly, K. Ataka's article titled, "Psychology of Zen," is considered the first reference with "Zen" as a keyword in the PsycINFO database (Kato 2005), one of the most popular psychology databases today. Other Japanese psychologists (e.g., Kasamatsu and Hirai 1966) also focused on empirically and scientifically investigating the psychophysiological effects of Zen practice (Muramoto 1984, 2003).

On the other hand, prominent psychoanalysts in the 1950s and 1960s—Fromm (1960), Fromm, Suszuki, & Demartino (1960), Horney (1945, 1952), and Kelman (1960) all became ambassadors of Western intellectual thought who

[1]The equivalence of "Zen" in Chinese Buddhism is "Chan," or "禅". "Chan" and "Zen" are not identical due to the influence of indigenous culture, Taoism (China) and Shintoism (Japan), respectively.

participated in dialogues with Japanese Zen scholars, teachers, and philosophers (Cooper 2010). They exhibited deep interest in studying Zen and incorporated it into their writings and practice. In particular, Fromm's collaboration with D.T. Suzuki left behind the volume on *Zen Buddhism and psychoanalysis* (Fromm et al. 1960), perhaps the earliest and most influential work that has inspired ongoing dialogues between the East and the West on this topic. Another historical moment for Zen and psychotherapy was the visit of Shin'ichi Hisamatsu, a well-known scholar affiliated with the Kyoto School of Philosophy, paid to Jung in 1958 (Muramoto 1998, 2003). This encounter continues to be reflected and contemplated upon among Japanese and Western scholars even today (Miller 2009; Muramoto 1998), despite reported miscommunication and lack of agreement between Hisamatsu and Jung (Meckel and Moore 1992; Shore 2002; Young-Eisendrath and Muramoto 2003).

These intellectual exchanges were further nourished by a few significant international symposiums and conferences, including the 1957 symposium on Zen and Psychoanalysis in Mexico (Kato), the 1999 Kyoto Conference on Buddhism and Psychotherapy (Young-Eisendrath and Muramoto 2003), and the 2006 Kyoto Conference on Self and No self in Psychotherapy and Buddhism (Mathers et al. 2009). The last two conferences have led to the publication of two edited volumes of rich scholarship discussions regarding the synthesis and divergence between Zen and psychotherapy (see Mathers et al. 2009 and Young-Eisendrath and Muramoto 2003 for contributions).

Vibrant dialogues that explore the relationship between Zen and psychotherapy continue to evolve today. Bobrow's (2010) *Zen and Psychotherapy: partners in liberation*, and Cooper's (2010) *The Zen Impulse and the Psychoanalytic Encounter* are among the more recent examples. Meanwhile, in the practice community, direct and explicit applications of Zen in psychotherapy, such as "Zen therapy" developed by Brazier (1997, 2001) and Rosenbaum's articulation of Zen in psychotherapy (Rosenbaum 2015), have also been established. In fact, Zen therapy is affiliated with the Institute for Zen Therapy based in UK, which offers training in Zen therapy and is affiliated with larger international community, Instituto Terapia Zen International (IZTI).

However, despite the growing popularity of Zen in popular culture and the realm of psychotherapy, it is rare for a discussion about Zen and psychotherapy to consider Zen as a religion in addition to a philosophy and practice. It is worth to note that "religion" in the context of Zen differs from a conception of religion as "a sect or creed or doctrine" (Uchiyama et al. 2004, p. 109), or concerns a relationship to an authority that people worship with complete submission, which is common to many monotheistic religions. Zen does not endorse any authority even the founder Shakyamuni Buddha, outside of the teaching of the true self that is connected to all things. Thus, Zen is a religion in the sense that it teaches an attitude and a way of life that honors the true reality of the self through ceaseless practice. This means to live each moment with a vow to look after everything around us with genuine care just as taking care of our own life (Uchiyama et al. 2004). This orientation to life inherently involves an ethical dimension, which yet cannot be realized simply by deferring to a prescribed set of rules and regulations, also common to monotheistic religions.

This religious and ethical aspect of Zen is often ignored or glossed-over in the academic discourse. In fact, some scholars argued that Buddhism is more a form of psychology than a religion (Christopher 2003; Robins 2002). This has raised the concern that the Western application of Zen may leave out the spiritual nature of Buddhism and its true essence of enlightenment, which goes deeper than being a technique or the focus of symptom relief (Muramoto 2003). Cooper (2010) discussed the general resistance to embracing Zen as a religion observing that "many Zenists, in order to be taken seriously by their scientifically oriented colleagues, tend to distance themselves from religiosity of the tradition and present Zen exclusively as a science, technique, or philosophy" (p. 53). We will return to this important critique in our later discussion.

Resonance Between Zen and Psychotherapy

We will now turn to a closer examination of the relationship between Zen and psychotherapy. On the surface, the two disciplines may seem incompatible. For example, psychology is primarily concerned with how "self" is developed and optimized (e.g., self-concept, self-esteem, and self-identity), which presupposes an ontological assumption of self as something that *exists* and exists independently, similar to an entity. In contrast, (Zen) Buddhism teaches the notion of "no self" and "nirvana," and the detachment from a fixed sense of self. The incompatibility seems to be as follows: Psychotherapy wants to develop the self, whereas Zen tries to get rid of the self. But do these two schools of thought truly contradict each other? To answer this question, we need to unpack basic assumptions embedded in those claims. For instance, what is what we call "self"? What constitutes existence and non-existence? Does "no self" signify a simple negation of the self?

These questions further reveal a dualistic framework that all incompatibility arguments seem to dwell on. That is, self and no self are contrasted on a plane of existence that already presupposes a dichotomous relation of existence and non-existence, assuming "existence" as a thing that can be accumulated (Uchiyama et al. 2004). The notion of "existence" itself is thus taken for granted and left out of our interrogation. This was Eric Fromm's insight when he pointed out, "the assumption of incompatibility between Zen Buddhism and psychoanalysis results only from a superficial view of both" (Fromm 1960, p. 81). If we can resist the trap of dualistic thinking, we may better access a deeper resonance between Zen and psychotherapy. It is with this intention we will discuss a few key concepts that draw synergy from both Zen and psychotherapy, including the notion of suffering, nature of the self, and the understanding of enlightenment and liberation.

On Suffering

First of all, both Zen and psychotherapy attend to direct human experiences with suffering (Gunn 2009), and focus on gaining perspectives and skills that "alleviate personal suffering in everyday life, and an increase of compassion for self and others" (Young-Eisendrath 2003, p. 65). In Buddhism, suffering is foregrounded in its basic teaching of the Four Noble Truths (Rahula 1959). The First Noble Truth, *dukkha*, refers to any conditioned state that is subject to change, which is usually translated as "suffering" in English. The Second Noble Truth states the origination of *dukkha* is ignorance, which includes desire, greed, craving, thirst for sense-pleasures, existence, becoming, and even death. The Third Noble Truth, *Nirodha*, suggests that "there is emancipation, liberation, freedom from suffering, from the continuity of *dukkha*" (Rahula 1959, p. 35). Such emancipation is commonly referred to as "*nirvana,*" the extinction of ignorance and desire. The Fourth Noble Truth is known as the "Middle Way" that further points to a Noble Eightfold Path that includes eight categories: Right Understanding, Right Thought, Right Speech, Right Action, Right Livelihood, Right Effort, Right Mindfulness, and Right Concentration (Rahula 1959). The path to the cessation of *dukkha* emphasizes practicing this Eightfold Path that cultivates virtue, compassion, wisdom, and equanimity.

Similarly, psychotherapy grows out of concerns for human suffering (Miller 2009). One of the formal definitions describes psychotherapy as "the treatment of emotional or physical ills by psychological means, implying a belief in the influence of the mind on the mind and of the mind on the body" (Cautin 2011). Similar to Zen, psychotherapy helps people transform their own suffering by deep introspective search and by analyzing their anguish. It is important to acknowledge the challenging nature of discussing psychotherapy as a whole since it has evolved from its origination in psychoanalysis into diverse and complex systems of knowledge with more than 500 modes of orientations (Lambert 2004). Those systems vary not only on specific forms and structures but also on each one's understanding of the very nature of psychotherapy (more discussion below). Nonetheless, they seem to share an underlying impetus to understand basic human conditions and sources of human suffering, and through therapeutic dialogues and reflection, to open up potentials for increased awareness, autonomy, and freedom.

Psychotherapy at its core focuses on layered and deep hermeneutic interpretations to understand and clarify distorted self-narratives. It is as much a process as an outcome, during which false consciousness is accessed and overcome, which allows opportunity for the alienated life history to be revived and reappropriated into one's consciousness (Freud 1921). The "patient" becomes aware of what were formerly regarded as external forces acting upon her and then can take responsibility for them and integrate them into a broader conception of who she is (Habermas 1971).

In this sense, Zen and psychotherapy converge on understanding, encountering, and transforming suffering. They both "seek to overcome a sense of alienation and to recover an original vitality that has got lost or has been buried under social conditioning and non-facilitating environments" (Gunn 2009, p. 19). This means to wrestle with "fundamental anxiety" that perpetuates the sense of alienation from the self, others, and the world, and rigid attachment and identification out of fear of the transient nature of life (Cooper 2010; Ogden 2007). However, Buddhism holds a broader conceptual understanding of suffering, which transcends the dualistic assumptions embedded in psychotherapy, for example, the dichotomy between happiness and suffering.

In Buddhism, *dukkha*, or "suffering," is not limited to its negative connotation of suffering and pain but also encompasses the notion of joy and pleasure (Rahula 1959). In fact, *dukkha* will arise whenever there is a distinction between the knower and what is known. This means *dukkha* arises when there is any use of words or concepts, or thinking, since such activities presuppose separation and distinction. Even experiencing a positive emotion suggests the separation of awareness and what is being aware of. Therefore, being a conscious human comes with suffering on this deeper level. In Buddhism, the ultimate cessation of *dukkha* is *nirvana*, which is regarded as the "Absolute Truth." However, *nirvana* can never be fully expressed using language for the very reason we just articulated. What *nirvana* means is beyond any dualistic view that distinguishes between "yes" and "no." Buddhist philosophy uses the term "empty" to describe this insight that the nature of existence is beyond simple yes and no.

In this sense, *nirvana* does not have a nihilist connotation that negates existence (i.e., self as pure nothingness) because nihilism also operates on the dualistic foundation (i.e., existence and non-existence) that Buddhism aims to transcend. For this very reason, Buddhism does not have an answer to the question about the cause of suffering, which essentially asks for an explanation of the origin of everything (e.g., the Big Bang theory). Although the Second Noble Truth states the connection between ignorance and *dukkha*, Shakyamuni Buddha himself avoided addressing the validity of questions about the cause of ignorance because everything has interdependent origination, and thus, these questions cannot be answered linearly or logically or in the form of language.

In contrast to Buddhism's resistance to simple cause-effect, psychotherapy from its very beginning tends to reify suffering as symptoms that can be alleviated via treatment. It foregrounds the need to inquire about the "cause" of suffering, assuming that understanding the cause will lead to proper choices of cure—a rather linear logic similar to what is embedded in the medical model. Today, with the prevalence or persistence of a positivist[2] psychology, symptoms are further reduced to observable and measurable behaviors,

[2]Positivism is a form of empiricism, a tradition of philosophy that considers the highest or only form of knowledge is the description of sensory phenomenon. This type of knowledge is considered "positively" given assuming we do not speculate it as the ground for truth.

and treatment is truncated to specific techniques and manualized procedures (e.g., Chambless et al. 1995). A poignant passage by Eric Fromm highlighted this concern long before the rise of contemporary psychotherapy:

> …the aim for the cure of the neurotic character were not radical enough; that well-being, freedom from anxiety and insecurity, can be achieved only if the limited aim is transcended, that is, if one realizes that the limited, therapeutic aim cannot be achieved as long as it remains limited and does not become part of the a wider, humanistic frame of reference. (Fromm 1960, p. 104).

This suggests that symptomatic relief is not sufficient for healing to be taken seriously and holistically. Healing on a deeper level is about understanding and transcending the most basic alienation underneath one's suffering and manifesting symptoms, and attending to one's whole being and wellness (Ando 2009). It is exactly what Zen may offer for a radical transformation of psychotherapy given its "spiritual humanistic orientation" (Fromm 1960, p. 102) and a deep understanding of suffering beyond a dualistic framework. Again, Fromm precisely articulated this possibility:

> Zen, different as it is in its method from psychoanalysis, can sharpen the focus, throw new light on the nature of insight, and heighten the sense of what it is to see, what it is to be creative, what it is to overcome the affective contaminations and false intellectualizations which are the necessary results of experience based on the subject-object split. In its very radicalism with respect to intellectualization, authority, and the delusion of the ego, in its emphasis on the aim of well-being, Zen thought will deepen and widen the horizon of the psychoanalyst and help [her] to arrive at a more radical concept of the grasp of reality as the ultimate aim of full, conscious awareness. (Fromm 1960, p. 108).

Our discussion so far compared and contrasted the aims and processes of psychotherapy and Zen, which already alludes to two other basic concepts that are pertinent to both psychotherapy and Zen: self and freedom—What is the nature of the self? How can we achieve liberation and freedom? It is evident that to understand and mitigate suffering requires an inquiry into the nature of the self (Ando 2009; Fromm et al. 1960) and finding ways to move "from bondage to freedom" (Fromm et al. 1960, p. 114). In the following section, we will continue to examine how Zen and psychotherapy take up the notion of self, as well as their convergence and divergence.

Self and No Self

Buddhism differentiates and embraces two aspects of the "self": self and no self, or in Sanskrit, *atman* and *anatman*, respectively. Buddhism considers *Atman* delusional and understands self as an ever-changing collection of five aggregates, like all existence. Self is thus essentially "empty" and lacks permanence and essentiality. From this perspective, no self, or *anatman*, is the "True Self" (Mathers et al. 2009) or the "universal self" (Uchiyama et al. 2004). The two aspects are not contradictory in Buddhism; rather, they are internally connected through the understanding of the "Middle Way"[3] (in Chinese, 中道). Basically, the Middle Way speaks of a paradoxical approach to concepts such as self and no self, form and emptiness, or phenomenal truth and absolute truth, and the "interpenetration" of these seemingly opposing aspects (Hanh 2009). The "Middle Way" can be understood as the free movement between any two opposites, which transforms the opposition into something new. From this perspective, self is both *atman* and *anatman*.

At the same time, we can also say that self is neither *atman* nor *anatman*. To be a self, one has to be responsible for her own life as an independent individual going through birth and death in the phenomenal world. Meanwhile, this individual self is "empty" because it is interconnected with

(Footnote 2 continued)
Positivism also comes with a strong optimism that science can help to solve all problems (Hollis 1994).

[3]The idea of the "Middle Way" originated from Shakyamuni Buddha and was further philosophized in a systematic way by an early Mahāyāna Buddhist master and philosopher named Nāgārjuna (ca 150–250 AD).

all beings and things. Thus, we may say that self is itself a dialectical[4] relationship and perhaps can be most closely expressed as self and no self within the limit of language, which inherently relies on distinctions and thus at bottom is incapable of escaping duality as discussed previously. By crossing out the words "self and no self" we apply French philosopher Jacques Derrida's use of *sous rature*[5] (Derrida 1997). This is a concept and practice characteristic of Derrida's theory and writing. It means that we both have to understand a concept and understand that it is not in the end the correct concept. The "correct concept" is both the one used and the simultaneous understanding of why it is misleading.

This dialectical or paradoxical view certainly can be difficult to comprehend from a linear dualistic mind-set, much prevalent in the Western intellectual history. Although the understanding of the self has been emphasized in Western philosophies beginning with Aristotle and Plato and evolving through the Enlightenment, transcendental philosophy, the language turn, existentialism, post-structuralism, feminist theory, and critical theory (Tugendhat 1989), dialectical thinking was only prominent in the work of Hegel's dialectics (1977, 1991) and Marx's dialectical materialism (Marx 1988), and mostly in the domain of philosophy and social theory. Psychotherapy, as a Western invention, is no exception in terms of falling prey to dualistic thinking.

Despite the wide range of psychological theories that have provided rich and complex understanding about the self (e.g., developmental theories, psychoanalysis, psychodynamics, individual psychology, object-relation theory, self psychology, attachment theory, humanistic psychology, and transpersonal psychology), most of these approaches tend to model self as a lone actor and view human motivation in the context of instrumental action based on a subject–object relation. That is, the actor acts with the motivation to achieve a certain goal, or strategically evaluates multiple courses of action and acts to achieve the maximal outcome (Habermas 1990). Such individual-based view sharply contrasts with the emphasis on the interconnective and trans-subjective feature of the self in Zen.

However, it is important to acknowledge that certain psychotherapy traditions have successfully resisted an individual-based understanding of the self by embracing an intersubjective, transpersonal, and humanistic vision, which is congruent with, although not fully identical to, the Zen perspective. For example, Jung's exploration of the psyche and collective consciousness (Heisig 2002; Jung 1969/1916); Adler's attempt to tie self-development to the development of social interest (Adler 1964); William James' conception of self as a stream of thought (Ando 2009; James 1892), and more recently, the development of intersubjective psychoanalysis (Stolorow et al. 1987), all aim to exceed the limited view of the self *only* as an isolated individual.

Zen Buddhism is even more radical in this aspect (Fromm 1960). It directly penetrates dualistic thinking through a vision that integrates "fundamental singularity on the one hand and bedrock intersubjectivity on the other" (Bobrow 2010, p. 103). In this sense, Zen is better able to offer a more encompassing framework[6] to further cultivate a non-dualistic development of psychotherapy through dynamic movements

[4]The term "dialectical" or "dialectics" originated in Hegel's dialectical philosophy, in which truth is understood as an ongoing movement within and for itself. Each of those movements involves two opposing aspects, thesis and antithesis, which together transform themselves onto a new level through their movement against each other, and another movement is on the horizon. Each new movement thus also has the previous movement embedded. See Hegel (1977, 1991) for more explanation.

[5]See Gayatri Chakravorti Spivak's preface to Derrida's *Of Grammatology* (1997) for the original explanation of this term. This application will appear in later sections of this chapter as well.

[6]A continuous application of Derrida's use of *sous rapture* to capture the dialectical thinking of Zen in our writing. In this example, "framework" itself would create a dualistic separation: inside and outside of a framework. By crossing it out, it suggests that this framework itself needs to be undermined and transcended, which is the essence of Zen. We will apply this linguistic strategy to undermine the dualistic nature of language itself throughout this chapter.

between deconstruction and reconstruction. For instance, since Zen does not negate the individual aspect of the self and the fact that only one self can be responsible for her life, it coincides with psychotherapy's aim for self-development and increased autonomy and self-determination. Meanwhile, Zen also reminds us that self is beyond the individual self.

Quite contrary to a popular understanding of Zen that equates Zen's notion of detachment and no self to a cynical attitude toward life, Zen foregrounds the ethical and moral necessity in one's self-development. Zen's teachings of no self and emptiness illuminate the interdependent origination of all beings and things. This is a "positive" manifestation of emptiness (Cook 1977), which points toward the communal elements of human life: connection, empathy, compassion, gratitude, and loving kindness—all qualities that psychotherapy aims to facilitate at heart beyond the instrumental aim of symptom reduction. Bobrow (2010) beautifully articulated that Zen "provides psychotherapy a trans-subjective framework in which emotions and emotional relatedness find their place as a subset of a more fundamental and vaster mutual belonging" (xxxvi). Therefore, the vision of Zen has the potential to expand and transform the very framework of psychotherapy to better include the growth of the whole person, community development, social justice, and human-nature sustainability among its fundamental aims and responsibilities. This reveals an underlying emancipatory orientation for both Zen and psychotherapy and lends itself to further questions: how do Zen and psychotherapy comprehend and achieve de-repression (Fromm 1960), liberation, and freedom? This will be our focus in the following section.

On Liberation and Enlightenment

Zen and Enlightenment. In Zen, the understanding of the self and the notion of liberation are inherently connected; both are essential. The latter is often articulated in context of "enlightenment." In contrast to the common view that Buddhist practice is the path to enlightenment as the ultimate goal of self-development, fourteenth-century Zen master Dōgen Zenji, perhaps the single most important influence on Japanese Zen, resisted any means-to-an-end interpretation of the relationship between practice and enlightenment (i.e., practice leads to enlightenment). Contemporary Zen master Kodo Sawaki Roshi also stated, "gaining is delusion; losing is enlightenment" (Uchiyama et al. 2004, p. 139). This is based on the understanding that if our action is guided by the motivation of gaining enlightenment, we still act out of our desire—even when the desire is enlightenment itself.

To deconstruct the temporal separation of practice and enlightenment, Zen teachings articulate that the two are essentially identical and thus not separated in time. In *Genjokoan*, the first essay in *Shōbōgenzō*,[7] Dōgen pointed out "enlightenment" is not an external attainment *through* practice but *is* practice itself. This teaching has had profound impact on the historical development of Zen, which privileges ceaseless practice as enlightenment (Okumura 2010). The ultimate reality is that all what we have is *Now*, the current moment where past and future both reside. The Now is the gateway to timeless reality to which we always have access.

With this understanding of "enlightenment," many Zen traditions emphasize "zazen,"[8] or "just sitting," as the central practice. Unlike other forms of meditation practiced among various Buddhist schools, which focus on mental concentration and use different techniques that facilitate concentration (e.g., mantras, visualizations, counting breaths, and chanting), zazen tries to refrain from techniques or even the connotation of mental concentration because those

[7]In Chinese "正法眼藏," literally translated as "Treasury of the True Dharma Eye." There are multiple versions of *Shōbōgenzō*, but four scholarly compilations are commonly considered: 60, 75, 12, or 28 books in chronological order (Bodiford 2012).

[8]"Zazen" is the Japanese pronunciation of two Chinese characters, "打禅," which is commonly referred to in Japanese as *shikantaza* and often translated as "just sitting." During zazen, one simply maintains an upright posture, breathing deeply, and letting go any thoughts that come up, again and again (Uchiyama et al. 2004).

concepts already imply a dualistic separation between practice and goals. Whenever we focus on something, it becomes a goal to attain and we are still in the realm of "gaining mind."

Zen also stresses that zazen is not stopping or eliminating thinking, as thinking is part of the reality and the natural function of being a human. Our effort to eliminate thinking becomes yet another goal to attain and perpetuates the dualism between thinking and not thinking. For Dōgen, zazen is not thinking and it is not non-thinking; it is beyond thinking (Uchiyama et al. 2004). "Beyond thinking" transcends any attempt to conceptually grasp what zazen is, similar to the Derrida's use of *sous rapture* described above. The moment we think we grasp the truth and realization, we miss it. Therefore, we can only keep practicing without a goal, which includes letting go of the goal of reaching enlightenment; practice itself is already an expression of enlightenment (Okumura 2010). Enlightenment and practice are one: Enlightenment "is only manifested within the process of practice, moment by moment" (Okumura 2010, p. 92).

Dōgen uses the expression "dropping off body and mind" (in Japanese *shinjin-datsuraku*, or in Chinese, "身心脱落") to describe what zazen is (Okumura 2010). Metaphorically, zazen means we take off any "coverings" of the self, such as fixed identity claims that we habitually maintain in our everyday life; fears and desires that create alienation and separate us from people around us; and the discriminating thinking mind itself. When we "drop off" our body and mind, we open ourselves to the truth of the self: That is, self is not our possession and does not have independent existence. Instead, we experience that our very existence sits on the ground of interdependent origination—the ultimate ground of being. In this sense, the teaching of zazen conveys a deep meaning of freedom: we are completely free when dropping off our body and mind in zazen.

Psychotherapy and Liberation. In contrast to Zen, psychotherapy's understanding of liberation, broadly speaking, is closely related to the process of self-reflection and gaining new self-knowledge, insight and new experience through therapeutic dialogues, which centers on transformation in time. What occurs during an authentic experience of self-reflection is "a cognitive, affective, and practical transformation as moments of a single process" (Bernstein 1978, p. 204). This echoes a common understanding shared by therapists that cognitive understanding is necessary but not sufficient (e.g., Teyber 2005). Self-knowledge is not only a *know-what* type of knowledge that can be explicitly articulated, but also a *know-how* type of knowledge that enables us to gain access to a deeper sense of being and basic attitude, and thus opens up opportunity for reconstruction (Carspecken 2009). True self-reflection makes us aware of our denial and resistance cognitively, affectively, and experientially.

In this way, awareness and new understanding have the potential to immediately transcend being itself, where knowing and being can be integrated in a single moment. Such moments are often experienced by a therapy dyad as a "critical moment," which helps the client gain a sense of freedom from a repressing power that was previously unknown. This growing freedom and increased autonomy and responsibility occur side by side—we become more autonomous in a deep way as we are willing to take more responsibilities to act in the world in new ways. Through the practice of self-reflection, alienated aspects of the self become fully reintegrated into a new self: The object becomes a new part of the subject—a great insight articulated by Freud (1921).

Therefore, there is also an underlying orientation toward liberation and freedom in psychotherapy: a deep interest to repair distorted communication and sustain a continuous self-formative process that permits open dialogues intrapersonally and interpersonally. On an intrapersonal level, truncated or distorted relation of self to self leads to false self-knowledge and self-deception. To reflect on the truncation and distortion makes it possible for reintegration toward a fuller self-realization. Similarly, on an interpersonal level, misunderstanding and distorted power relations hinder our fundamental existential need for mutual recognition and perpetuate the clinging to fixed identity claims. Repairing misunderstanding and distortion in relationships facilitates identity development, because it expands the ways we can be a valid person who is genuinely accepted and respected by more people (Habermas 1981).

Liberation: A Zen and Psychotherapy Comparison. This is clear that both Zen and psychotherapy have inherent impetus toward liberation and freedom through the grasp of and the unification with the authentic self or universal self. For Zen, enlightenment is freedom, but it is not a goal external to the self; freedom ultimately resides in practice (e.g., zazen) moment by moment. In zazen, there is no longer a separation between the knower and what is attained as knowledge: Being, doing, and knowing are united; the separation between subject and object breaks down. We can approach ourselves, others, and everything in the world with great compassion and care because they are us just as much as we are them. Similarly, in psychotherapy, freedom is facilitated by an integration of knowing, being, and doing: a moment of convergence of cognitive self-understanding, affective and experiential experience, and the impetus for transformative actions. In self-reflection facilitated by a therapeutic dialogue, one becomes aware of previous self-alienation and alienation from others, which are exposed for reintegration and reconstruction. When alienation is continuously being resolved, we develop a fuller and deeper connection with the authentic self along with an increased acceptance and compassion toward others.

A few additional similarities stand out. First of all, both Zen and psychotherapy rely on one central practice, zazen and talk therapy, respectively, both of which reconfigure one's understanding of and experience with self-relation and relation with others. The trajectory of this reconfiguring process points toward a self that is beyond the confined and alienated individual self, but a self that is more open, fluid, expansive, and boundless, which cannot be captured by a single world or concept although we can intuit it as "no self," "universal self," "unconsciousness," or "authentic self."[9] On the surface, zazen and talk therapy are two very different practices: one is completely silent, mostly solitary, whereas the other is communicative and relational. However, they do form a complimentary relationship, like yin and yang in Taoism, or like the thesis and antithesis of a dialectal relation in Hegelian philosophy (Hegel 1977, 1991). Both sides of such complimentary relationships are constitutive of the same truth, and yet as opposites transform together toward a larger whole.

Secondly, we consider the shared emphasis on the present moment. Open awareness and transformative potential reside in the Now for both Zen and psychotherapy. While Zen's notion of "dropping off body and mind" can be seen as a radical and thorough expression of embracing the Now, many psychotherapy approaches such as Gestalt therapy, existential therapy, psychodynamic, emotional-focused, and mindfulness-based therapies all seem to value the power of Now. It is in the present moment that one may become acutely and more accurately aware of the reality away from a self-centered and delusional view. Such awareness makes it possible to create distance from more rigid and habitual patterns in our thoughts, feelings, and actions. This process of de-identification creates space, fluidity, and vitality, which make us feel freer and more connected to larger life forces beyond individual will. This form of awareness has gained tremendous popularity in the realm of psychotherapy, often in the name of "mindfulness."[10]

---

[9]Continuous application of Jacques Derrida's use of *sous rature*[9] (Derrida 1997).

[10]The English word "mindfulness" can be traced back to the Pali term *sati,* the Sanskrit term *smrti*, the Tibetan term *trenpa*, and the Chinese term *nian* (Wynne 2007). The Sanskrit word *satipaṭṭhāna* combines *sati* (mindfulness) and *upatthana* (applications) to convey the practice of mindfulness. Chinese has an equivalent expression called *nian chu* (*nian* means being mindful and *chu* means being in the present) (Hanh 2006). As the combination of meditative absorption and the practice of mindfulness through meditation (in Sanskrit: *vipassana*), mindfulness also the seventh fold of the Noble Eightfold Path that leads to the development of wisdom (Rahula 1959).

Mindfulness is described by Kabat-Zinn (1994, 2005) as purposefully paying attention to the present moment through our experiences without judgment. It encourages us to realize that our perception is processed by associating the input (e.g., images and sounds) to preference judgments (e.g., likes and dislikes; Thera 1996). So, by having a more receptive attitude, we can begin to welcome change and allow it to become an accepted part of human existence, which helps to transcend our suffering. The practice of mindfulness also helps to cultivate deeper objectivity in our perception, which is beyond the subject–object separation (Hanh 2006; Nanda 2009), because the ultimate objectivity is not conceptualized as contrast to subjectivity but the ability to apprehend in experience the inseparability of subject and object.

Therefore, practicing mindfulness returns us to our senses and bodily sensations in the moment, so that we are *being* instead of *thinking* (Kabat-Zinn 2005). In this sense, "mindfulness" has a close connection to Zen's notion of "dropping off body and mind," although the use of mindfulness in the West has been largely stripped of its religious context. Interestingly, Zen teaching rarely emphasizes the term "mindfulness," either as a state of mind, a form of awareness, or a concentration technique, outside of its teaching of zazen. Perhaps the notion of mindfulness has been fully embodied in any moment of "dropping off body and mind" without the need to name another concept that creates further separation.

Thirdly, both Zen and psychotherapy reveal the ever-ending nature of self-development and practice. Given its understanding of self and reality, Zen supports enlightenment as ceaseless practice and the idea that any understanding of the self has to remain open and cannot be totalized. This idea is beautifully articulated by Dōgen as "there is a trace of realization that cannot be grasped," and yet "we endlessly express this ungraspable trace of realization" (Okumura 2010, p. 75). In psychotherapy, the idea that the process of treatment and the nature of self-reflection have to stay open is much more implicit, although seasoned therapists often experience that psychotherapy does not have an end point (Jennings and Skovholt 1999). Reflecting on Freud's work, philosopher Jürgen Habermas precisely articulated, "the interpretation of a case is corroborated only by the successful continuation of a self-formative process, that is by the completion of self-reflection" (Habermas 1971, p. 232). The only criterion for successful therapy is the client's experience of true self-reflection, which is always open to further development and thus cannot be totalized or fully objectified.

This suggests that there is an internal limit to the form of knowledge generated through psychotherapy: the experience of self-reflection or the self-formative process is not fully communicable. It is a form of knowledge, that is, a process and ultimately non-communicable (Carspecken 2009). This precisely points toward the experience of zazen, which may not be fully described due to the breakdown of subject–object separation and thus the use of language. However, this process involves a continuous transformation that one can directly experience and feel certain about moment by moment, although it can always be called into question. Thus, the validity of self-reflection cannot be grounded simply in observations of behavioral changes or even in the self-reports of the patient due to the possibility of self-deception. This open nature poses challenges to both Zen and psychotherapy because we are not able to tell with certainty whether a Zen practitioner experiences "enlightenment," or whether psychotherapy "succeeds." We will return to this limitation in our final reflection.

With these overarching similarities and differences between Zen and psychology in mind, we will now feature some specific examples of psychotherapy traditions in terms of their convergence with Zen. This includes a few classical orientations such as psychoanalysis, existential and Gestalt therapy, and rational emotive-based therapy (REBT), as well as the representatives of contemporary mindfulness-based psychotherapy movements featuring DBT, MBSR, MBCT, and ACT. In this section, we would like to "zoom in" and shift our attention from overarching themes to more specific relationships between Zen and the specific psychotherapy tradition on the level of methods and techniques. We will then return to a meta-level reflection on and critique of this content-level comparison in a later section.

The Crossroads of Psychotherapy and Zen: Specific Examples

Zen and Psychoanalysis

In this section, we will start with highlighting a few resonances between psychotherapy and Zen in psychoanalytical practices including the notion of "transference," "psychoanalytical listening," and "total exertion." First of all, psychoanalysis's approach to transference[11] assembles the concept of *katto* (in English, vine) in Zen. Working through *katto* is an essential part of the teacher–student relationship, where a student could experience deep communal experience with the teacher without losing her own individuality (Young-Eisendrath 2003). This aspect of Zen practice manifests Zen's understanding of the true self as the Middle Way between the individual and universal self, which we discussed previously. The relationship of a Zen teacher and the disciple provides an intimate context for the dyad to foster the coexistence of individuality and interdependence of the self. This is similar to the emphasis on working through transference and countertransference as a major vehicle for healing in psychoanalysis. It aims to cultivate new ways of understanding and experiencing the self, simultaneously honoring an authentic connection with others and a true interdependence of the self (Muramoto 2003).

Nonetheless, the intention and scope of such processes differ between Zen and psychoanalysis. While psychoanalysis focuses on recognizing and reconfiguring unconscious habitual patterns that lead to relieve psychological suffering, Zen intends for a broader scope of personal and spiritual growth. It carries a more radical orientation toward deeply understanding and experiencing the true self and the identity of practice and enlightenment. Zen thus consciously aims for moving beyond a dualistic conception of the self through the teacher–student relationship. This intention is mostly implicit or underdeveloped in the conception of therapeutic relationship in psychoanalysis. In this sense, Zen's approach to *katto* may help to enrich the potency of relational interventions in psychoanalysis by encompassing continuous transformation in *both* the client and the therapist, and the development of their whole being. Such potential echoes Eric Fromm's insight about the transformative power of Zen in relation to psychotherapy discussed previously.

Secondly, the emphasis on psychoanalytical listening echoes Zen's focus of zazen on full awareness in the present moment. Psychoanalytical listening, referred to by Freud (1912) as a state of "evenly suspended attention," is a therapist's attention to the patients' verbal discourse, voice tone, and nonverbal expressions from posture to gestures. Freud did not articulate specific ways to cultivate such a state. Zen meditative practices such as zazen may help analysts hone their psychoanalytical listening because Zen meditation aims for a "deeper level of awareness of self and others" (Cooper 2014) which in turn encourages a compassionate stance on analysands' current experiences in a neutral and nonjudgmental way.

Open awareness may help the therapist temporarily relinquish the expert role to share her feelings, which is important for trust and transference, to develop an effective therapeutic relationship. With such modeling, analysands learn to contain tensions and avoid conflicts, thereby eluding good/bad dichotomies in their perception (Jung 1969/1916; Young-Eisendrath 2003). Practicing zazen may also help analysts approach unevenness in their attention (e.g., a moment of inattentiveness) with acceptance and compassion, instead of reacting with self-judgment that would further interfere with psychoanalytical listening (Cooper 2014).

[11]Transference is defined as the transmission of a feeling about a particular context from an analysand to the therapist, but the analysand believes that the feeling originated with the therapist (Young-Eisendrath 2003).

Psychoanalytical listening is also closely related to another concept in psychoanalysis called "total exertion," meaning focusing on "our full energy and attention to the task at hand" (Cooper 2011, p. 592). Through total participation, our experience can be more fully discovered (Cooper 2011). For analysts, total exertion means giving analysands their full attention, experiencing everything analysands share without judgment. Thus, working with total exertion can create new flows of thoughts and feelings, which could encourage people to enjoy their moment-to-moment daily events, experiencing life more fully (Cooper 2011). It also helps analysts refrain from a "thinking ahead mind" (Cooper 2014, p. 600), which may impair their connection with their patients. Overall, what psychoanalysts try to cultivate in themselves is beyond a set of technique or skills that are external, but at bottom a practice within the self, which approximates the practice and experience of zazen in Zen. Thus, zazen may help to transform the reminiscence of an instrumental connotation of "psychological listening" and "total exertion" into a way of *being* (in contrast to *doing*) that is congruent with the true self.

Zen and Existential/Gestalt Therapy

An existential approach to therapy focuses on increasing self-awareness, encouraging clients to search for meaning, and helping them deal with anxiety as a condition of living and the fear of death that implicitly perpetuates anxiety (MacHovec 1984). This general goal is achieved by engaging in a journey of self-discovery for both client and therapist. Though not a technique-oriented approach, existential therapy does intend to assist clients in clarifying their assumptions and beliefs. Overall, existential therapy and Zen share several commonalities, primarily revolving around the focus on the present moment, a holistic approach to human experience, prioritizing experience over intellectualization, and the mind–body connection. MacHovec (1984) even calls the *Four Noble Truths* "an existential therapy system" (p. 93).

A good Zen student intends to achieve nothing, except being present and available to learn from the awareness of life. Similarly, existential therapists work against the psychologization of the human experience (Bazzano 2010). When a therapist judges a client's narrative, classifying their insights by what is perceived by the therapist as superficial or authentic, the therapist's own judgment becomes constricted. Existential therapy thus digresses from symptom relief by focusing on the "being" part of living. In like manner, Zen does not prescribe a structured system of beliefs, which can help therapists to refrain from creating theories and systems to relieve a client's anxiety (Bazzano 2010). Zen also does not offer an absolute path to happiness; rather, it directs us to the "sublime in the everyday" (Bazzano 2010). As a result, both Zen teachers and existentialist therapists move away from the expert role and encourage students' and clients' own discovery.

Gestalt therapy is closely related to the existential approach because it fosters personal responsibility, observes change as part of the human nature, and focuses on how people act in the "now" through a phenomenological approach instead of interpretation and intellectualization (Crocker and Philippson 2005). This "present-centeredness" (Naranjo 1970) helps clients realize how their experience to a large extent depends on their own perceptions and helps them experiment in sessions with how they deal with life. This approach resembles Zen's focus on seeing reality as it is, and its experimental orientation toward practice "moment by moment." The idea of "dropping off mind and body" in Zen also finds echo in Gestalt therapy's focus on bringing therapist and clients to their senses by "losing" their minds, encountering immediate feelings and the unknown in the Now. In fact, the influential Gestalt therapist, Fritz Perls, studied Zen himself and advocated the use of *koans*[12] or parables to facilitate the present

[12]Koans are usually parables and metaphors used by Zen masters to encourage students to seek insights and a deeper understanding of truth (Bodiford 2006; Young-Eisendrath and Muramoto 2003). For examples, see Cleary and Cleary (1977). Different Japanese Zen

focus (Crocker and Philippson 2005; MacHovec 1984; Williams 2006). Overall, the existential and Gestalt therapies and Zen converged on their motivation to engage primarily in a state of being than doing, and liberating people to experience life in the present moment and with attuned awareness toward "touching our full humanity" (Williams 2006, p. 16).

REBT and Zen

Rational emotive behavior therapy (REBT), first developed by Albert Ellis, is one of the first representatives of the school of cognitive behavioral therapy (CBT). REBT asserts that what is considered rational for some can be irrational for others. The main objective of a REBT practitioner is to encourage clients to try something they fear doing, to break their irrational thoughts that impair the enjoyment of experience (Ellis 1962). REBT is known for its A-B-C model, which argues that it is the irrational beliefs (B) that lead to negative behavioral and emotional consequences (C), instead of the activating event itself (A). This model suggests that therapeutic work should focus on the teaching of techniques that challenge clients' most basic core assumptions, or irrational beliefs, which modify their perception of activating events on ways that create distress (Ellis 1992; Kwee and Ellis 1998).

REBT also shares some characteristics with Zen, especially surrounding *koan* and *satori*,[13] two related Zen practices prominent in certain Japanese Zen schools such as the Rinzai sect (Griffith 2000). Through the use of *koan*-like parables or metaphors, a REBT therapist, similar to a Zen master, encourages clients to move way from intellectualizing, which weakens their defense mechanisms, and to focus on the development of insights grounded in experiences in the present moment (Kwee and Ellis 1998). This leads to the experience of *satori*, a mode of experiencing the world through the real self without intellectualization (Maupin 1962). Also, *koan* is recurrently experienced as a humorous intervention, embraced by both Zen and REBT to lighten the path to illumination (Kwee and Ellis 1998).

However, in Zen, *koan* is more than a means-to-the-end method to achieve a moment of enlightenment. In fact, the notion of *satori* as a goal for one to "achieve" has been deconstructed from within the Zen tradition itself, for example, in the work of Zen Master Dōgen, which was discussed previously. More fundamentally, *koan* helps to engage Zen students in wrestling with the limitation of thinking that is inherently dualistic. By having a direct experience with a simultaneous mode of knowing and being, which is beyond thinking, students grasp a glimpse of the nature of the truth self. Such practice does not position enlightenment as a goal but is identical to the process practicing itself. Again, this seems to be a more radical vision beyond borrowing *koan* and *satori* simply as a therapeutic applications articulated by some REBT scholars. This suggests that if therapists can move beyond primarily applying *koan* and *satori* as tools to achieve certain therapeutic outcomes, such Zen practices may lead to more profound and holistic impact on healing envisioned by Fromm (1960).

Another commonality between Zen and REBT lies in their shared rejection of dogmatism (Christopher 2003). Zen never claims to be better than other contemplative practices offered by other religions and spiritual traditions. Instead, it encourages an attitude of critical inquiry by constantly asking questions without the need to derive a totalizing answer, as well as a ceaseless practice that helps us to view the reality with more depth and clarity. Similarly, REBT finds itself aligned with a postmodernist and

(Footnote 12 continued)
traditions have different emphases on koan practice. For example, it is widely practiced in the Rinzai tradition but not essential for the Soto Section.

[13]Satori is commonly understood in Japanese culture as the equivalent of "enlightenment," a moment of awakening to the true reality with full awareness and free from any attachment, or in other words a moment of *nirvana*. It is closely related to the experience of *Kenshō*; *Ken* means "seeing," *shō* means "nature" or "essence" (Kapleau 1989). As discussed previously, many Zen teachers and practitioners such as Dōgen negate the idea of achieving satori as the essence of Zen (Uchiyama et al. 2004).

constructivist philosophical orientation (Kwee and Ellis 1998), which defies any dogmatic view on truth and reality. Through challenging rigid and irrational beliefs in provocative therapeutic dialogues, REBT aims to help clients to restore distorted perceptions of reality and gain access to enlightenment through a "more rational lifestyle" (Christopher 2003, p. 286).

Nonetheless, we need to be aware that a rejection of dogmatism or holding a philosophical stance such as postmodernist or constructivist does not automatically make such orientations equivalent to Zen. As we discussed earlier, Zen carries an epistemological view, that is, dialectical and non-dualistic, which actually deconstructs itself as anything that can be fully expressed in language like what we are attempting in this sentence. Therefore, Zen is more than taking a non-dogmatic perspective but a radical way of *being with* truth and reality that cannot be intellectualized. It is most important for therapists to learn how to *be* with clients and themselves in a deep way than claiming a philosophical stance.

In addition, REBT encourages clients to "abandon" the self, when clinging to the self prevents growth and self-reflection. REBT articulates a multifaceted view of the self (Lazarus 1977) and suggests a new way to understand the self as many "selves," as well as the use of "i" instead of a singular "I" to honor the fluidity and non-fixed nature of the self. This treatment of the self resonates with Zen's understanding of self as "no self" and its support for developing detachment from any fixation in our sense of identity. This is well captured in Suzuki and Fromm's insight that "if a person is identified with nothing more than an act, then the person is not a living human being at all, but a concept of the mind" (1960, p. 46). Again, it is worth to note that Zen's understanding of the true self cuts right through any dichotomous plane based on which any conceptualization of the self is constituted. Self as many "selves" or self as non-fixed is very insightful and yet they may fall short to thoroughly break through the assumption about "existence" itself as an accumulative entity. Experience with the true self in Zen resides in zazen.

Zen and Mindfulness-Based Psychotherapies

After discussing the intersection between Zen and a few traditional forms of psychotherapies, we will shift our focus to comparisons on more contemporary crossroads between the two disciplines, which certainly concerns the application of mindfulness. As eluded to earlier in this chapter, mindfulness has become a buzz in the world of Western psychotherapy. Mindfulness has had a deep impact on what is known as the third wave of behavioral therapy (Harris 2006), which comprises a series of psychotherapy modalities, including dialectical behavior therapy (DBT), mindfulness-based stress reduction (MBSR), mindfulness-based cognitive therapies (MCBT), and acceptance and commitment therapy (ACT). In fact, mindfulness-based psychotherapies as a whole are projected to be the single most popular form of psychotherapy orientation in 2022 (Norcross et al. 2013). We already offered some definitional and contextual information about this movement previously, and in the following section, we will provide a brief sketch of each of those mindfulness-based approaches.

Dialectical Behavior Therapy. DBT was first established by Linehan (1993) to help women who struggle with suicidality exacerbated by conditions of borderline personality disorder. DBT addresses those difficulties using strategies that range from cognitive restructuring and assertiveness training to mindfulness training to enhance the capacity to accept themselves and others (Linehan 1993; Robins 2002). This last technique in particular drew on Linehan's own experience with Zen, which might have served an inspiration for the dialectical thinking and mindfulness-based interventions used in DBT.

The foundation of DBT is based on a holistic and dialectical worldview. Linehan emphasized interrelatedness, wholeness, dialectical relation between polarity, fluidity in identity, and the nature of continuous change in her theory (Linehan 1993; Robins 2002). It uniquely postulates that positive change occurs through movement between support and challenge, two seemly opposing aspects that can be synthesized into new movement through therapist's skillful implementation of dialectical conceptualization and interventions (Linehan 1993). This approach is congruent with the premises of Zen teachings, especially the notion of Middle Way, the balance between two extremes and the transcendence of dichotomies, which we described previously.

DBT also infused mindfulness-based techniques such as nonjudgmental observation, meditation, and awareness of sensations to enhance distress tolerance, emotion regulation, and interpersonal effectiveness (Linehan 1993). By gaining more mindful self-awareness, clients may act less impulsively as they become aware of the self as separate from the emotional states. They develop increased capacity to stay connected with their present experiences instead of preoccupied in rumination or repeating destructive patterns. Again, this general therapeutic orientation echoes Zen's emphasis on developing openness and non-attached awareness of whatever arises in the moment, which helps us apprehend true reality in a less self-centered way. Thus, both DBT and Zen facilitate a process of decentering and de-identification, which can in turn lead to more fluidity and flexibility in how people view themselves and others.

In addition, DBT assumes that people always have wisdom in themselves and the potential to change. Connecting to such inner wisdom could lead to tremendous opening and transformation. This is why DBT therapists do not view their clients as "having" a disorder, but as "acting, at times, in disordered ways" (Robins 2002). This attitude is aligned with Buddhist understanding of Buddha nature; that is, the seed of enlightenment is always within every person, which can grow with facilitating conditions. In fact, Dōgen expressed a more radical view on this insight that all people are already Buddha, but they will always need to practice (Okumura 2010).

Mindfulness-Based Stress Reduction. MBSR was founded by Jon Kabat-Zinn, perhaps the single most influential individual in the history of mindfulness study in the Western world. In 1979, he established the world-renowned Stress Reduction Clinic at the University of Massachusetts Medical Center, which was highly successful in managing chronic pain through a program called mindfulness-based stress reduction (MBSR) (Kabat-Zinn 2005). In 1990, Kabat-Zinn began writing about his experiences and successes in using MBSR (Kabat-Zinn 1990, 1994). He wrote in a highly accessible manner in an effort to legitimize mindfulness practices for the scientifically oriented layperson. Following the work of Kabat-Zinn, the study of mindfulness exploded in the 1990s (e.g., Moore 1997; Santorelli 1999; Thynn 1995). Since then, MBSR has gained increasing credibility and is now being implemented in a number of settings including medicine, psychotherapy, performance-enhancement, parenting, and education.

MBSR is an eight-week mindfulness training program infused with didactic teaching. More importantly, it provides direct practice with mindfulness such as mindfulness breathing, body scan, and yoga practice (Kabat-Zinn 1990, 1994). In this sense, MBSR resembles Zen's emphasis on ceaseless practice of "dropping off mind and body" and refraining from over intellectualization. However, at the same time, MBSR completely stripped away the explicit religious and spiritual context of Zen. It may be fair to say that MBSR is a secularized and Westernized from of Buddhist practice.

The evolution of MBSR has also drawn increasing research interest since the 1990s in the fields of psychology, neuroscience, and cognitive science (e.g., Kabat-Zinn 2003; Shapiro et al. 2006; Williams and Kuyken 2012). This trend has been thus far marked by a constant tension between science and spirituality. Emerging researchers differ in the level of respect and attention they pay to the religious origins and spiritual underpinnings of mindfulness practice. There is often a struggle to meet the standards of the empiricist-science dogma in academia without ignoring spiritual issues. We will return to this issue in our final reflection.

Mindfulness-Based Cognitive Therapy. Cognitive behavioral therapies have also been riding the current of mindfulness along the "third wave" of behavioral therapy, which features a commitment to mindfulness, openness, and an emphasis on inviting emotional depth in the moment (Hayes 2004; Johanson 2006). In particular, Segal et al. (2002) have developed a mindfulness-informed modification of cognitive behavioral therapy, called mindfulness-based cognitive therapy (MBCT), which has shown significant success in preventing relapse in depression. Since then, MBCT has also been successfully applied to treat a myriad of mental difficulties including social phobia, panic attacks, and anxiety disorder (Chiesa and Malinowski 2011).

MBCT draws on traditional CBT techniques (Chiesa and Malinowski 2011) but combines them with its own mindfulness-directed technique referred to as the "three-minute breathing space" (Segal et al. 2002, p. 173). This technique bridges a formal meditation practice to a three-step exercise to address negative feelings and thinking patterns. This exercise foregrounds the awareness of thoughts, feelings, and sensations in the moment, focusing on attention in breathing and then expanding it to a broader awareness of the surroundings. It is noticeable that this technique is similar to the experience of zazen, although the latter does not prescribe attention on any particular thing throughout. Both approaches encourage people to increase their self-awareness and distance themselves from their own thoughts, committing to redirecting perception from thought-provoking to thought-observing (Robins 2002).

Acceptance and Commitment Therapy. Acceptance and commitment therapy (ACT) has been considered a groundbreaking progress in Western psychotherapy (Harris 2006). Developed by Steve Hayes in 1986, ACT has accumulated a significant amount of empirical studies that support its efficacy treating a myriad of psychological difficulties, such as depression (Zettle and Raines 1989), anxiety (Harris 2006), stress (Dahl et al. 2004), substance abuse (Hayes et al. 2006), OCD (Twohig et al. 2006), and schizophrenia (Bach and Hayes 2002). Deviating from traditional cognitive behavioral therapy, ACT does not encourage clients to fight negative feelings; instead, it encourages clients to cultivate acceptance toward negative thoughts and feelings (Chiesa and Malinowski 2011) and practice mindfulness.

ACT believes that the use of language is the basis of human suffering (Harris 2006) and thus takes a non-pathologizing view of symptoms. The primary focus of ACT is not on symptom reduction but on helping clients develop new ways off viewing their relation to their symptoms while increasing acceptance and compassion toward their situations, which, paradoxically, leads to symptom relief (Hayes 2004). Therefore, both ACT and Zen see suffering as an inherent and inevitable part of the human experience.

ACT and Zen also view language similarly. Language perpetuates anxiety or melancholy when it drives people from direct experience with the Now as they cope with fear and uncertainty via various means of avoidance. ACT addresses such existential avoidance directly through the development of nonjudgmental awareness of clients' language use that permits avoidance and enables stuckness (Harris 2006). Likewise, the teachings and practice of Zen facilitate observation and awareness of our habitual or fixated patterns, which at bottom can be traced to the discriminating nature of language. ACT encourages the use of metaphors as a more holistic language tool to reveal and undermine the dualistic nature of language, through illuminating paradoxes in clients' experiences in order to help clients elicit insights to liberate themselves from their suffering. Similarly, the use of metaphors such as *koans* is a common practice in Zen teachings for the very same reasons.

In sum, this series of mindfulness-based psychotherapies all manifest aspects of Zen on different levels. For example, MBSR, MBCT, DBT, and ACT all aim at helping people distance from ruminating patterns that perpetuates anxiety, or the recurrence of depression (Segal et al. 2002; Robins 2002). Nonetheless, all of those approaches have the explicit and implicit goal of attaining certain efficacy of treatment in a positive direction and thus differ from Zen in the most fundamental way. Zen, as a religion and a system of philosophical and spiritual practices, does not lead toward attaining a specific goal, not even enlightenment. By now we have compared and contrasted Zen and psychotherapy on general and specific levels, and we would like to close the chapter with a critical reflection on some important issues that have emerged throughout the chapter.

A Brief Case Discussion

Thus far our discussion has stayed mostly on a theoretical level. To illustrate how a Zen-informed therapy process may unfold in practice, in the following we introduce a brief clinical case discussion. Our focus here is not about the complexity of the case, but how some Zen principles may manifest in the therapeutic process. The client, "Melissa," is a white woman in her early thirties, born and raised in a small affluent community in the northeast. She moved to a large city to attend college and secured a well-paid job in a large corporation. She reported feeling "depressed" and "empty," and experiencing a lack of closeness in both her friendships and romantic relationships. Observing her distress, a colleague referred her to a therapist.

To work with Melissa, the Zen therapist did not prioritize symptom reduction as the primary or ultimate goal, but instead encouraged and supported her to sit with her problems, depressed feelings, and anxious thoughts. To do so, the therapist educated Melissa about some basic Zen and Buddhist principles concerning the nature of suffering and "self" in relation to our attachment to false perceptions and self-defeating thinking patterns. The Zen therapist also suggested the possibility of an alternative way of being, moving Melissa toward liberation and transformation, developed through deep self-acceptance and compassion and detached from fixed and false scripts about the self, so that she developed genuine connections between self, others, and the world. Lin and Seiden (2015) translated this process into a four-step approach, comprised of "facing it," "accepting it," "dealing with it," and "letting it go" (p. 325).

Specifically, the therapist first encouraged Melissa to face the roots of her depression, to "look in" and examine what could have contributed to her depression. Through this self-led exploration, Melissa discovered the self-fulfilling nature of her thinking and certain past conditions that could have shaped such a pattern. This led to her increased self-compassion and willingness to take responsibility to change while recognizing her limitations. It is important to note that Zen's focus here is not just to identify and challenge core beliefs (as in the case of traditional CBT) or to submerge in the unconscious roots of Melissa's predicament (as often occurs in a psychoanalytical approach). Zen goes beyond that—encouraging Melissa to be friends with her thoughts and difficulties instead of "getting rid of" them, and to understand the "cause-effect" between the past and the present but also focus on reconfiguring her relationship to changeable or unchangeable conditions in the present lived experience. For instance, the therapist guided Melissa to be conscious of the feelings and thoughts that arise when relating to other people, and to practice being present with how challenging feelings felt in her body. With such conscious experiential encounters, Melissa began to learn *how to* relate to her thinking and feeling with more space, flexibility, and compassion. This is a non-dualistic way to relate to her self and experiences, which in turn helped soften painful feelings and ruminations that had perpetuated her depression and relational difficulties.

In terms of "strategies," the therapist used *koans* to help Melissa cultivate understanding and direct encounter with the impasse of dichotomous thinking that fuels her underlying rumination and self-judgment. The therapist also encouraged her to develop a *zazen* practice, structured to her level and physical capacity, during and outside of therapy sessions. In this practice, *zazen* is not conceptualized simply as a "tool" that is external to her but part of her true being, which she learns to gain access to herself through this very practice and understands that by practicing she is already reaching this "goal." This is the paradoxical or dialectical basis of Zen teaching: The goal is the process and the process is the goal. Most importantly, the therapist helped Melissa understand that practice does not stop at the termination of therapy, or the disappearance of her problems. Instead, it is a process of a life-long learning and practice that she will continue to cultivate and deepen. Only by staying alive and awake, and engaging in ongoing practice, will we not forfeit our potential to become and transform, even though we also know that we are already our true self. Elliot (1944) elegantly captures this paradoxical process of self-development in his *Little Gidding*:

> What we call the beginning is often the end
> And to make an end is to make a beginning.
> The end is where we start from.
> ...
> We shall not cease from exploration
> And the end of all our exploring
> Will be to arrive where we started
> And know the place for the first time.

A Critical Reflection

Mutual Fertilization Between Zen and Psychotherapy

To return to our starting point of the presumed incompatibility between Zen and psychotherapy, our exploration seems to suggest the opposite. Although the two traditions grew out of drastically diverging historical roots and manifest in varying forms, at their core they share some underlying understanding and aims related to the nature of the self and the process of self-development toward liberation. There is much ground for their mutual fertilization if they are viewed as "partners in liberation" (Bobrow 2010). Cooper (2010, p. 52) formulated a very pertinent question on this issue: "How do psychoanalysis and Zen as lived and living disciplines remain open and contribute to creative ways of effectively addressing suffering and human potential?" We have a few thoughts on this question.

Zen and psychotherapy, to a large extent, form a dialectical relation where they complement each other. For example, whereas psychotherapy places significant weight on tracing the development of the self (e.g., family of origin, past history, and early childhood experiences), and on future-oriented positive change, Zen centers on practicing being in the present moment. If we imagine the former as a spiral[14] inspired by Hegelian philosophy (Hegel 1977), which constantly develops as repetition and transcendence simultaneously, the latter can be seen as the origin where the spiral both stems from and returns to—a single "point" that is timeless and yet is equally true as a dialectical development in time within and for itself. These two aspects are the two sides of the same coin. This means that Zen practitioners may benefit from tuning into their own internal resistance (Freud 1921) and gaining more self-understanding by exploring narratives and karmic conditions that have shaped the constitution of their self and patterns of attachment (Ando 2009). Such opportunities for de-identification and de-alienation may further facilitate one's experience of dropping off mind and body in zazen. On the other hand, psychotherapy can benefit from the therapeutic potency of the Now through expanding open awareness in the therapist and the client through Zen practice such as zazen, which may lead to profound transformation during the course of therapy.

Similarly, Zen and psychotherapy address a dialectically related understanding of the self—self as emptiness and self as an evolving individual—again, both sides of the same coin, which is in fact a basic understanding of Zen. In this sense, Zen seems equipped with a larger capacity to embrace both sides of the truth and thus may help broaden and deepen the understanding of the self in psychotherapy that goes beyond any dualistic conceptualization (e.g., individual and collective, unique and universal, specific ingredient, and common factor). Self has

[14]The caveat in this analogy is its inability to exceed the limitation to fully express inexpressible truth as expressed in Dōgen's quote at the beginning of this chapter. But the holistic quality of a metaphor may help us to gain insight and understanding within this limitation. We cross out spiral in the text, another application of Derrida's use of *sous rapture*, to contest the limitation of using a metaphor to convey something that is beyond the metaphor itself.

to be *both-and and beyond* as it is interconnected with all things. This conceptual shift may have profound ethical and moral implications, which may redefine psychotherapy as the means to relieve individual sufferings but also comes with an inherent ethical and moral dimension.

Such a conceptual shift calls for taking responsibility to address local and global issues and limiting social conditions that perpetuate injustice, prejudice, and privilege. All of those issues and conditions create alienation from the true self that we all share and are part of. Meanwhile, Zen can develop immunity to better resist a nihilist orientation in Zen practice by embracing the humanistic and affective aspects of the self, which are more foregrounded in psychotherapy. In this way, the impetus to negate and escape can be resolved and one can whole-heartedly embrace the suffering and joy in the phenomenal world, experiencing the vitality of life through ordinary experiences, as well as working toward positive social changes.

In addition, Zen and psychotherapy may benefit from reaching a more fine-tuned balance between the emotional/affective and cognitive aspects of practice by borrowing from each other. Cultivated in Chinese and Japanese cultures, the language of Zen teachings tend to privilege "thinking" in describing experiences, which creates separation from the moment. Although the word "thinking" in the Zen context does signify all sensual experiences, including feelings and emotions, Zen has little reference to handling emotional and affective qualities in practice. It is easy to imagine that strong emotional reactions may surface as one sits in silence for a long period of time facing the "demon" within the self as defense mechanism and distractions are no longer available.

For this reason, attending to one's emotional health and learning from intense affective experiences can be very valuable for Zen practitioners to work through the barriers for dropping off body and mind. On the other hand, psychotherapy can truly benefit from the Zen's notion of "beyond thinking" and refrain from excessive intellectualization, conceptualization, and theorization, and just sit with whatever experience comes up in the moment and be present with fears, uncertainty, and insecurity that are more easily masked by "thinking." Therefore, these two traditions can nurture and complement each other to offer hope for salvation and liberation in the midst of suffering.

An Epistemological Critique

As we close up the chapter, we would like to return to a few discussions left unfinished earlier on, which could benefit from a more holistic and critical examination. The first concern raised earlier is about the tendency for both psychotherapy and Zen to become subjugated to the domain of science, a trend that is prevalent in social sciences in general under the banner of positivism (Hollis 1994; Habermas 1990). This trend has manifested itself in the increasing focus on symptom reduction and prevention in the realm of psychotherapy (Young-Eisendrath 2003). For instance, Vasquez (2010) in the influential *Handbook of Multicultural Counseling* defines psychotherapy as:

> …a change process designed to provide symptom relief, personality change, and prevention of future symptomatic episodes and to increase the quality of life, including the promotion of adaptive functioning in work and relationships, the ability to make healthy and satisfying life choices, and other goals arrived at in the collaboration between client/patient and psychotherapist (p. 129).

This definition seems to leave out psychotherapy's emancipatory mission of developing self-knowledge, overcoming alienation, and facilitating growth toward authenticity and meaning. It has a narrower focus on observable and quantifiable changes on symptomatic and functional levels. Similarly, contemporary mental health care prioritizes short-term therapy approaches joined by the prescription of psychotropic medications, which stresses diagnosis based on which "patients" are treated with medication and brief therapy sessions oriented toward ameliorating symptoms, most often without addressing the real (and hidden) source of suffering (Young-Eisendrath 2003). In line with this tendency to medicalized psychotherapy, "biological determinism" (Young-Eisendrath 2003, p. 68) also prevails, which attempts to explain and predict psychological problems solely based on genetics, and consequently advances the logic that medication is the most effective means for treatment. We are concerned that this general orientation may further perpetuate the very alienation that psychotherapy aims to overcome, where one no longer has direct knowledge of herself but relies on specialized knowledge from the experts (e.g., physicians and therapists), and attribution and methods for healing become externalized and fall largely outside of her own agency and responsibility. Instead of transforming the "object" (the alienated aspect of the self) into consciousness and free the subject, we may position the subject toward further objectification.

Meanwhile, Zen may also experience a force of objectification, perhaps most visible in the development of mindfulness in psychotherapy and the popular culture. Mindfulness has been increasingly treated as a tool, a means to an end, and is stripped away its essence in (Zen) Buddhism as a way of being that is beyond a subject–object separation. With such (mistaken) reduction of mindfulness, it becomes a skill to be learned (Nanda 2009) instead of an essential aspect of being human (Cavill 2010). Also in the realm of scientific research, mindfulness has been operationalized into a variable, which assumes a "positive" ontological stance as something that exists and is measurable. With this treatment, a large volume of empirical studies[15] across the spectrum of psychology and cognitive and neurosciences have studied the "effectiveness" of mindfulness and its correlation to brain functions and neurological activities. There is no doubt that this line of research can be incredibly valuable and insightful, although it also seems to converge on an underlying instrumental and technocratic orientation toward understanding mindfulness. We have to ask: Is that all that mindfulness is? What is the epistemological nature of mindfulness? What are the forces that steer the current mindfulness movement, as both enabling and limiting conditions?

With some philosophical contemplation, we may notice that a common understanding of mindfulness today (e.g., as a skill or technique) follows the logic of *instrumental action*, that is, the actor acts with the motivation to achieve a certain goal, or strategically evaluates multiple courses of action and acts to achieve the maximal outcome (Habermas 1990). This leads to the therapeutic and research focus placed on "what works?"; "what conditions lead to desired outcomes?"; and "how can we spread the success?" (e.g., effectiveness and efficacy studies in counseling research). What is foregrounded in instrumental action is a *technical interest* oriented toward control and prediction based on a subject–object relation, which has found fertile ground in natural sciences and technology (Habermas 1971). In contrast, what occurs during psychotherapy is primarily *communicative action,* that is, oriented to *mutual understanding* through phenomenological and hermeneutic means instead of instrumental ones. What is foregrounded in communicative action is a social interest toward self-understanding and communality based on a *subject–subject* relation (Habermas 1981, 1990).

And there is yet another fundamental interest underneath both psychotherapy and Zen. Emancipatory in nature, this interest guides internal self-reflection and self-critique and corresponds to a form of knowledge aimed at recognizing and critically examining ideological distortions in knowledge claims (McCarthy 1981). This type of knowledge falls into the realm of critical social sciences that examine the conditions and limitations of freedom. This interest is an *emancipatory interest*, which is deeply connected to our earlier discussion on liberation and enlightenment, which aims at exceeding the limitation of subject–object thinking and moving toward the intersubjective and trans-subjective realm. Given this unique epistemological status of knowledge, it is categorically mistaken to believe that an empirical-analytical framework alone is capable

[15]For examples for this line of research, see a wonderful ongoing aggregate of mindfulness research archived by American Mindfulness Research Association, retrievable via https://goamra.org/publications/mindfulness-research-monthly/.

of fully understanding mindfulness. In fact, insisting such belief could make us commit scientism, a prevalent self-belief in the empirical-analytic sciences that equates science with knowledge and turns it into a dogma. This risk concerns various Zen scholars and therapists (e.g., Bazzano 2015; Cooper 2010). Thus, preserving the most essential identity for Zen and psychotherapy as a critical and emancipatory science instead of an instrumental can be an important shared goal for both disciplines.

In addition, the nature of emancipatory knowledge also suggests that there is fundamental uncertainty related to the validity criteria for evaluating "change" and "success" in both psychotherapy and Zen practice, an issue that we already eluded to in an earlier discussion. This is because what occurs in genuine self-reflection or zazen blurs the boundary between the knower and what is known. During the moment of reflection or zazen, knowing and the being of the person become identical; being becomes the knowledge of itself (Carspecken 2009). Validity for such moments is essentially equivalent to the notion of freedom itself—knowing what freedom is and being free at the same time. This understanding coincides with Dōgen's emphasis on "ceaseless practice" and the "untraceable trace" for realization discussed previously. It suggests that we may need a broader and yet more precise perspective to conceptualize "change," "success," and "outcome" in psychotherapy, which cannot be fully captured in observable and measurable changes in behaviors and functions. Our understanding of change orientated toward emancipation has to stay open to new transcendence within itself on the horizon. In accordance with Zen, our very impetus to achieve such understanding needs to be further softened into the experience of being in the present moment because that is where immeasurable and perhaps uncommunicative freedom resides.

Lastly, we would like to take a moment to examine the larger sociocultural contexts and system forces that might have simultaneously given rise to mindfulness while subjecting it to the truncation outlined above. At the very beginning of the chapter, we postulate the possible connection between the soaring epidemics of mental health concerns such as anxiety and depression in today's society and the increasing popularity of Eastern ideas such as mindfulness. From a sociological perspective, this parallel is accompanied by ever increasing societal complexity coupled with growing desire for certainty and control (Habermas 1981). It brings the triumph of instrumental rationality that rests on a means-to-the-end logic and focuses on problem solving, which further fuels society's thirst for certainty and lack of tolerance of ambiguity (Weber 1978).

The interaction between the over-reliance on instrumental rationality and changes in social structure (e.g., increasing complexity) also gives rise to a form of "managerialism," which shifts the ideal of an open and experimenting society to a managing and assessing one (Schwandt 2008). This managerialist approach has its roots in the instrumental reasoning, that is, salient in the economic domains and the accompanying management models driven by consumerism. The rise of managerialism provides a fertile ground for the insurance industry and the managed care organizations in medicine and mental health. This development is further complicated by their close tie to the pharmaceutical industry, all driven by the system's needs for technical and instrumental tools for assurance (i.e., effectiveness, efficiency, and accountability) and the underlying profit-driven consumerism. Meanwhile, the pressure from the system ruled by system imperatives (i.e., market, money circulation, efficiency, and corporate interests) inevitably forms intimate relationships with the political system (Schwandt 2008). One of the outcomes of this enterprise is to produce differentiated labor force for the market, which in turns reproduces the status quo of the social order (Marx 1988).

This is what Max Weber foresaw as an "iron cage" of the capitalistic society (Weber 1978), reinforced by the codependence of the economic, political, and instrumental rationality with one another, which suppresses the society, forcing it to become increasingly scientized, manageralized, specialized, and technologized, oriented toward means, ends, profit, effectiveness, and efficiency. This leaves out a more inclusive rationality that encompasses values, norms, communication, social relation, ethics, and morality (Schwandt 2008). This systemic analysis reveals some hidden forces embedded in the system that have likely shaped current trends in psychotherapy to become a more instrumental operation while being subjected to managerialist scrutiny. It also provides some clues about why mindfulness quickly became a new tool to sooth pervasive collective anxiety and despair, growing out of modern society's tremendous fear of uncertainty, discomfort with ambiguity, and growing sense of alienation.

Conclusion

As we have seen throughout this chapter, Zen and psychotherapy share many underlying traits and one broad common goal, to transcend human suffering through compassion and interconnectedness with oneself, others, and beyond. Undoubtedly, Zen and psychotherapy will continue to dialogue with one another and shape each other, a process that has enriched both disciplines. However, even though many studies are proving the positive benefits of mindfulness for the alleviation of symptoms (Kabat-Zinn and Hanh 2009), it seems that such focus of mindfulness may be narrowing the scope of potential influence of Zen on psychotherapy (Bazzano 2015). Perhaps leaving out the spiritual and emancipatory aspect of Zen's insight for psychotherapy, mindfulness has been largely reduced to a "thing" like skill or technique. In our view, this is at best a limited understanding of mindfulness and Zen and a utilitarian application of what Zen and Buddhism have to offer. This likely will be an ongoing enigma for us to contemplate: How Zen and psychotherapy can both be made stronger by feeding off each other, without losing essential elements?

As we close up the chapter, our discussions and reflection have likely stirred up more concerns and unsolved questions than provided answers, which we hope is congruent with the Zen spirit. We would like to leave with a few final questions for the readers to ponder. We came across a video[16] of Kabat-Zinn (2007) giving a talk to Google employees about how to create a better environment for productivity through five-minute mindfulness sessions. We could not help but wonder: Is this the ultimate meaning of staying present? Can someone be present for a few minutes, when the main purpose of those minutes is to be more effective for someone else's profit? Is mindfulness immune from social and economic power and privilege? If it is not, do we need to engage in a broader ethical reflection on where we are going with it? How can we truly honor Zen's non-gaining mind and its essence as "good for nothing" (Uchiyama et al. 2004), to go beyond "mindfulness skill training" and turn inward to cultivate one's being *in and for itself* toward more freedom? Many opportunities remain for the partnership between Zen and psychotherapy during these interesting times.

Acknowledgements The authors greatly appreciate Meadow Didier for insightful discussions and comments on earlier versions of this manuscript.

References

Adler, A. (1964). *Social interest: A challenge to mankind.* New York: Capricorn Books.

Ando, O. (2009). Psychotherapy and Buddhism: A psychological consideration of key points of contact. In D. Mathers, M. E. Miller, & O. Ando (Eds.), *Self and no-self: Continuing the dialogue between Buddhism and psychotherapy* (pp. 8–18). New York: Routledge.

Bach, P., & Hayes, S. (2002). The use of acceptance and commitment therapy to prevent the rehospitalisation of psychotic patients: A randomized controlled trial. *Journal of Consulting and Clinical Psychology, 70,* 1129–1139.

Bazzano, M. (2010). A true person of no status. Existential analysis. *Journal of the Society for Existential Analysis, 21*(1), 51–62.

Bazzano, M. (2015). Before and after mindfulness. *Self & Society, 43*(1), 3–5.

[16]This video can be retrieved from www.youtube.com/watch?v=3nwwKbM_vJc. The part that we address here occurs between 48:20 and 49:25 of the video.

Bernstein, R. J. (1978). *The restructuring of social and political theory*. Philadelphia: University of Pennsylvania Press.

Bobrow, J. (2010). *Zen and psychotherapy: Partners in liberation*. New York: WW Norton & Company.

Bodiford, W. M. (2006). Koan practice. In J. D. Loori (Ed.), *Sitting with koans*. Somerville, MA: Wisdom Publications.

Bodiford, W. M. (2012). Textual genealogies of Dōgen. In S. Heine (Ed.), *Dōgen: Textual and historical studies*. New York: Oxford University Press.

Brazier, D. (1997). *Zen therapy: Transcending the sorrows of the human mind*. New York: Wiley.

Brazier, D. (2001). *Zen therapy: A Buddhist approach to psychotherapy*. London: Robinson.

Carspecken, P. (2009). Limits to knowledge with existential significance: An outline for the exploration of post-secular spirituality of relevance to qualitative research. In R. Winkle-Wagner, C. Hunter, & D. H. Ortloff (Eds.), *Bridging the gap between theory and practice in educational research: Methods at the margins*. New York: Palgrave Macmillan.

Cautin, R. L. (2011). A century of psychotherapy, 1860–1960. In J. C. Norcross, G. R. VandenBos, & D. K. Freedheim (Eds.), *History of psychotherapy: Continuity and change* (2nd ed., pp. 3–38). Washington, DC: American Psychological Association.

Cavill, M. (2010). Mindfulness, nothing special. *Existential Analysis, 21*(1), 37–40.

Chambless, D. L., Babich, K., & Crits-Christoph, P. (1995). Training in and dissemination of empirically-validated psychological treatments: Report and recommendations. *The Clinical Psychologist, 48*(1), 3–24.

Chiesa, A., & Malinowski, P. (2011). Mindfulness-based approaches: Are they all the same? *Journal of Clinical Psychology, 67*(4), 404–424.

Christopher, M. S. (2003). Albert Ellis and the Buddha: Rational soul mates? A comparison of rational emotive behaviour therapy (REBT) and Zen Buddhism. *Mental Health, Religion & Culture, 6*(3), 283–293.

Cleary, T., & Cleary, J. C. (1977). *The blue cliff record*. Boston: Shambhala Publications.

Cook, F. H. (1977). *Hua-yen Buddhism: The jewel net of Indra*. University Park: Penn State Press.

Cooper, P. C. (2010). *The Zen impulse and the psychoanalytic encounter*. New York: Routledge/Taylor & Francis Group.

Cooper, P. C. (2011). Total exertion: Zen, psychoanalysis, life. *Journal of Religion and Health, 50*(3), 592–601.

Cooper, P. (2014). Zen meditation, reverie, and psychoanalytic listening. *The Psychoanalytic Review, 101*(6), 795–813.

Crocker, S., & Philippson, P. (2005). Phenomenology, existentialism, and eastern thought in gestalt therapy. In A. Woldt & S. Toman (Eds.), *Gestalt therapy: History, theory, and practice* (pp. 65–81). Thousand Oaks, CA: SAGE Publications Inc.

Dahl, J., Wilson, K. G., & Nilsson, A. (2004). Acceptance and commitment therapy and the treatment of persons at risk for long-term disability resulting from stress and pain symptoms: A preliminary randomized trial. *Behavior Therapy, 35,* 785–802.

Derrida, J. (1997). *Of grammatology*. Baltimore: The Johns Hopkins University Press.

Elliot, T. S. (1944). *Four quartets*. London, England: Faber and Faber.

Ellis, A. (1962). *Reason and emotion in psychotherapy*. Secaucus, NJ: Citadel.

Ellis, A. (1992). The revised ABCs of rational-emotive therapy (RET). In J. K. Zeig & J. K. Zeig (Eds.), *The evolution of psychotherapy: The second conference* (pp. 79–99). Philadelphia, PA: Brunner/Mazel.

Freud, S. (1912). *Recommendations to physicians on practicing psychoanalysis* (pp. 111–120). London: Hogarth Press.

Freud, S. (1921). *A general introduction to psychoanalysis*. New York: Boni and Liveright.

Fromm, E. (1960). Psychoanalysis and Zen Buddhism. In E. Fromm, D. T. Suzuki, & R. Demartino (Eds.), *Zen Buddhism and psychoanalysis* (pp. 1–76). New York: Harper & Brothers.

Fromm, E., Suzuki, D. T., & De Martino, R. (1960). *Zen Buddhism and psychoanalysis*. New York: Harper & Brothers.

Griffith, F. T. (2000). The form and function of koan literature. A historical overview. In S. Heine & D. S. Wright (Eds.), *Texts and contexts in Zen Buddhism.* Oxford: Oxford University Press.

Gunn, R. J. (2009). Two arrows meeting in mid-air. In D. Mathers, M. E. Miller, & O. Ando (Eds.), *Self and no-self: Continuing the dialogue between Buddhism and psychotherapy* (pp. 19–24). New York: Routledge.

Habermas, J. (1971). *Knowledge and human interests* (J. J. Shapiro, Trans.). Boston: Beacon Press.

Habermas, J. (1981). *The theory of communicative action. Volume I: Reason and the rationality of society*. Boston: Beacon Press.

Habermas, J. (1990). *On the logic of the social sciences*. Cambridge, MA: The MIT Press.

Hanh, T. N. (2006). *Transformation and healing: Sutra on the four establishments of mindfulness*. Berkeley, CA: Parallax Press.

Hanh, T. N. (2009). *Peaceful action, open heart: Lessons from the Lotus Sutra*. Berkeley, CA: Parallax Press.

Harris, R. (2006). Embracing your demons: An overview of acceptance and commitment therapy. *Psychotherapy in Australia, 12*(4), 2–8.

Hayes, S. C. (2004). Acceptance and commitment therapy, relational frame theory, and the third wave of behavioral and cognitive therapies. *Behavior Therapy, 35*(4), 639–665.

Hayes, S. C., Luoma, J. B., Bond, F. W., Masuda, A., & Lillis, J. (2006). Acceptance and commitment therapy: Model, processes and outcomes. *Behaviour Research and Therapy, 44*(1), 1–25.

Hayes, S. C., Strosahl, K. D., & Wilson, K. G. (1999). *Acceptance and commitment therapy: An experiential approach to behavior change*. Guilford Press.

Hegel, G. F. (1977). *The phenomenology of spirit* (A. V. Miller, Trans.). Oxford: Clarendon Press.

Hegel, G. F. (1991). *Hegel's science of logic* (A. V. Miller, Tans.). New York: Humanity Books.

Heisig, J. W. (2002). Jung, Christianity and Buddhism. In P. Young-Eisendrath & S. Muramoto (Eds.), *Awakening and insight: Zen Buddhism and psychotherapy* (pp. 149–171). New York, NY, USA: Brunner-Routledge.

Hollis, M (1994) *The philosophy of social science: An introduction*. New York: Cambridge Press.

Horney, K. (1945). *Our inner conflicts*. New York: Norton.

Horney, K. (1952). The paucity of inner experiences. *The American Journal of Psychoanalysis, 12*(1), 3–9.

James, W. (1892). *Psychology: Briefer course*. New York: H. Holt, and Company.

Jennings, L., & Skovholt, T. M. (1999). The cognitive, emotional, and relational characteristics of master therapists. *Journal of Counseling Psychology, 46*(1), 3–11.

Johanson, G. J. (2006). The use of mindfulness in psychotherapy. *Annals of the American Psychotherapy Association, 9*(2), 15–24.

Jung, C. G. (1969/1916). The transcendent function. In *The collected works of C.G. Jung* (vol. 8, R. F. C. Hull, Trans.). Princeton, NJ: Princeton University Press.

Kabat-Zinn, J. (1990). *Full catastrophe living: Using the wisdom of your body and mind to face stress, pain, and illness*. New York: Bantam Dell.

Kabat-Zinn, J. (1994). *Wherever you go, there you are*. New York: Hyperion.

Kabat-Zinn, J. (2003). Mindfulness-based interventions in context: Past, present, and future. *Clinical Psychology: Science and Practice, 10*(2), 144–156.

Kabat-Zinn, J. (2005). *Coming to our senses. Healing ourselves and the world through mindfulness*. London: Piatkus.

Kabat-Zinn, J. (2007, November 12). Mindfulness with Jon Kabat-Zinn. [Web log comment]. Retrieved from https://www.youtube.com/watch?v=3nwwKbM_vJc

Kabat-Zinn, J., & Hanh, T. N. (2009). *Full catastrophe living: Using the wisdom of your body and mind to face stress, pain, and illness*. New York: Delta.

Kapleau, P. (1989). *The three pillars of zen: Teaching, practice, and enlightenment*. New York: Anchor.

Kasamatsu, A., & Hirai, T. (1966). An electroencephalographic study on the Zen meditation (Zazen). *Psychiatry and Clinical Neurosciences, 20*(4), 315–336.

Kato, H. (2005). Zen and psychology. *Japanese Psychological Research, 47*, 125–136.

Kelman, H. (1960). Psychoanalytical thought and Eastern wisdom. In J. Ehrenwald (Ed.), *The history of psychotherapy*. New York: Jason Aronson.

Kessler, R. C., Brandenburg, N., Lane, M., Roy-Byrne, P., Stang, P. D., Stein, D. J., & Wittchen, H. U. (2005). Rethinking the duration requirement for generalized anxiety disorder: Evidence from the National Comorbidity Survey Replication. *Psychological Medicine, 35*, 1073–1082.

Kwee, M., & Ellis, A. (1998). The interface between rational emotive behavior therapy (REBT) and Zen. *Journal of Rational-Emotive & Cognitive-Behavior Therapy, 16*(1), 5–43.

Lambert, M. J. (2004). *Bergin and Garfield's handbook of psychotherapy and behavior change* (5th ed.). New York: Wiley.

Lazarus, A. A. (1977). Toward an egoless state of being. In A. Ellis & R. Grieger (Eds.), *Handbook of rationalemotive therapy* (pp. 113–118). New York: Springer.

Lin, P., & Seiden, H. M. (2015). Mindfulness and psychoanalytic psychotherapy: A clinical convergence. *Psychoanalytic Psychology, 32*(2), 321–333.

Linehan, M. M. (1987). Dialectical behavioral therapy: A cognitive behavioral approach to parasuicide. *Journal of Personality Disorders, 1*(4), 328–333.

Linehan, M. M. (1993). *Cognitive-behavioral treatment of borderline personality disorder*. New York: Guilford Press.

Linehan, M. M. (1995). *Treating borderline personality disorder: The dialectical approach*. New York: Guilford Publications.

Linehan, M. M. (2013). *Dialectical behavior therapy*. Phoenix, AZ, USA: Milton H. Erickson Foundation.

MacHovec, F. J. (1984). Current therapies in the ancient East. *American Journal of Psychotherapy, 38*(1), 87–96.

Marx, K. (1988). *Economic and philosophic manuscripts of 1844* (M. Milligan, Trans.). Amherst, NY: Prometheus Books.

Masis, K. V. (2002). American Zen and psychotherapy, and ongoing dialogue. In P. Young-Eisendrath & S. Muramoto (Eds.), *Awakening and insight: Zen Buddhism and psychotherapy* (pp. 147–168). New York, NY, USA: Brunner-Routledge.

Mathers, D., Miller, M. E., & Ando, O. (Eds.). (2009). *Self and no-self: Continuing the dialogue between Buddhism and psychotherapy*. New York: Routledge.

Maupin, E. W. (1962). Zen Buddhism: A psychological review. *Journal of Consulting Psychology, 26*(4), 362–378.

McCarthy, T. (1981). *The critical theory of Jürgen Habermas*. MIT Press.

Meckel, D. J., & Moore, R. L. (Eds.). (1992). *Self and liberation: The Jung/Buddhism dialogue*. New York and Mahwah, NJ: Paulist Press. Ford Press.

Miller, M. E. (2009). Buddhism and psychotherapy: A dialogue. In D. Mathers, M. E. Miller, & O. Ando (Eds.), *Self and no-self: Continuing the dialogue between Buddhism and psychotherapy* (pp. 3–7). New York, NY, USA: Brunner-Routledge.

Moore, D. W. (1997). *The accidental Buddhist*. Chapel Hill, North Carolina: Algonquin Books of Chapel Hill.

Muramoto, S. (1984). On the relationship of psychology to Zen Buddhism (2): Psychologia and Koji Sato. *Zengaku-Kenkyu (Studies in Zen Buddhism), 63*, 69–93.

Muramoto, S. (1998). The Jung-Hisamatsu conversation. In A. Molino (Ed.), *The couch and the tree: Dialogues in psychoanalysis and Buddhism*. New York: North Point Press.

Muramoto, S. (2003). Buddhism, religion, and psychotherapy in the world today. In P. Young-Eisendrath & S. Muramoto (Eds.), *Awakening and insight: Zen Buddhism and psychotherapy* (pp. 15–28). New York, NY, USA: Brunner-Routledge.

Nanda, J. (2009). Mindfulness. *Existential Analysis: Journal of the Society for Existential Analysis, 20*(1), 147–162.

Naranjo, C. (1970). Present-centeredness: Technique, prescription, and ideal. In J. Fagan & I. L. Shepherd (Eds.), *Gestalt therapy now* (pp. 47–69). Palo Alto, CA: Science and Behavior Books.

Norcross, J. C., Pfund, R. A., & Prochaska, J. O. (2013). Psychotherapy in 2022: A Delphi poll on its future. *Professional Psychology: Research and Practice, 44* (5), 363.

Ogden, T. H. (2007). *This art of psychoanalysis: Dreaming undreamt dreams and interrupted cries*. New York: Routledge.

Okumura, S. (2010). *Realizing Genjokoan: The key to Dōgen's Shōbōgenzō*. Boston: Wisdom Publications.

Rahula, W. (1959). *What the buddha taught*. Oxford: Oneworld Publications.

Robins, C. J. (2002). Zen principles and mindfulness practice in dialectical behavior therapy. *Cognitive and Behavioral Practice, 9*(1), 50–57.

Rosenbaum, R. (2015). *Zen and the heart of psychotherapy*. New York: Routledge.

Santorelli, S. (1999). *Heal thyself: Lessons on mindfulness in medicine*. New York: Bell Tower.

Schwandt, T. A. (2008). Educating for intelligent belief in evaluation. *American Journal of Evaluation, 29*(2), 139–150.

Segal, Z. J., Williams, M. G., & Teasdale, J. D. (2002). *Mindfulness-based cognitive therapy for depression: A new approach to preventing relapses*. New York: Guilford Press.

Shapiro, S. L., Carlson, L. E., Astin, J. A., & Freedman, B. (2006). Mechanisms of mindfulness. *Journal of Clinical Psychology, 62*(3), 373–386.

Shore, J. (2002). A Buddhist model of the human self. In P. Young-Eisendrath & S. Muramoto (Eds.), *Awakening and insight: Zen Buddhism and psychotherapy* (pp. 149–171). New York, NY, USA: Brunner-Routledge.

Stolorow, R. D., Brandchaft, B., & Atwood, G. E. (1987). *Psychoanalytic treatment: An intersubjective approach*. Hillsdale, NJ: Analytic Press.

Teasdale, J. D., & Segal, Z. V. (2007). *The mindful way through depression: Freeing yourself from chronic unhappiness*. New York: Guilford Press.

Teyber, E. (2005). *Interpersonal process in therapy: An integrative model*. Brooks Cole.

Thera, N. (1996). *The heart of Buddhist meditation*. Boston: Weiser Books.

Thynn, D. T. (1995). *Living meditation, living insight: The path of mindfulness in daily life*. Carmel, NY: The Buddhist Association of the United States.

Tugendhat, E. (1989). *Self-consciousness and self-determination*. Cambridge, MA: MIT Press.

Twohig, M. P., Hayes, S. C., & Masuda, A. (2006). Increasing willingness to experience obsessions: Acceptance and commitment therapy as a treatment for obsessive compulsive disorder. *Behavior Therapy, 37*(1), 3–13.

Uchiyama, K., Wright, T., Warner, J., & Okumura, S. (2004). *Opening the hand of thought: Foundations of Zen Buddhist practice*. New York: Simon and Schuster.

Vasquez, M. J. (2010). Ethics in multicultural counseling practice. In J. G. Ponterotto, J. M. Casas, L. A. Suzuki, & C. M. Alexander (Eds.), *Handbook of multicultural counseling* (pp. 127–145). Thousand Oaks, CA: Sage Publications.

Weber, M. (1978). *Economy and society: An outline of interpretive sociology*. Oakland, CA: University of California Press.

Williams, J. M. G., & Kuyken, W. (2012). Mindfulness-based cognitive therapy: A promising new approach to preventing depressive relapse. *British Journal of Psychiatry, 200,* 359–360.

Williams, L. (2006). Spirituality and Gestalt: A Gestalt-transpersonal perspective. *Gestalt Review, 10* (1), 6–21.

World Health Organization. (2012). Depression. Retrieved on June 20, 2015, from http://www.who.int/mediacentre/factsheets/fs369/en/

Wynne, A. (2007). *The origin of Buddhist meditation*. Oxford: Routledge.

Young-Eisendrath, P. (2003). The transformation of human suffering. In P. Young-Eisendrath & S. Muramoto (Eds.), *Awakening and insight: Zen Buddhism and psychotherapy* (pp. 149–171). New York, NY, USA: Brunner-Routledge.

Young-Eisendrath, P., & Muramoto, S. (2003). *Awakening and insight: Zen Buddhism and psychotherapy*. New York, NY, USA: Brunner-Routledge.

Zettle, R. D., & Raines, J. C. (1989). Group cognitive and contextual therapies in treatment of depression. *Journal of Clinical Psychology, 45,* 438–445.

Zen's Thoughts on Psychopathology and Wellness

Akihiko Masuda and Kayla Sargent

Keywords
Zen · Buddhism · Psychopathology · Mindfulness · Behavioral health

Putting my right and left hands together as one, I just bow.
Just bow to become one with Buddha and God.
Just bow to become one with everything I encounter.
Just bow to become one with all the myriad things.
Just bow as life becomes life.
Uchiyama (2004).

Behavioral health is an interdisciplinary enterprise that emphasizes the mutual relationship between the holistic view of human behavior and the well-being of the body as a whole entity. In recent years, the field has begun to pay greater attention to the wisdom and teachings of Zen Buddhism more so than ever before. Mindfulness, acceptance, nonjudgment, and compassion, the terms said to be equivalent to or originated from the teachings of Zen and Buddhism, have gained the status of buzzwords among behavioral health professionals and scholars (Germer and Neff 2013; Monteiro et al. 2015; Neff 2003). Experts predict that the influence of mindfulness and related approaches is likely to continue as a dominant force in psychotherapy at least for the next several years (Norcross et al. 2013). The expansion of mindfulness- and acceptance-based cognitive behavioral therapies (Hayes et al. 2004, 2011), such as acceptance and commitment therapy (ACT; Hayes et al. 1999), dialectical behavior therapy (Linehan 1993), mindfulness-based cognitive therapy (Segal et al. 2002), and mindfulness-based stress reduction (Kabat-Zinn 1990), has contributed substantially to this movement. Additionally, other major psychotherapies such as interpersonal psychotherapy have incorporated mindfulness and compassion into their theories and practices (Mathers et al. 2009; Norcross et al. 2013; Young-Eisendrath and Muramoto 2002).

The field of behavioral health has integrated mindfulness and Zen practices into its mainstream practice because of their salutary effects found on health (Brown et al. 2007; Chiesa 2009). Whereas

A. Masuda (✉) · K. Sargent
University of Hawaii at Manoa, Honolulu, USA
e-mail: amasuda4@hawaii.edu

K. Sargent
e-mail: kaylansargent@gmail.com

A. Masuda and W.T. O'Donohue (eds.), *Handbook of Zen, Mindfulness, and Behavioral Health*,
Mindfulness in Behavioral Health, DOI 10.1007/978-3-319-54595-0_16

this effort is generally encouraging, Zen Buddhism practitioners and scholars caution us to practice Zen while being explicit about the purpose of doing so (Suzuki 1994, 1997; Uchiyama et al. 2004). For Zen Buddhists, the incorporation of Zen practices into mainstream behavioral health care can be problematic only if such integration intends to promote what Zen Buddhism calls "return to the original wholeness" (Tanahashi and Levitt 2013), or "pure subjectivity" (Suzuki 1996), the heart of Zen Buddhism. The original wholeness or pure subjectivity is the process of perfecting self with an earnest endeavor for the benefit of mankind and all sentient beings (Japan Buddhist Federation 1978).

Kosho Uchiyama (内山 興正; 1912–1998), a monk internationally recognized for his efforts to disseminate Soto Zen Buddhism to the West, used the term *bonpu zen* (i.e., utilitarian Zen; Common-person *Dhyana*) to refer to Zen practices for the sake of bettering or improving one's own condition or circumstances. Although never criticizing utilitarian Zen, Uchiyama made a clear distinction between practicing Zen unconditionally for the Buddha Way (i.e., the original wholeness, pure subjectivity) and Zen for utilitarian purposes. Practicing Zen unconditionally is to practice Zen for the sake of it alone—something entirely consistent with Zen's focus on focus—with an attitude of letting go of all thoughts of how Zen could benefit the self and refraining from acting on them.

Kodo Sawaki (沢木 興道; 1880–1965), Uchiyama's teacher, also stated that "Zen is good for nothing" (Uchiyama and Okumura 2014, p. 138). What we often want from Zen and mindfulness practice in the context of psychotherapy is the cessation of discontent, suffering, or psychopathology (e.g., depression, anxiety) or the improvement of self (e.g., enlightenment, pursuit of a better being). However, as Sawaki's saying implies, Zen may not be good for seeking these utilitarian ends (e.g., symptom reduction), especially when one practices Zen for these. Shohaku Okumura (奥村 正博; 1948–present), an internationally recognized Soto Zen monk and a student of Uchiyama, also stated the following:

> We practice not to get somewhere better. We practice here and now, transcending the distinction between samsara and nirvana (Uchiyama and Okumura 2014, p. 17).

Samsara refers to the pain and suffering as well as the joy and happiness that our lives bring us. Nirvana refers to the experience of enlightenment or tranquility as well as that of living hell (Bobrow 2010; Rahula 1974; Suzuki 1970). For Zen, the transcendence of the distinction between samsara and nirvana is to become less entangled by our habitual way of thinking (e.g., categorization, differentiation, judgment) as well as to become fully open to the events unfolding here and now. Statements like these can be confusing or seem illogical from such an analytic perspective; thus, we will explain the nuance in detail below.

Epistemological Standpoints of Zen and Behavioral Health

Scholars have pointed out many similarities between behavioral health practices and Zen (de Silva 1984; Kurak 2003; Shapiro and Zifferblatt 1976). However, the two may be fundamentally different from each other at an epistemological level. We do not argue that the epistemological standpoint of behavioral health is superior to that of Zen Buddhism, or vice versa. Rather, we simply say that their different worldviews yield fundamentally different "ways of knowing" (see the introductory chapter of this volume). In general, the field of behavioral health is epistemologically analytic, categorical, and mechanistic (Masuda and Nisbett 2001), although such an overgeneralization like this is misleading. In fact, there are several behavioral perspectives of Western origin that seem to overlap epistemologically with Zen Buddhism, such as B.F. Skinner's radical behaviorism (Skinner 1971, 1974), J.R. Kantor's interbehaviorism (Hayes and Fredericks 1999; Kantor 1959), and S. C. Hayes' functional contextualism (Hayes et al. 2012; Wilson et al. 2014). Epistemologically, Zen Buddhism is perhaps more holistic, inclusive, and transient, although such a Western classification is not suitable for faithfully capturing the heart of Zen (Dogen et al. 2011; Tanahashi and Levitt 2013).

Importance of Elucidating Epistemological Standpoint

There are at least three critical reasons for the importance of elucidating the epistemological positions of Zen, behavioral health, and the person of interest (e.g., a given therapist, client, or the reader of this chapter). First, we form an idea and engage in a particular practice based upon a set of particular epistemological and metaphysical assumptions, collectively called a worldview (Gergen 1983). As noted below extensively, it is not surprising that elaborated classification systems of psychopathology emerged from a Western sociocultural context as its worldview is largely analytic, logical, and categorical. Similarly, because of its worldview, it is not surprising that Zen does not develop such classification systems for understanding or treating mental health or any other human activities. Instead, Zen often makes seemingly illogical statements about human nature (e.g., "Zen is to study the self, and studying the self is to not study the self"). Relevant to the topic of present chapter, differences between Zen and behavioral health in their accounts of psychopathology are not empirical ones, but philosophical ones.

Second, a person's epistemological assumptions influence the way he or she interacts with the world, including the ideas and practices of others. For example, a given statement (e.g., "life is suffering") can be interpreted differently, depending on one's epistemological position. Some may interpret the statement "life is suffering," from a holistic and inclusive perspective as if it evokes the feelings of interrelatedness with, or even compassion toward, the self and others as a whole (Dogen et al. 2011; Okumura 2010). For others, the statement is the description of a set of discrete events in a logically consistent manner (Nisbett et al. 2001). As such, the meaning of a given statement is not in the statement itself, but in the *perceiver* of that statement. This point is also crucial for practicing Zen and mindfulness. The nature of Zen and mindfulness practices largely depends upon the person who practices these (Bien 2006; Dogen et al. 1997).

Third, although a worldview plays a pivotal role in how we think, feel, and use our language, it is also often unnoticed. Szasz (1960) stated that when a worldview underlying certain activities is widely shared, those who participate in these activities often lose sight of it. Thus, what begins as conscious consensus or agreement among participants in a social or cultural group slowly evolves into an assumption or guiding framework for life (i.e., a worldview). In behavioral health, we as professionals do what we do (e.g., procedures in assessment, psychotherapy, consultation) as if it is *the way* it is without intentionally becoming cognizant of the underlying presumptions of what we do. For example, the construct of psychopathology may be the product of a particular worldview we hold, which happens to be culturally shared by many of us in our sociolinguistic and cultural context (Hayes et al. 1988; Szasz 1960; Uchiyama et al. 2004).

Aims of the Present Chapter

In this chapter, we present Zen's thoughts on what we call psychopathology and wellness. To do so, we first present a Western analytic perspective that serves as the underlying epistemological framework for Western behavioral health. We then present how this framework is embedded within its own theory and classification system for psychopathology and health. Subsequently, we will delineate a Zen's epistemological perspective and its thoughts on psychopathology and behavioral health. Finally, we will present the aim of Zen, which is to "live fully here and now while transcending psychopathology and psychological well-being."

The Field of Behavioral Health: Its Worldview and Trends

Western culture is known for its analytic and logical way of thinking (Nisbett et al. 2001; Uchiyama et al. 2004), and Western behavioral health is no exception. Analytic worldviews assume that the world, or the phenomenon of interest, is reducible to its parts with unique properties (e.g., the collection of distinct objects) and that these distinct parts interact with one other in a systematic fashion (Hayes et al. 1988; Masuda and Nisbett 2001; Nisbett et al. 2001). This "way of knowing" may be considered mechanistic (Hayes et al. 1988); that is, its application can be likened to the metaphor of a machine in that specific and discrete concepts relate to other specific and discrete concepts in some systematic way, set in motion by an observable force. In Western cultures, this way of thinking shapes the way we make sense of the self and the world through formal processes like science as well as informal like common discourses in popular culture.

The analytic way of thinking is at the core of Western science and technology, and it is the major vehicle of advancing Western society as well as globalization. Through understanding, predicting, and influencing parts of the world, the analytic way of thinking has advanced our society in the areas of medicine, communication, chemistry, physics, astronomy, cellular biology, to name a few. As a result, we have longer life expectancy and greater mobility than ever before.

The relation between this analytic way of thinking and linguistic practices warrants additional explanation. As linguists posit (e.g., Maynard 1997), our cultural beliefs and practices (e.g., worldviews) shape the way we use language and vice versa. In the West, language serves to identify, categorize, and differentiate phenomena of interest by using words and sentences corresponding to them. For example, in discussing psychological knowledge in Western cultures, Gergen (1983) describes the role of language as follows:

> To "understand" a given phenomenon in present-day psychology essentially requires that its property be synthesized into a linguistic framework. At a minimum, such a framework also requires the imposition of a category system onto the phenomena of interest. In this sense, language lends itself to an atomistic approach to understanding; language requires that the phenomena be broken into disparate segments (p. 133).

The analytic worldview is also logical (Nisbett et al. 2001). In Western thinking, simply categorizing events is incomplete; it is necessary to make sense of the relations among events by understanding them through law-like principles (e.g., prediction-and-control). In Western behavioral health, a set of symptoms is framed into a given mental disorder through a principle of association as a demonstration of this systematic way of thinking. A causal model of psychopathology also exemplifies this systematic approach: Severe conditions (e.g., war) cause a set of particular symptoms that are collectively categorized as posttraumatic stress disorder (PTSD) because war and these symptoms relate to one another.

It is important to note that the analytic worldview is not limited to Western sociolinguistic contexts (Maynard 1997). According to Suzuki (1997), this way of thinking is built within every linguistic practice, including Japanese and other Asian cultures (Markus and Kitayama 1991, 2010): It is simply more noticeable among Westerners than among Easterners (Nisbett et al. 2001; Peng and Nisbett 1999).

Western Analytic Account of Psychopathology

In behavioral health literature, psychopathology is often defined as the scientific study of the development and maintenance of mental disorders, including efforts to identify their genetic, biological, psychological, and sociocultural causes as well as the development of effective classification schemes (nosology) and treatment interventions (Follette and Houts 1996). The term psychopathology also refers to the presentation of behaviors (i.e., symptoms) that indicate the presence of a mental disorder.

The construct and practice of psychopathology reflects Western analytic way of thinking. One of the most commonly used classification systems of psychopathology is the Diagnostic and Statistical Manual of Mental Disorders (DSM; American Psychiatric Association 2013). The DSM dichotomizes human experiences into normal versus abnormal behaviors as if they are mutually exclusive entities, subsequently dividing the abnormal into over 300 distinct disorders. Following an analytic worldview, we presuppose that there are *crystalized and distinct entities*, called mental illnesses (e.g., "binge eating disorder is a medical condition"; Szasz 1960). Whether the DSM is a valid classification system is not a central topic here (Follette and Houts 1996; Frances 2013b; Lasalvia 2015; Wakefield 2015). Rather, we intend to highlight the ways in which our presuppositions behind our professional activities, such as our adherence to the DSM, are analytic and often unnoticed.

Symptom reduction and problem-solving are quintessential goals of therapies (Hayes et al. 1996) as well as a core competency for clinicians (Whaley and Davis 2007) in Western behavioral health. As discussed extensively elsewhere (Weisz et al. 1984), once a given event is viewed as something unwanted (e.g., the entity that is inherently problematic), making efforts to eliminate it is considered the most logical solution (Anderson et al. 1997). For example, when a binge eating is considered pathological, behavioral health intervention is implemented to reduce its occurrence.

Finally, Western behavioral health is known for its intrapsychic approach, although the field has recognized the importance of integrated care and the organism–environment relationship more so than ever before (Cummings and O'Donohue 2012; Cummings et al. 2001; O'Donohue and Maragakis 2015). The greater focus on one's internalizing issues in Western behavioral health (e.g., the use of psychotropic mediation to alleviate emotional sufferings) is said to stem from the sense of self derived from an analytic and logical way of thinking. As Markus and Kitayama (1991) stated, we, as Westerners, tend to view the self as an independent, self-contained, autonomous entity that "(a) comprise[s] a unique configuration of internal attributes (e.g., traits, abilities, motives, and values) and (b) behave[s] primarily as a consequence of these internal attributes" (Markus and Kitayama 1991, p. 224). As such, many of what we call a mental disorder, such as depression and anxiety, and well-being are often attributed largely to an individual's internal characteristics, such as symptoms and self-esteem, and treatments often focus on these intrapsychic phenomena exclusively.

In sum, the Western behavioral health often treats and conceptualizes psychopathology as a set of discrete entities that are essentially problematic and may be caused and maintained by other intrapsychic entities. Following this line of reasoning, efforts to eliminate these entities are common directions in the treatment for promoting the client's functioning and behavioral adaptation (Mennin et al. 2013). Therefore, for Western behavioral health, psychopathology (e.g., the presence of psychiatric symptoms, such as depression and anxiety) is viewed as the direct contrast with well-being and the event to be removed from the self. In other words, one's health is often understood as the extent to which these symptoms are absent from the person.

Zen's Worldview

Zen Buddhism is holistic, inclusive, and transient in its worldview: The world is seen as a whole that is constantly changing. Its worldview transcends categorization and differentiation, including analytic versus holistic distinctions (Suzuki 1970). As the opening quote by Uchiyama says, the aim of Zen is to realize and embody this holistic and transient nature of life as oneself, called *buddhadharma*, the Buddha Way (Dogen et al. 2011; Uchiyama et al. 2004). For Zen, to learn the Buddha Way is to learn this experience of the self (Dogen et al. 2011; Okumura 2010). In the opening of *Genjokoan* in *Shobogenzo*, Dogen Zenji (道元禅師; 1200–1253), the founder of Japanese Soto Zen, stated:

> To practice and learn about the Buddha Way is to practice and learn about *jiko*. To practice and learn about *jiko* is to forget *jiko*. Forgetting about *jiko*, one is affirmed by all things, all phenomena (all dharmas). To be affirmed by all things means to be made to let go of all concepts and artificial divisions of one's body and mind, as well as the body and mind of others, by those very things that affirm us (see Uchiyama et al. 2004, p. xxiv).

In Zen literature, the term "self" is a rough translation of Japanese term *jiko* (自己), with its meanings going beyond the self as an independent and discrete entity. More specifically, the term *jiko* simultaneously reflects what Westerners think of as the self and the universe (one's entire subjective experience) more broadly.

Prior to interpreting the quote by Dogen Zenji further in detail, it is important to present key features of linguistic practice in Zen Buddhism. From our conventional and literal perspective, the quote by Uchiyama appears quite analytic and linear. That is, it appears to present a Zen Buddhism version of how to live one's life: "the Buddha Way is a study of self, which learns to see the self as the sum of all experiences that person encounters in his or her life, as well as all living beings in the world." If we interpret the quote literally, it is also quite bizarre. From a conventional as well as natural science standpoint, the self is inherently distinct from the rest of the world: For example, if your friend says that she is bringing herself to your house tomorrow, you do not think that she will bring the entire universe with her.

Zen Buddhism uses words and language much less literally than the way we typically use our language (Kasulis 1981; Wright 1992). For Zen, the transient wholeness (e.g., one's entire personal experience) is the basic unit of knowing, and epistemologically speaking, Zen Buddhism makes sense of the world though the *subjective experience* of this wholeness (Suzuki 1994), not from the perspective of the whole as the sum of distinct parts. Once again, we do not argue that Zen's perspective is superior to that of Western behavioral health. Rather, Zen Buddhism and Western behavioral health happen to have distinct ways of understanding the world. Because of its epistemological standpoint being holistic and transient, linguistic practice in Zen Buddhism is also holistic and transient.

In Zen Buddhism discourse, a given word (e.g., "insect") is used as if it refers to a point through which one experiences the whole. For example, the term "insect" is a word that refers not only to a distinct entity, but also to the entire wheel of life. Furthermore, the linguistic context of Zen Buddhism encourages the user of the word to become blended with the word as well as what the word refers to, experientially. The following quote by D.T. Suzuki makes this point further, and he called this way of experiencing the world as "pure subjectivity." He stated:

> When I began to study Zen, mountains were mountains: when I thought I understood Zen, mountains were not mountains; but when I came to full knowledge of Zen, mountains were again mountains (Suzuki 1996, p. 240).

In this quote, we can see the transition from how we typically perceive the world (i.e., the first part), and what we may think of what enlightened experience is (i.e., the second part) to what D.T. Suzuki means by "pure subjectivity" (i.e., the third part). The first part, "When I began to study Zen, mountains were mountains," describes how we typically relate to the world and ourselves. We tend to perceive and construe an event we see, hear, or touch as what our mind says it is as a unique and essential entity (Magid 2002). There is one-to-one correspondence between a word (i.e., "mountain") and what it refers to (what we refer to as a mountain). When we see mountains, they are "mountains" that are differentiated from "us," the perceivers, as well as other objects we perceive (e.g., sky, birds, the sun).

The second part, "when I thought I understood Zen, mountains were not mountains," is the stance of complete rejection of concepts or differentiations, which is often believed to be the state of enlightenment. When we hear the perspective of wholeness and oneness as an alternative to our Western worldview, we quickly try to reject any perception framed with a word as a delusion (e.g., "everything is formless, so there is no such thing as a mountain or self"). According to D.T. Suzuki, such an attitude is also a sign of our habitual way of thinking ("e.g., formlessness is good" and "labeling and classification is bad").

In the last part of the quote, D.T. Suzuki demonstrates the experience of a mountain as if it is an aspect of the whole into which D.T. Suzuki himself is also blended experientially. In this experience, there is no distinction between the perceiver and the perceived (e.g., "the absence of subject–object duality), and the word "mountains" is used accordingly as the reflection of this wholeness.

Another feature of Zen language and discourse is its dialectical stance, which is slightly different from that of the West (Miyamoto and Ryff 2011; Peng and Nisbett 1999; Zhang et al. 2015). Take the idiom "Life is sweet and sour." For Westerners, this idiom implies that life is the sum of multiple parts: Some aspects of life are sweet, and some aspects are sour. Dialectical efforts for Westerners include attempts to synthesize contradicting parts that are fundamentally distinct from one another. For Zen Buddhism, this idiom suggests that life is sweet and sour as *one,* that sweet and sour is life (e.g., the entire universe as a whole). Furthermore, Zen encourages the perceiver of the idiom to blend into the here-and-now experience with the idiom (e.g., the blending of subject–object in perceiver's experience). This Zen Buddhist's way of dialectical thinking is not the point of compromise or the coexistence of distinct entities. Rather, it is the experience of one (Suzuki 1970).

Here is Dogen Zenji's (1200–1253) quote again. It says:

> To practice and learn about the Buddha Way is to practice and learn about *jiko*. To practice and learn about *jiko* is to forget *jiko*. Forgetting about *jiko*, one is affirmed by all things, all phenomena (all dharmas). To be affirmed by all things means to be made to let go of all concepts and artificial divisions of one's body and mind, as well as the body and mind of others, by those very things that affirm us (see Uchiyama et al. 2004, p. xxiv).

From Zen's perspective, this quote is not linear or logical. It does not describe a systematic relation of distinct entities. It simply points to the transient wholeness by using different terms one after another (e.g., Buddha Way, *jiko*, dropping of body–mind"). Furthermore, this quote also encourages the perceiver of this quote (e.g., the reader of this chapter) to notice whether she or he feels the sense of oneness (Tanahashi and Levitt 2013; Uchiyama et al. 2004), including "becoming one with this quote." For many of us, this is a very strange linguistic and experiential practice (Wright 1992).

The Self as a Whole: The Fundamental Unit of Knowing

From a Zen Buddhist perspective, what Western behavioral health seems to overlook in mindfulness and Zen-like practices is this universal, interdependent, and transient sense of wholeness. Once again, we do not say that Zen Buddhism is better than the Western behavioral health because of its holistic perspective. Rather, we simply state that the difference between Zen and Western behavioral health is simply the difference in their epistemological positions. For Zen, the wholeness is the self becoming one with everything that the self encounters *experientially*. As with all the myriad things, a person experiences the self along with the transient and interdependent nature of life. Okumura (Dogen et al. 2011) observed the following concrete examples of embodying the true self:

> Concretely speaking, we should accept everything as the contents of our "self." We should meet everything as part of ourselves. "To study the self," means to awaken to such a self. For instance, many people visit my house or write me letters. Many of these people talk or write about their troubles and anguish and ask for my advice. I never feel troubled by such requests. As soon as I am asked about such troubles, they become my own. I meet people and problems in such a way. As long as I have such an attitude, these problems are my own. And they enrich my life. If I reject other people's problems saying, "That's not my business," my life becomes poorer and poorer. Therefore, to meet everything, without exception, as part of my life is most essential in the Buddha Way. This is what Dogen Zenji meant by saying, "To study the Buddha Way is to study the self" (p. 182).

Additional explanations for Okumura's statement just above are warranted. This quote does not mean that we are responsible for solving our own problems as well as those of others. Or, this quote does not say that one should experience what others experience exactly. We never know or feel exactly what it is like be this person who recently lost his loved one. Instead, what Okumura states here is the importance of perspective taking, empathy, compassion, and relatedness directed toward the self and others as a whole.

Ordinary Living and the Buddha Way

The experience of Buddha Way is to do what the self does every day wholeheartedly (Poceski 2015). As such, there is nothing sensational or enlightening about the Buddha Way. Rather, the Buddha Way is quite ordinary and yet quite extraordinary at the same time (Magid 2002; Uchiyama et al. 2004). It can be expressed in everyday activities, such as brushing teeth, preparing a meal, cleaning, working, communicating with peers, farting, and watching TV.

Qualitatively, the Buddha Way is to live fully from moment to moment, while *embracing* two fundamental principles of life in any given moment that capture the transient, holistic, and inclusive stance of living: impermanence (*mujo*: 無常) and interdependence (e.g., *engi*: 縁起, dependent arising). Ancient and contemporary Buddhism and Zen texts often describe impermanence as the Buddhist notion that everything is constantly changing and that all of conditioned existence, without exception, is transient, or in a constant state of flux. Uchiyama (Uchiyama et al. 2004), however, described the principle of impermanence rather boldly. He stated:

> Impermanence, *shogo mujo* [諸行無常], means that every living thing dies. In other words, everything that has life loses life. Moreover, no one, least of all the living thing itself, knows exactly when its life will end. Life has a limit, and it is always in a state of uncertainty. This is the first undeniable reality. I have mentioned that many people think that simply pursuing material happiness or riches is most important in life. But stand that way of life next to the reality of death and it completely falls apart. When a person who thinks he is happy because of his material situation has to face death, he's likely to fall into the depths of bitterness and despair. If happiness means having plenty of money and good health, then by that very definition, you're only going to hit rock bottom when it's your time to die. When you are faced with death, what good is being healthy or wealthy? That is why all of these materialistic pursuits only end in despair in the face of the undeniable reality of death… What exactly is it that we have to learn from this first undeniable reality? We have to clarify what life and death really are. We have to know clearly just what it means to be alive and what it means to die… It means knowing clearly just what death is, and then really living out one's life (pp. 7–8).

The principle of interdependence (e.g., dependent co-arising) states that "all concrete entities occur in accordance with various conditions, that they always happen based on conditions and never apart from or separate from such factors, and that all abstract entities have meaning because of their mutual relations" (Uchiyama et al. 2004, p. 98). Put together, all phenomena result from causation and are without permanent and independent substance. Nothing is completely isolated, and nothing is completely still. The Buddha Way is to live with the attitudes of embracing impermanence and interdependence from moment to moment As noted above, the impermanence and interdependence happen in here and now as the person's experience, not there as the knowledge. It is to experientially let one's own life to be part of this impermanence fully as well as part of this wholeness (e.g., the self becoming one with all the myriad things) while undermining arbitrarily created categorization and differentiation. Uchiyama called this whole process of full living as "opening the hand of thought" (Uchiyama et al. 2004).

Zen's View of Psychopathology and Health

The heart of Buddhism is sometimes said to be summed up in the Four Noble Truths. The contents of Four Noble Truths vary across Buddhist scholars and practitioners, but they generally follow this framework:

(1) All life is inevitably sorrowful,
(2) Sorrow emanates from attachment to self-absorbed and egocentric desire,
(3) Sorrow can only be stopped by the detachment from desire, and
(4) This can only be done by a course of careful conduct (as cited in Masuda and O'Donohue 2009, p. 234)

Interestingly, Barry Magid, a Zen teacher and psychoanalyst, stated that the Original Buddha (i.e., Gautama Buddha) could have stopped with the First Noble Truth: All life is inevitably sorrowful (Magid 2008, p. 69). This makes sense given that potential pitfalls present themselves when we are exposed to the second, third, and fourth truths. That is, if we interpret the Four Noble Truths through the framework of an analytic worldview, we end up understanding them as the Buddhism version of "how to get rid of struggle and suffering." As mentioned extensively elsewhere (Broughton 2009; Uchiyama et al. 2004), this is not what Zen Buddhism is for. Zen Buddhism is not for fulfilling an ego-protective desire (Uchiyama and Okumura 2014), including the cessation of suffering or the pursuit of happiness and enlightenment. If we expect something in return by practicing Zen and maintain the conventional sense of self and world, we are unlikely to awaken to the true self.

Zen and Psychopathology

Given its transient, inclusive, and holistic perspective, it is not surprising that Zen Buddhism does not have a concept equivalent to the Western notion of psychopathology. Similarly, Zen Buddhism does not have a specific practice comparable to psychotherapy, either. From this standpoint, Zen does not make an ontological claim of whether psychopathology exists. For example, Zen Buddhism does not affirm or negate the existence of a major depressive disorder with a specific biological origin(s). Zen Buddhism does not attempt to categorize particular forms of behavior into a syndrome or to exclude them as being normal. This is simply because Zen Buddhism has its unique epistemological position distinct from the Western analytic thinking. For Zen, in the pursuit of the Buddha Way with an earnest endeavor for the benefit of mankind and all sentient beings (Japan Buddhist Federation 1978; Suzuki 1994), the concept and practice of psychopathology is not necessary. However, Zen Buddhism can say about how our perception of psychopathology (e.g., "people with a mental illness are unpredictable") or personal experience of psychopathology (e.g., "I can't stop being anxious") affects the practice of the wholeness.

Zen does not minimize all of human sufferings by saying that they are all illusions. There are certainly personal, social, and cross-national issues in our life that should be resolved (e.g., interpersonal conflicts evoked from utilitarian desires). Nevertheless, some of what we identify as problematic (e.g., the lack of confidence, feeling of emptiness, severe depression, fear, anger, obsessive thoughts) may not have to be treated as a problem (Uchiyama and Okumura 2014). For Zen, functional impairments due to common mental disorders, such as depression and anxiety, seem to lighten indirectly if we promote the experience of transient and interdependent wholeness. Magid describes Zen practice and its effect on what we call psychopathology and suffering below:

> … the end of suffering that we realize we can achieve through practice turns out to be an end of *separation* from suffering. Suffering ceases to exist when it is no longer something we experience as impinging on our life, as an unnecessary, avoidable intrusion that we finally learn to exclude from our lives once and for all. Instead, what we realize deeply is that suffering is inseparable from life. I like to describe what happens by saying that suffering doesn't disappear *from* our life, but *into* our life. When we live our life as a whole, there is no longer an aspect that gets singled out as "suffering".
>
> Magid (2008, p. 70)

Once again, what Magid suggests here is the epistemological shift, a shift from an analytic worldview to the worldview of wholeness and impermanence. Although the aim of Zen is not the elimination of suffering, the pursuit of embracing wholeness and impermanence naturally blends suffering into life. This pursuit, at least, begins to dissolve the arduous struggle that coincides with an analytic desire to eliminate suffering completely.

To some extent, Western cultural practices may maintain a sense of separateness from others, exploiting the feelings of difference that underlie many forms of suffering or distress. For example, attachment to particular identities, in the form of "I am a depressed person," or demographically related identities like "I am a sexual minority," is pervasive in the field of behavioral health both in terms of theories and treatments of psychopathology. These various identities are conceptualized as somehow distinct with unique predictors, corresponding to unique treatments, corresponding to unique outcomes. Paradoxically, this way of thinking about the self seems to foster a sense of separateness and permanence: *I am different from others; my difference is a permanent.* In this regard, a Zen perspective on psychopathology and the way in which we identify ourselves with suffering and with our environment may inherently reduce suffering caused by this categorization, without intending to do so.

Zen and Living Fully

As the quote by Magid appears too simplistic for many Westerners, additional explanation will warrant. To do so, we will focus on the last sentence of his quote: "When we live our life as a whole, there is no longer an aspect that gets singled out as "suffering"." First, it is important for us to know that the last sentence is not of how to get rid of suffering or how to ease ourselves from suffering. Instead, it is of facing one is encountering openly and fully as a whole person whatever it is. For example, being a parent of a child with autism spectrum disorder is joyful and challenging at the same time (Blackledge and Hayes 2006). Some parents of children diagnosed with autism report the strong sense of guilt and shame ("I feel terrible hoping that my child is not autistic") in raising their children. Living one's life as a whole (i.e., living fully) in the context of raising a child diagnosed with autism is to raise the child unequivocally while being open to a whole range of emotional experiences, including shame, guilt, and joy. For the child with autism, living fully is to expose himself or herself to the natural and social environment and learn what he or she is capable of learning. Living fully, from a Zen perspective, is not to achieve a certain developmental or interpersonal milestones (e.g., living independently) or having a life better than those of others. Rather, it is to strive to fulfill one's potential set for each one of us (Okumura 2010; Uchiyama and Okumura 2014).

Zen and Behavioral Health

As noted above, Zen is concerned about its underlying assumptions of psychopathology (e.g., mental disorders) more so than the concept of psychopathology itself. In other words, some of what we call psychopathology (e.g., abnormalization of emptiness, depression, anxiety, substance use) are no longer events to be removed, but the ones to be acknowledged, if we incorporate the wisdom of impermanence and interdependence into our lives. This experiential and epistemological standpoint is not necessarily unique to Zen, and it is historically well supported across the world (Masuda and O'Donohue 2009). However, as our society becomes increasingly industrialized, we as a culture become increasingly unwilling to accept the transient and interdependent nature of our lives (Suzuki 1998; Szasz 1960; Uchiyama et al. 2004). A salient example is the increased risk of overpathologizing human experiences as seen in the most recent DSM, which obscures the difference between mental disorder and normality further than its predecessors (Frances 2013a; Lasalvia 2015). Similarly, our culture inflames our egocentric desires by promoting ideas of happiness that are contingent upon particular, often arbitrary, life domains such as body shape, relationships, and lifestyle (Frances 2013b;

Magid 2008; Uchiyama and Okumura 2014). Zen Buddhism does not say that we should stop pursuing our desires. Instead, it says that once we experience the self as the interdependent and transient whole, such experience of self naturally directs us to the pursuit of desires at an optimal level. In Buddhism, this optimal range of conducts is called the Middle Way (*chudo*: 中道).

An additional discussion of the Middle Way is warranted here. According to Zen Buddhism, the shift in personal priority occurs once we become to identify ourselves that go beyond our conventional sense of self as unique and isolated beings. For example, some people begin to endorse less on individual achievement in fame and profit (Uchiyama et al. 2004), spending more times with family and loved ones. Others may continue to endorse time for individual achievements, but not because of the fear of losing them, but because of the intrinsic joy of pursing these ends. Similarly, many Zen practitioners begin to practice Zen for the sake of bettering or improving one's own condition or circumstances at least initially (Uchiyama and Okumura 2014; Uchiyama et al. 2004). However, once they become closer to the experience of wholeness, these agendas are no longer the aim of practice.

This slight shift in perceived sense of self appears to contribute to healthy lifestyle change (Magid 2000; Uchiyama and Okumura 2014). The following is a clinical case that the first author (A.M) supervised as a licensed psychologist in a university psychology clinic. The client was a 40-year-old mother with chronic pain, and she was seen by one of his graduate supervisees. As she identified herself with the experience of chronic pain, one piece of advice that the first author gave the supervisee was to help the client expand her sense of self. In particular, the student supervisee (the therapist) encouraged her to get in touch with the sense of self as a woman with chronic pain, as well as a loving and caring mother of three daughters, and the person who enjoys a sunny day as a whole. Then, he advised the supervisee to help the client identify the activities that she would like to engage from the sense of that larger self. Following the discussion with the supervisee along with the approval from her physician, the client took her daughters to a local amusement park for the first time in 3 years, despite pain and anticipated fears of pain getting worse. In the following session, the clients reported the experience of pain while she was in the amusement park with her daughters, and she also presented the sense of aliveness and accomplishment by taking her daughters to the park. She stated that it was her sense of self as a mother and the daughters' smiles that made it worth experiencing pain. This was the turning point of the therapy, and since that episode, the client gradually increased her activity levels despite the presence of chronic pain. Two months after the episode, the case was successfully terminated.

Morita Therapy: A Zen-Based Psychotherapy

Whereas the majority of psychotherapies today have been developed within Western sociocultural contexts (Messer and Gurman 2011), therapies have been developed within the context of a Zen worldview and inside of non-Western linguistic cultures (Reynolds 1989). One such example is the work of Dr. Shoma Morita (1874–1938), a Japanese psychiatrist whose Zen practice greatly influenced his work, developed what is known as Morita Therapy (Kato 2005; Kondo 1953; Morita et al. 1998) in the early 1900s. Morita Therapy continued to develop in Japan and subsequently evolved to influence Western psychoanalysts such as Karen Horney and Erich Fromm (Molino 1998). Dr. Morita summarized how his own personal experiences influenced the development of Morita Therapy below:

> When I came to Tokyo at age 18 [in 1892], I was afflicted with paralytic beri-beri. Soon after matriculation in the medical school I was diagnosed as having both beri-beri and neurasthenia, after which my life became inseparable from medications, and I had difficulties with my studies. Further, at one point my living expenses from home stopped inexplicably. I was frustrated, angry, and desperate [the late 19th century ethos in Japan was such that there was little possibility for college students to self-support if the funding stops]. At

> the moment of desperation, I decided to "go for broke." I abandoned all the medications and regimens and plunged into studying day and night. Incredibly, all the symptoms of beri-beri and neurasthemia vanished. Today I often see patients with similar complaints (Chang 2011, pp. 135–136).

At the time, *beri-beri* referred to symptoms associated with vitamin B1 deficiency, including weight loss, sensory and motor impairments, edema, and mood difficulties. *Neuroasthenia*, however, was a vague medical and psychological term that referred to general fatigue, anxiety, headache, hypertension, depression, etc. Interpreting these symptoms within present-day understandings of psychopathology, it is safe to say that these are common symptoms of patients presenting with "mental illnesses" and seeking treatment.

Individuals suffering with "anxiety-based" disorders, or *Shinkeishitsu* in Japanese, were the original population for which Morita Therapy was intended; however, this category of "anxiety-based" mental illnesses included symptoms from what we know of today as trauma and physical injury to depression and social anxiety. Dr. Morita's approach attempted to alter patients' perceptions of the self within the world through four stages that bring them into the present moment, avoiding judgment and intellectualization, and moving from being a "feelings-centered" person to a "purpose-centered" person (Reynolds 1984, p. 174). The first stage begins with a period of complete seclusion and isolation, secondly followed by light physical activity (e.g., walking, observing the outdoors) in silence to reorient the patient to the present moment and immediate experiential reality. Third, strenuous physical activity (e.g., chopping wood) offers practice in creativity and healing of the body–mind from within the self. The final phase reintegrates patients back into society in an effort to maintain their fresh, more authentic perspective of self in the presence of social influences. Ultimately, Dr. Morita recognized that the treatments available (e.g., hypnosis) during his time were ineffective for more than brief symptom relief and sought to create a holistic approach to treatment that addresses how patients relate to their social environments as well as how they relate to themselves. In this sense, personal development is not achieved by eliminating painful or unwanted experiences; rather, it is achieved by cultivating awareness, decentralizing the self, and honoring both the self and the natural environment, including honoring difficult feelings and experiences. In other words, rather than treating an isolated symptom of "anxiety," the target of change is broadened from a single symptom to include the whole person and the way in which the whole person relates to their whole environment.

In applying Zen to behavioral health care today, it is important to focus on the ways in which we can take a step back from the exclusive focus on symptom reduction in order to find a more holistic "solution," if you will, to human suffering. Rather than viewing Zen as a distinct technique to apply with suffering patients via acute application of mindfulness or meditation techniques, we can instead utilize the concept of interrelated and transient wholeness within various theoretical orientations and practices. As we will discuss in more detail below, utilitarian implementation of Zen for the purpose of symptom reduction requires that Zen be molded into and employed within an analytic worldview.

Cautions in Applying Zen to Behavioral Healthcare Practice

The overarching goal of Western behavioral health is the promotion of client's greater functioning and behavioral adaptation (Mennin et al. 2013; O'Donohue and Maragakis 2015). In recent years, the field of behavioral health is influenced by cultural pressures that favor the unrealistic pursuit of happiness (e.g., self-confidence, self-esteem) and the complete elimination of pain and discomfort (Frances 2013a, b), which do not necessarily yield greater functioning, however. Under this sociocultural atmosphere, behavioral health professionals have incorporated Zen and mindfulness into theories and practices, perhaps with the hope of fulfilling this unrealistic utilitarian agenda.

As the principle of Middle Way suggests, the moderate pursuit of utilitarian desire appears to yield optimal health outcomes. However, if the unrealistic pursue of happiness and complete cessation of discomfort and suffering become dominant voices, inevitable are falling into pitfalls through pathologizing inevitable, often "normal," aspects of our lives such as the pain of loss or anxiety associated with various aspects of life (Frances 2013b; Lasalvia 2015; Maj 2014; Wakefield 2015).

For example, a large body of evidence demonstrates the clinical effectiveness of acceptance and commitment therapy (ACT; Hayes et al. 1999) and a mindfulness- and acceptance-based behavioral therapy, for improving daily functioning among patients with chronic pain (see McCracken and Vowles 2014 for comprehensive review of ACT for patients with chronic pain). Incorporating mindfulness and Zen meditative practice, ACT aims to promote patients' greater functioning and the pursuit of meaningful life regardless of chronic pain. More specifically, patients are taught to experience pain and other difficult internalizing events openly as they come and go, while shifting their focus on activating and engaging in activities which become intrinsically reinforcing (e.g., taking a child to school, going shopping, attending a social gathering, and preparing for meals).

However, if clinicians remain faithful to the utilitarian agenda (e.g., complete elimination of pain), patients practice a mindfulness exercise as a new tool to down-regulate chronic pain (e.g., "if you practice mindfulness, your pain will go away"). Paradoxically, a growing body of evidence demonstrates a positive association between pain intensity and efforts to eliminate or down-regulate pain in patients with chronic pain (Scott et al. 2016): That is, the more a person with chronic pain is trying to eliminate his or her pain, the greater pain intensity become. This vicious cycle inevitably leads to greater disability.

From Zen's standpoint, the reality of our living is life delineated by the principles of interdependence and impermanence (Uchiyama et al. 2004). As Szasz (1960) addressed, there will always be "problems in living," and individuals cannot be distinguished by whether they have problems or not. Furthermore, within the principle of interdependence and impermanence, there are problems in our lives that are transient and can be resolved in a conventional sense. For example, with proper diet and moderate exercise, we can lower blood pressure. At the same time, we also have problems, such as the inevitability of death and separation with loved ones, which we cannot overturn despite our best efforts. As noted above, living fully means to choose the course of action that becomes intrinsically nurturing the self and others, while changing the things that the self can change and letting things that self cannot change come and go freely. This wisdom is fundamental and universal, but typically overlooked or denied (Masuda and O'Donohue 2009).

Zen and Traditional Cognitive Behavior Therapies

Cognitive behavior therapy (CBT), a family of psychotherapies, is well recognized as an effective approach for promoting greater behavioral adaptation (Herbert et al. 2013; Mennin et al. 2013; O'Donohue and Fisher 2009). In fact, today CBT is considered a treatment of choice for individuals with various forms of psychological disorders across the globe (Hofmann 2006; Nathan and Gorman 2015). Despite its effectiveness, Zen Buddhism is concerned about some of the premises and directions of therapy that *clinicians* may endorse when practicing a CBT or other psychotherapies.

It is important first to clarify how the present authors view CBT. In behavioral health literature, a CBT is often viewed as a set of particular therapeutic techniques (e.g., psychological education, cognitive reappraisal, behavior activation) tailored to a particular mental disorder. A manual-based or module-based treatment delivery is an exemplar of this way of understanding. Alternatively, we view CBT as a dynamic series of purposeful *acts of a clinician* in therapeutic contexts that are both principle-informed and experientially guided (Masuda 2016). Viewing a CBT as a therapist's skill set is useful for understanding individual differences in the delivery of CBT across therapists (Norcross and Goldfried 2005) and therapists' clinical and cultural competency (Masuda 2014).

In behavioral health literature, the opponents of traditional CBTs express concern about its overemphasis on intellectual and cognitive aspects of human activities (Mirea 2013). More specifically, traditional CBTs are often criticized for narrowly focusing on what are referred to as *mind* and other intrapsychic phenomena, meanwhile overlooking the physical, sociocultural, and interpersonal domains of the individual. Once again, the claim such as this is overgeneralized and misleading. When clinicians have a tendency to make sense of the world analytically, inevitable is greater vulnerability to the pitfalls of analytic thinking. That is, clinicians treat clients' presenting concerns as discrete entities dichotomously and somewhat rigidly as either good or bad, rational or irrational (e.g., "feeling confident is good, but anxiety is bad"), and the therapy is directed toward the elimination of these events.

Categorizing and evaluating a given event is not inherently problematic so long as the people are well aware of the process of doing so and their actions are not dictated exclusively by verbal categorization and judgment. Similarly, for individuals to have meaningful lives, some of the events we consider problematic (e.g., auditory hallucination, tinnitus symptoms) do not need to be eliminated per se (Gaudiano 2015; Hesser et al. 2012; Westin et al. 2011), whereas other events may be high priority for elimination (e.g., domestic violence, substance use). For the former, all we need is an alternative way to relate to these events. One such alternative is to let these events come and go freely while engaging in whatever action one does or values in that moment fully (Uchiyama et al. 2004).

What may be overlooked by traditional CBT is that analytic way of thinking can add additional layers of suffering to life. More specifically, these layers of suffering can arise out of the linguistic process of differentiation and evaluation: Our linguistic process is a two-edged sword: Whereas flouring our life, it could hinder our well-being. Given these iatrogenic aspects of human linguistic process, D.T. Suzuki teaches us to take what our minds say lightly (Suzuki 1994, 1996).

Zen and Mindfulness- and Acceptance-Based Psychotherapies

Mindfulness- and acceptance-based psychotherapy is an emerging force in contemporary psychotherapy practice and theory (Hayes et al. 2004; Norcross et al. 2013). This movement often distinguishes itself from traditional therapeutic approaches by incorporating acceptance, mindfulness, nonjudgment, and decentering perspectives into therapy, particularly in the areas of internalizing experiences (e.g., cognition, emotion, and physiological responses). Some mindfulness- and acceptance-based psychotherapies explicitly state that their theories and practices are based on Zen or Buddhism (Kabat-Zinn 2003; Robins 2002).

However, from a Zen perspective, there are several notable slippery slopes in this approach. Problems of mindfulness- and acceptance-based psychotherapies are tricky, because they appear to parallel Zen teaching and practice (Masuda and O'Donohue 2009). The bottom line is that the application of Zen for utilitarian purposes can be problematic in that it prevents the self from experiencing the wholeness or pure subjectivity. The following are several pitfalls that are likely to be seen in mindfulness- and acceptance-based psychotherapy.

Mindfulness for What? A major concern regarding mindfulness-based psychotherapy is that the transient and interdependent nature of our lives is often overlooked. With respect to an Zen Buddhist account of impermanence and interdependence, mindfulness encompasses the entire life domain in a way that one lives fully in the complexity of life (Masuda and O'Donohue 2009). Living fully means to live actively with a purpose, which is derived from the sense of universal self (i.e., self becoming one with everything she encounters as well as becoming one with all the myriad things), not a conventional sense of self as a unique individual. In the process of active living, one will experience a range of experience. As Uchiyama noted, one then let an experience come and go one at a time and move forward. For Zen, mindfulness practice is a reminder that one can bring himself or herself to this universal sense of self and moves forward. As such, it is not a mental band-aid used only when we are upset.

Impermanence within the Self as Flux of Change. Early psychologists, such as Karen Horney and Erich Fromm, acknowledged the values of Zen Buddhism in relation to human suffering derived from our sense of self (see Molino 1998). As Magid (2002, 2008) suggested, Western cultures tend to facilitate and maintain a strong sense of self as an essential and distinct being that is separated from others and the world (Markus and Kitayama 1991). Contemporary mindfulness movements attempt to tackle self-related sufferings, but seem to maintain the standpoint of this narrowly perceived sense of self.

Whether one awakens to true self depends on whether he or she takes a leap of faith with the principles of interdependence and impermanence. Many of us are okay with the Buddhist principle of interdependence. Despite the primarily focus of autonomy and independence in our society, we still acknowledge the interdependent and social nature of human beings. And yet we are hesitant to bring the reality of impermanence to our every waking moment. However, for Zen Buddhism, keeping the transient nature of our life close to self is extremely important, especially for choosing the course of action one takes (Uchiyama and Okumura 2014; Uchiyama et al. 2004).

Having the reality of death close to the self certainly evokes intense fear in many of us. At the same time, by having the reality of death closer to the self, one can also clarify the direction and purpose of one's life. It is also likely to clarify the priority in one's limited lifetime. From this experiential standpoint, true compassion and empathy may emerge. Unless clients and therapists build this experience and expression of self, value-directed living and acceptance could fall into the Web of detrimental self-defense.

Zen and Therapy: The Two Can Co-occur

Throughout this chapter, we have explored a Zen account of psychopathology as well as the epistemological issues that underlie psychological and Zen practices in multiple contexts. From a Western perspective, categorization and dualism are married to psychological practice and research in ways that appear to be mutually exclusive with Zen. And while it is true that Zen and Western psychological practices are often epistemologically dissimilar, it is also true that any event or behavior that is experienced wholly and mindfully can unfold the Buddha Way.

In this sense, there are many ways in which categorization is an integral component of healing, and it need not always be seen as mutually exclusive from a Zen perspective. Rather, it is rigid, inflexible adherence to categories that Zen seeks to relieve us from. A psychologist working with children to reduce self-injurious behaviors will need to identify those behaviors in some way before creating a treatment plan. Thus, a "self-injurious behavior" must be distinct from "healthy behavior" for treatment purposes in some contexts. Further, an identified diagnosis of autism spectrum disorder may inform how the therapist interacts with the patient and family. Applying techniques and therapies with suffering patients may include strict behavioral contingencies—for example, administering reinforcement for every five-minute interval without self-injurious behavior present—but this does not mean that a therapists' relationship with the patient must focus solely on a single "problem" behavior. A therapist integrating Zen into treatment may also encourage patients and their families to acknowledge and embrace the transient nature of life, challenging the meanings we attach to "problem behaviors" such as *if my child bangs his head against walls, I am a bad parent*. Such a perspective could also be taken with other more specific or manualized treatments like exposure therapy for patients with obsessions and compulsions. It can be taken with patients reporting depression, anxiety, or loss. Ultimately, the Zen therapist asks the question "What does this client need in order to live a more vital, connected, and mindful life?" rather than "What can I do to relieve this client's suffering?" These are inherently different questions, for former addressing the person as a whole in his or her context and the latter merely addressing symptom reduction. It is important to bear in mind that whereas Zen should be avoided as a utilitarian technique, any action, even the use of categories, can unfold the Buddha Way.

Conclusion

Given its unique epistemological standpoint, Zen Buddhism does not have a concept equivalent to that of psychopathology as it is known in Western behavioral health. Instead, Zen teachings encourage students to build the experience of self as one with everything they encounter as well as all the myriad things (Dogen et al. 2011), which includes "psychopathology," and act according to this sense of self (Dogen et al. 1995; Uchiyama and Okumura 2014). From this standpoint, what we usually refer to as psychopathology (e.g., depression, anxiety) is an ordinary aspect of life. Many of them are not to be eliminated from our life, but to be blended into our life. As Sayama (1985) suggested, behavioral health professionals must also fully taste the bittersweet nature of life (i.e., continuous stream of change) as a whole.

As behavioral health professionals, we are prone to using therapeutic techniques as a mechanism to achieve a specific, isolated goal, preventing us from capturing our patients wholly as well as experiencing our own psychological sufferings and struggles. However, seeing and fully experiencing life as it is may be the first step to truly connecting with client problems. Buddhism and Zen say that if we are wise (i.e., living along with the stream of change in life), it does not matter which forms of action we take. The chosen form of action is always the way. Similarly, it does not matter what form of practice we may prefer or adhere to (e.g., CBT, ACT, psychoanalysis) per se; all forms of practice in behavioral health care can unfold the Buddha Way. Rather, the Zen practitioner is one that asks "How can I help my patient as a whole person in relation to their entire context?" as opposed to "How can I get my patient to stop having panic attacks?"

References

American Psychiatric Association. (2013). *Diagnostic and statistical manual of mental disorders* (5th ed.). Washington, DC: American Psychiatric Association.

Anderson, C. M., Hawkins, R. P., & Scotti, J. R. (1997). Private events in behavior analysis: Conceptual basis and clinical relevance. *Behavior Therapy, 28*(1), 157–179. doi:10.1016/s0005-7894(97)80040-8

Bien, T. (2006). *Mindful therapy: A guide for therapists and helping professionals*. Somerville, MA, US: Wisdom Publications.

Blackledge, J. T., & Hayes, S. C. (2006). Using acceptance and commitment training in the support of parents of children diagnosed with autism. *Child & Family Behavior Therapy, 28*(1), 1–18. doi:10.1300/J019v28n01_01

Bobrow, J. (2010). *Zen and psychotherapy: Partners in liberation*. New York, NY, US: W W Norton & Co.

Broughton, J. L. (2009). *Zongmi on Chan*. New York, US: Columbia University Press.

Brown, K. W., Ryan, R. M., & Creswell, J. D. (2007). Mindfulness: Theoretical foundations and evidence for its salutary effects. *Psychological Inquiry, 18*(4), 211–237.

Chang, S. C. (2011). Psychotherapy and culture Morita therapy: An illustration. *World Cultural Psychiatry Research Review, 6*(2), 135–145.

Chiesa, A. (2009). Zen meditation: An integration of current evidence. *Journal of Alternative & Complementary Medicine, 15*(5), 585–592. doi:10.1089/acm.2008.0416

Cummings, N. A., & O'Donohue, W. (2012). *Restoring psychotherapy as the first line intervention in behavioral care*. Dryden, NY, US: Ithaca Press.

Cummings, N. A., O'Donohue, W., Hayes, S. C., & Follette, V. (2001). *Integrated behavioral healthcare: Positioning mental health practice with*

medical/surgical practice. San Diego, CA, US: Academic Press.
de Silva, P. (1984). Buddhism and behaviour modification. *Behaviour Research and Therapy, 22*(6), 661–678.
Dogen, E., Leighton, T. D., & Okumura, S. (1995). *Dogen's Pure Standards for the Zen Community: A translation of Eihei Shingi*. Albany, New York: State University of New York Press.
Dogen, E., Nishiari, B., Okumura, S., Suzuki, S., & Weisman, S. M. (2011). *Dogen's Genjo Koan: Three commentaries*. Barkeley, CA, US: Counterpoint.
Dogen, E., Uchiyama, K., Okumura, S., & Leighton, T. D. (1997). *The wholehearted way: A translation of Eihei Dogen's Bendowa with commentary by Kosho Uchiyama Roshi*. North Clarendon, VT, US: Tuttle Publications.
Follette, W. C., & Houts, A. C. (1996). Models of scientific progress and the role of theory in taxonomy development: A case study of the DSM. *Journal of Consulting and Clinical Psychology, 64*(6), 1120–1132. doi:10.1037/0022-006X.64.6.1120
Frances, A. (2013a). The past, present and future of psychiatric diagnosis. *World Psychiatry, 12*(2), 111–112. doi:10.1002/wps.20027
Frances, A. (2013b). *Saving normal: An insider's revolt against out-of-control psychiatric diagnosis, DSM-5, Big Pharma, and the medicalization of ordinary life*. New York, NY, US: William Morrow & Co.
Gaudiano, B. A. (2015). *Incorporating acceptance and mindfulness into the treatment of psychosis: Current trends and future directions*. New York, NY, US: Oxford University Press.
Gergen, K. J. (1983). Zen Buddhism and psychological science. *Psychologia: An International Journal of Psychology in the Orient, 26*(3), 129–141.
Germer, C. K., & Neff, K. D. (2013). Self-compassion in clinical practice. *Journal of Clinical Psychology, 69* (8), 856–867. doi:10.1002/jclp.22021
Hayes, L. J., & Fredericks, D. W. (1999). Interbehaviorism and interbehavioral psychology. In W. O'Donohue, R. Kitchener, W. O'Donohue, & R. Kitchener (Eds.), *Handbook of behaviorism* (pp. 71–96). San Diego, CA, US: Academic Press.
Hayes, S. C., Barnes-Holmes, D., & Wilson, K. G. (2012). Contextual behavioral science: Creating a science more adequate to the challenge of the human condition. *Journal of Contextual Behavioral Science, 1*(1–2), 1–16. doi:http://dx.doi.org/10.1016/j.jcbs.2012.09.004
Hayes, S. C., Follette, V. M., & Linehan, M. M. (2004). *Mindfulness and acceptance: Expanding the cognitive-behavioral tradition*. New York, NY US: Guilford Press.
Hayes, S. C., Hayes, L. J., & Reese, H. W. (1988). Finding the philosophical core: A review of Stephen C. Pepper's world hypotheses: A study in evidence. *Journal of the Experimental Analysis of Behavior, 50*, 97–111
Hayes, S. C., Strosahl, K. D., & Wilson, K. G. (1999). *Acceptance and commitment therapy: An experiential approach to behavior change*. New York, NY US: Guilford Press.
Hayes, S. C., Villatte, M., Levin, M., & Hildebrandt, M. (2011). Open, aware, and active: contextual approaches as an emerging trend in the behavioral and cognitive therapies. *Annual Review of Clinucal Psychology, 7*, 141–168. doi:10.1146/annurev-clinpsy-032210-104449
Hayes, S. C., Wilson, K. G., Gifford, E. V., Follette, V. M., & Strosahl, K. (1996). Experiential avoidance and behavioral disorders: A functional dimensional approach to diagnosis and treatment. *Journal of Consulting and Clinical Psychology, 64*(6), 1152–1168.
Herbert, J. D., Gaudiano, B. A., & Forman, E. M. (2013). The importance of theory in cognitive behavior therapy: A perspective of contextual behavioral science. *Behavior Therapy, 44*(4), 580–591. doi:10.1016/j.beth.2013.03.001
Hesser, H., Gustafsson, T., Lundén, C., Henrikson, O., Fattahi, K., Johnsson, E., … Andersson, G. (2012). A randomized controlled trial of internet-delivered cognitive behavior therapy and acceptance and commitment therapy in the treatment of tinnitus. *Journal of Consulting and Clinical Psychology, 80*(4), 649–661. doi:10.1037/a0027021
Hofmann, S. G. (2006). The importance of culture in cognitive and behavioral practice. *Cognitive and Behavioral Practice, 13*(4), 243–245.
Japan Buddhist Federation. (1978). *Understanding Japanese Buddhism*.
Kabat-Zinn, J. (1990). *Full catastrophe living*.
Kabat-Zinn, J. (2003). Mindfulness-based interventions in context: Past, present, and future. *Clinical Psychology: Science and Practice, 10*(2), 144–-156. doi:10.1093/clipsy/bpg016
Kantor, J. R. (1959). *Interbehavoral psychology: A sample of scientific system construction*. Bloomington, IN, USA: Principia Press.
Kasulis, T. P. (1981). *Zen action Zen person*. Honolulu, HI, US: University of Hawaii Press.
Kato, H. (2005). Zen and psychology. *Japanese Psychological Research, 47*(2), 125–136. doi:10.1111/j.1468-5884.2005.00280.x
Kondo, A. (1953). Morita therapy: A Japanese therapy for neurosis. *The American Journal of Psychoanalysis, 13*, 31–37. doi:10.1007/BF01872067
Kurak, M. (2003). The relevance of the Buddhist theory of dependent co-origination to cognitive science. *Brain & Mind, 4*(3), 341–351. doi:10.1023/B:BRAM.0000005468.95009.86
Lasalvia, A. (2015). DSM-5 two years later: Facts, myths and some key open issues. *Epidemiology and Psychiatric Sciences, 24*(3), 185–187. doi:10.1017/S2045796015000256
Linehan, M. M. (1993). Cognitive-behavioral treatment of borderline personality disorder. New York, NY US: Guilford Press

Magid, B. (2000). The couch and the cushion: Integrating Zen and psychoanalysis. *Journal of the American Academy of Psychoanalysis, 28*(3), 513–526.

Magid, B. (2002). *Ordinary mind: Exploring the common ground of Zen and psychotherapy*. Somerville, MA, US: Wisdom Publications.

Magid, B. (2008). *Ending the pursuit of happiness: A Zen guide*. Somerville, MA, US: Wisdom Publications.

Maj, M. (2014). DSM-5, ICD-11 and 'pathologization of normal conditions'. *Australian and New Zealand Journal of Psychiatry, 48*(2), 193–194. doi:10.1177/0004867413518825

Markus, H. R., & Kitayama, S. (1991). Culture and the self: Implications for cognition, emotion, and motivation. *Psychological Review, 98*(2), 224–253.

Markus, H. R., & Kitayama, S. (2010). Cultures and selves: A cycle of mutual constitution. *Perspectives on Psychological Science, 5*(4), 420–430. doi:10.1177/1745691610375557.

Masuda, A. (2014). *Mindfulness and acceptance in multicultural competency: A contextual approach to sociocultural diversity in theory and practice*. Oakland, CA, US: Context Press/New Harbinger Publications.

Masuda, A. (2016). Principle-based cultural adaptation of cognitive behavior therapies: A functional and contextual perspective as an example. *Japanese Journal of Behavior Therapy, 42*(1), 11–19.

Masuda, A., & O'Donohue, W. T. (2009). Buddhism: It's chic, but they could have it wrong. In N. Cummings, W. O'Donohue, & J. Cummings (Eds.), *Psychology's war on religion* (pp. 229–253). Phoenix, AZ US: Zeig, Tucker & Theisen.

Masuda, T., & Nisbett, R. E. (2001). Attending holistically versus analytically: Comparing the context sensitivity of Japanese and Americans. *Journal of Personality and Social Psychology, 81*(5), 922–934.

Mathers, D., Miller, M. E., & Ando, O. (2009). *Self and no-self: Continuing the dialogue between Buddhism and psychotherapy*. New York, NY, US: Routledge/Taylor & Francis Group.

Maynard, S. K. (1997). *Japanese communication: Language and thought in context*. Honolulu, HI, US: University of Hawaii Press.

McCracken, L. M., & Vowles, K. E. (2014). Acceptance and commitment therapy and mindfulness for chronic pain: Model, process, and progress. *American Psychologist, 69*(2), 178–187. doi:10.1037/a0035623

Mennin, D. S., Ellard, K. K., Fresco, D. M., & Gross, J. J. (2013). United we stand: Emphasizing commonalities across cognitive-behavioral therapies. *Behavior Therapy, 44*(2), 234–248. doi:10.1016/j.beth.2013.02.004

Messer, S. B., & Gurman, A. S. (2011). *Essential psychotherapies: Theory and practice* (3rd ed.). New York, NY, US: Guilford Press.

Mirea, D. (2013). Review of Developing resilience: A cognitive-behavioural approach. *Existential Analysis, 24*(2), 342–346.

Miyamoto, Y., & Ryff, C. D. (2011). Cultural differences in the dialectical and non-dialectical emotional styles and their implications for health. *Cognition and Emotion, 25*(1), 22–39. doi:10.1080/02699931003612114

Molino, A. (1998). *The couch and the tree: Dialogues in psychoanalysis and Buddhism*. New York, NY, US: North Point Press.

Monteiro, L. M., Musten, R. F., & Compson, J. (2015). Traditional and contemporary mindfulness: Finding the middle path in the tangle of concerns. *Mindfulness, 6*(1), 1–13. doi:10.1007/s12671-014-0301-7

Morita, S., Kondo, A., & LeVine, P. (1998). *Morita therapy and the true nature of anxiety-based disorders (shinkeishitsu)*. Albany, NY, US: State University of New York Press.

Nathan, P. E., & Gorman, J. M. (2015). *A guide to treatments that work* (4th ed.). New York, NY, US: Oxford University Press.

Neff, K. D. (2003). Self-compassion: An alternative conceptualization of a healthy attitude toward oneself. *Self and Identity, 2*(2), 85–101. doi:10.1080/15298860309032

Nisbett, R. E., Peng, K., Choi, I., & Norenzayan, A. (2001). Culture and systems of thought: Holistic versus analytic cognition. *Psychological Review, 108*(2), 291–310. doi:10.1037/0033-295X.108.2.291

Norcross, J. C., & Goldfried, M. R. (2005). *Handbook of psychotherapy integration* (2nd ed.). New York, NY, US: Oxford University Press.

Norcross, J. C., Pfund, R. A., & Prochaska, J. O. (2013). Psychotherapy in 2022: A Delphi poll on its future. *Professional Psychology: Research and Practice, 44*(5), 363–370. doi:10.1037/a0034633

O'Donohue, W. T., & Fisher, J. E. (2009). *General principles and empirically supported techniques of cognitive behavior therapy*. Hoboken, NJ, US: Wiley.

O'Donohue, W. T., & Maragakis, A. (2015). *Integrated primary and behavioral care: Role in medical homes and chronic disease management*. Cham, Switzerland: Springer International Publishing.

Okumura, S. (2010). *Realizing Genjokoan: The key to Dogen's Shobogenzo*. Boston MA, US: Wisdom Publications.

Peng, K., & Nisbett, R. E. (1999). Culture, dialectics, and reasoning about contradiction. *American Psychologist, 54*(9), 741–754. doi:10.1037/0003-066X.54.9.741

Poceski, M. (2015). *The records of Mazu and the making of classical Chan literature*. New York, USA: Oxford University Press.

Rahula, W. (1974). *What the Buddha taught*. New York: Grove Press.

Reynolds, D. K. (1984). *Playing ball on running water: The Japanese way to building a better life*. New York, NY, US: William Morrow & Co.

Reynolds, D. K. (1989). On being natural: Two Japanese approaches to healing. In A. A. Sheikh, K. S. Sheikh, A. A. Sheikh, & K. S. Sheikh (Eds.), *Eastern and Western approaches to healing: Ancient wisdom and*

modern knowledge (pp. 180–194). Oxford, England: Wiley.
Robins, C. J. (2002). Zen principles and mindfulness practice in dialectical behavior therapy. *Cognitive and Behavioral Practice, 9*(1), 50–57.
Sayama, M. K. (1985). *Samadhi: Self development in Zen, swordsmanship, and psychotherapy*. Albany, New York: State University of New York Press, Albany.
Scott, W., McCracken, L. M., & Norton, S. (2016). A confirmatory factor analysis of facets of psychological flexibility in a sample of people seeking treatment for chronic pain. *Annals of Behavioral Medicine, 50* (2), 285–296. doi:10.1007/s12160-015-9752-x
Segal, Z. V., Williams, J. M. G., & Teasdale, J. D. (2002). *Mindfulness-based cognitive therapy for depression: A new approach to preventing relapse*. New York, NY, US: Guilford Press.
Shapiro, D. H., & Zifferblatt, S. M. (1976). Zen meditation and behavior self-control: Similarities, differences, and clinical applications. *American Psychologist, 31*(7), 519–532.
Skinner, B. F. (1971). *Beyond freedom and dignity*. New York, NY, US: Knopf/Random House.
Skinner, B. F. (1974). *About behaviorism*. Oxford, England: Alfred A. Knopf.
Suzuki, D. T. (1994). *Essays in Zen Buddhism*. New York, US: Grove Press (original work published in 1949).
Suzuki, D. T. (1996). *Zen Buddhism: Selected writings of D. T. Suzuki*. New York, US: An Image Book.
Suzuki, D. T. (1997). *Eastern perspective [Toyoteki na mikata]*. Tokyo, Japan: Iwanami Shoten.
Suzuki, D. T. (1998). The Zen doctrine of no-mind. In A. Molino (Ed.), *The couch and the tree: Dialogues in psychoanalysis and Buddhism* (pp. 26–36). New York, NY, US: North Point Press.
Suzuki, S. (1970). *Zen mind, beginner's mind: Informal talks on Zen meditation and practice*. Boston, MA USA: Weatherhill.
Szasz, T. S. (1960). The myth of mental illness. *American Psychologist, 15*(2), 113–118. doi:10.1037/h0046535
Tanahashi, K., & Levitt, P. (2013). *The essential Dogen: Writings of the great Zen master*. Boulder, CO, US: Wisdom Publications.
Uchiyama, K., & Okumura, S. (2014). *The Zen teaching of homeless Kodo*. Somerville, MA, US: Tuttle Publications.
Uchiyama, K., Wright, T., Warner, J., & Okumura, S. (2004). *Opening the hand of thought: Foundations of Zen Buddhism practice*. Somerville, MA, US: Wisdom Publications.
Wakefield, J. C. (2015). DSM-5, psychiatric epidemiology and the false positives problem. *Epidemiology and Psychiatric Sciences, 24*(3), 188–196. doi:10.1017/S2045796015000116
Weisz, J. R., Rothbaum, F. M., & Blackburn, T. C. (1984). Standing out and standing in: The psychology of control in America and Japan. *American Psychologist, 39*(9), 955–969. doi:10.1037/0003-066X.39.9.955
Westin, V. Z., Schulin, M., Hesser, H., Karlsson, M., Noe, R. Z., Olofsson, U., ... Andersson, G. (2011). Acceptance and commitment therapy versus tinnitus retraining therapy in the treatment of tinnitus: A randomised controlled trial. *Behaviour Research and Therapy, 49*(11), 737–747. doi:10.1016/j.brat.2011.08.001
Whaley, A. L., & Davis, K. E. (2007). Cultural competence and evidence-based practice in mental health services: A complementary perspective. *American Psychologist, 62*(6), 563–574. doi:10.1037/0003-066x.62.6.563
Wilson, D. S., Hayes, S. C., Biglan, A., & Embry, D. D. (2014). Evolving the future: Toward a science of international change. *Behavioral and Brain Science, 37*(4), 395–416.
Wright, D. S. (1992). Rethinking transcendence: The role of language in Zen experience. *Philosophy East & West, 42*(1), 113–138.
Young-Eisendrath, P., & Muramoto, S. (2002). *Awakening and insight: Zen Buddhism and psychotherapy*. New York: NY, US.
Zhang, B., Galbraith, N., Yama, H., Wang, L., & Manktelow, K. I. (2015). Dialectical thinking: A cross-cultural study of Japanese, Chinese, and British students. *Journal of Cognitive Psychology, 27*(6), 771–779. doi:10.1080/20445911.2015.1025792

modern knowledge (pp. 180–194). Oxford, England: Wiley.

Robins, C. J. (2002). Zen principles and mindfulness practice in dialectical behavior therapy. *Cognitive and Behavioral Practice, 9*(1), 50–57.

Sayama, M. K. (1985). *Samadhi: Self development in Zen, swordsmanship, and psychotherapy*. Albany, New York: State University of New York Press, Albany.

Scott, W., McCracken, L. M., & Norton, S. (2016). A confirmatory factor analysis of facets of psychological flexibility in a sample of people seeking treatment for chronic pain. *Annals of Behavioral Medicine, 50* (2), 285–296. doi:10.1007/s12160-015-9752-x

Segal, Z. V., Williams, J. M. G., & Teasdale, J. D. (2002). *Mindfulness-based cognitive therapy for depression: A new approach to preventing relapse*. New York, NY, US: Guilford Press.

Shapiro, D. H., & Zifferblatt, S. M. (1976). Zen meditation and behavior self-control: Similarities, differences, and clinical applications. *American Psychologist, 31*(7), 519–532.

Skinner, B. F. (1971). *Beyond freedom and dignity*. New York, NY, US: Knopf/Random House.

Skinner, B. F. (1974). *About behaviorism*. Oxford, England: Alfred A. Knopf.

Suzuki, D. T. (1994). *Essays in Zen Buddhism*. New York, US: Grove Press (original work published in 1949).

Suzuki, D. T. (1996). *Zen Buddhism: Selected writings of D. T. Suzuki*. New York, US: An Image Book.

Suzuki, D. T. (1997). *Eastern perspective [Toyoteki na mikata]*. Tokyo, Japan: Iwanami Shoten.

Suzuki, D. T. (1998). The Zen doctrine of no-mind. In A. Molino (Ed.), *The couch and the tree: Dialogues in psychoanalysis and Buddhism* (pp. 26–36). New York, NY, US: North Point Press.

Suzuki, S. (1970). *Zen mind, beginner's mind: Informal talks on Zen meditation and practice*. Boston, MA USA: Weatherhill.

Szasz, T. S. (1960). The myth of mental illness. *American Psychologist, 15*(2), 113–118. doi:10.1037/h0046535

Tanahashi, K., & Levitt, P. (2013). *The essential Dogen: Writings of the great Zen master*. Boulder, CO, US: Wisdom Publications.

Uchiyama, K., & Okumura, S. (2014). *The Zen teaching of homeless Kodo*. Somerville, MA, US: Tuttle Publications.

Uchiyama, K., Wright, T., Warner, J., & Okumura, S. (2004). *Opening the hand of thought: Foundations of Zen Buddhism practice*. Somerville, MA, US: Wisdom Publications.

Wakefield, J. C. (2015). DSM-5, psychiatric epidemiology and the false positives problem. *Epidemiology and Psychiatric Sciences, 24*(3), 188–196. doi:10.1017/S2045796015000116

Weisz, J. R., Rothbaum, F. M., & Blackburn, T. C. (1984). Standing out and standing in: The psychology of control in America and Japan. *American Psychologist, 39*(9), 955–969. doi:10.1037/0003-066X.39.9.955

Westin, V. Z., Schulin, M., Hesser, H., Karlsson, M., Noe, R. Z., Olofsson, U., … Andersson, G. (2011). Acceptance and commitment therapy versus tinnitus retraining therapy in the treatment of tinnitus: A randomised controlled trial. *Behaviour Research and Therapy, 49*(11), 737–747. doi:10.1016/j.brat.2011.08.001

Whaley, A. L., & Davis, K. E. (2007). Cultural competence and evidence-based practice in mental health services: A complementary perspective. *American Psychologist, 62*(6), 563–574. doi:10.1037/0003-066x.62.6.563

Wilson, D. S., Hayes, S. C., Biglan, A., & Embry, D. D. (2014). Evolving the future: Toward a science of international change. *Behavioral and Brain Science, 37*(4), 395–416.

Wright, D. S. (1992). Rethinking transcendence: The role of language in Zen experience. *Philosophy East & West, 42*(1), 113–138.

Young-Eisendrath, P., & Muramoto, S. (2002). *Awakening and insight: Zen Buddhism and psychotherapy*. New York: NY, US.

Zhang, B., Galbraith, N., Yama, H., Wang, L., & Manktelow, K. I. (2015). Dialectical thinking: A cross-cultural study of Japanese, Chinese, and British students. *Journal of Cognitive Psychology, 27*(6), 771–779. doi:10.1080/20445911.2015.1025792

What Is Measured by Self-report Measures of Mindfulness?: Conceptual and Measurement Issues

Sungjin Im

Keywords
Measurement · Mindfulness · Assessment · Behavioral health · Psychological assessment

Introduction

Over the past decades, there has been growing research interest in mindfulness (Bishop et al. 2004). As Fig. 1 shows, Google Scholar searches using mindfulness as a keyword returned 2820 published articles prior to 1990 compared to 48,100 since 2011, indicating a rapid increase in research attention to mindfulness. The growing volume of research on mindfulness led to investigation into its clinical applications and development of mindfulness-based interventions (MBIs). Some MBIs, such as mindfulness-based stress reduction (MBSR; Kabat-Zinn 1982) and mindfulness-based cognitive therapy (MBCT; Segal et al. 2002), focus on formal meditation practices, while other programs such as Acceptance and Commitment Therapy (ACT; Hayes et al. 1999) and Dialectical Behavior Therapy (DBT; Linehan 1993) incorporate key components of mindfulness (e.g., present-moment awareness and acceptance) into their treatment protocol without requiring regular meditation practice.

Such increase in research attention has been largely driven by empirical evidence that MBIs provide clinically meaningful improvements in psychological well-being (e.g., quality of life and positive affect) as well as symptoms of psychological disorders (e.g., depression, anxiety disorders, and substance abuse) (see Keng et al. 2011; Khoury et al. 2013 for review and meta-analysis). These symptom reductions have been shown to occur for a wide range of age-groups (Biegel et al. 2009; Creswell et al. 2012; Regehr et al. 2013) and for both clinical and non-clinical samples (Khoury et al. 2013). Furthermore, a recent meta-analysis on 209 studies of MBIs indicated that the overall effect sizes on physical (e.g., chronic pain) and psychological conditions (e.g., depression) were estimated to be moderate, and more importantly, the mean effect sizes for MBIs were not significantly different from those for conventional cognitive behavioral therapies and pharmacological treatments (Khoury et al. 2013). Considering their large scope of application and demonstrated clinical evidence, further research is warranted on the underlying mechanism by

S. Im (✉)
University of Nevada, Reno, USA
e-mail: m.sungjin@yahoo.com

A. Masuda and W.T. O'Donohue (eds.), *Handbook of Zen, Mindfulness, and Behavioral Health*,
Mindfulness in Behavioral Health, DOI 10.1007/978-3-319-54595-0_17

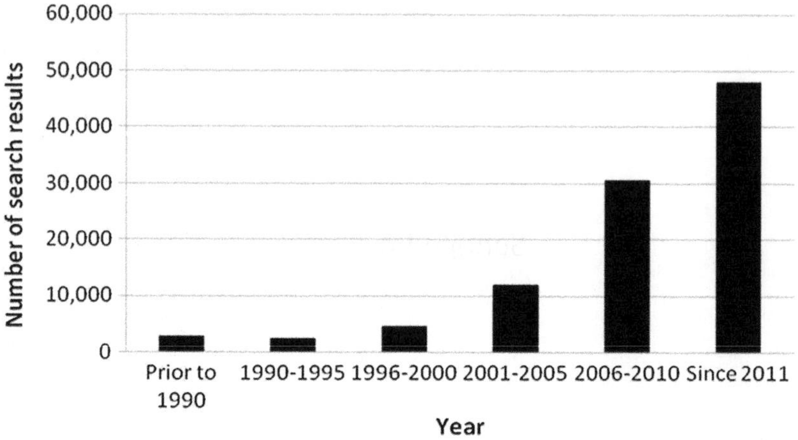

Fig. 1 Number of search results for mindfulness. *Note* Search was conducted on May 15, 2016 using Google Scholar

which MBIs produce clinically beneficial outcomes.

In fact, the increasing evidence base of MBIs has shifted the focus of mindfulness research toward the investigation into their mechanisms of change. The attempt to elucidate the underlying mechanism of mindfulness is critical for gaining direct evidence that improvement in clinical outcomes is due to change in mindfulness rather than other extraneous variables that may have confounded with MBIs. Furthermore, mindfulness has been proposed to comprise multiple components (Baer et al. 2006), and each aspect of mindfulness may have differential impacts on treatment outcomes. Such knowledge provides information about to which degree each element of mindfulness contributes to their known benefits and allows for a modification of current MBIs to meet treatment needs.

From a methodological point of view, the first step to investigating the mechanism of mindfulness involves operationalizing and assessing mindfulness before and after a MBI is delivered. If mindfulness mediates treatment outcomes, an increase in levels of mindfulness should be observed. Then, increased mindfulness in turn will lead to a change in treatment outcomes (Baron and Kenny 1986). However, if an MBI reliably changes clinical outcome but not measured levels of mindfulness, this indicates that the MBI is probably not effective through mindfulness but through other factors that are embedded in the MBI. In either case, assessing mindfulness with a valid and reliable instrument is essential. Of course, not all scholars and mindfulness teachers believe that mindfulness can be accurately measured via a self-report instrument (Gunaratana 2011), and measurement utility of mindfulness scales will be further discussed later.

This chapter aims to address the four aims with regard to the measurement of mindfulness. First, the chapter will review various conceptualizations and facets of mindfulness that have been proposed in the literature. In particular, this review will introduce how mindfulness has been conceptualized in traditional Buddhist texts and will examine secular conceptualizations proposed by contemporary Western scholars. Second, the chapter will review eleven self-report instruments of mindfulness available in the literature and will present how the identified facets of mindfulness map onto these instruments. Previous research found that the correlations between mindfulness measures vary widely from weak to strong, indicating their lack of concurrent validity (Baer et al. 2006). Since no established referent of mindfulness exists yet, the review will focus on linking key mindfulness facets identified in theoretical sources with mindfulness components specified in the instruments. Third, we will evaluate the psychometric properties and provide general guidelines for the use of these mindfulness measures. Finally, the chapter will address three important issues regarding the assessment of mindfulness:

measurement utility of mindfulness questionnaires, types of mindfulness, and implications for future research.

Conceptualization of Mindfulness: What Is Mindfulness?

Mindfulness has theoretical and methodological roots in Buddhism and has long been practiced in the form of meditation across Asia. The Buddha suggested practicing the Noble Eightfold Path as a means of liberating oneself from suffering, which includes Right View, Right Resolve, Right Speech, Right Action, Right Livelihood, Right Effort, Right Mindfulness, Right Concentration (Bodhi 2010). As the seventh element of the Noble Eightfold Path, mindfulness is translated from the Pali term, *Sati*, which means to "remember" or "to be aware" (Thera 2014). Unlike Western scientific approach to mindfulness, Buddhist psychology does not explicitly attempt to conceptualize mindfulness. This implies that an understanding of mindfulness must be attained through direct mindfulness practice, not through discursive, analytic, and didactic processes.

Despite the lack of a systematic analysis or conceptualization, Buddhist texts provide a detailed account of how to cultivate mindfulness. For instance, the 22nd text of the Collection of Long Discourses of the Buddha (Satipaṭṭhāna Sutta; Walshe 1995) lists four foundations of mindfulness: Mindfulness of the Body (kayanupassana), Mindfulness of Feelings (vedananupassana), Mindfulness of the Mind (cittanupassana), and Mindfulness of Mind-Objects or Phenomenon (dhammanupassana). It is noted that these four objects of mindfulness mostly involve internal events such as one's bodily sensations, perceptions, and feelings. Although mindfulness skills can be practically applied to deal with external phenomena (e.g., having a conversation with a friend in a mindful way), mindfulness in Buddhist tradition is primarily oriented toward internal experience with introspective nature.

As noted before, Buddhist texts primarily concern methods of mindfulness instead of explicating the meaning of mindfulness. However, these methods insinuate some essential characteristics of mindfulness. The first characteristic includes clear observation of the object of mindfulness. This point is illustrated as, "In what is seen there must be only the seen; in what is heard must be only the heard; in what is sensed there must be only what is sensed; what is thought there must be only what is thought" (Thera 2014; p. 171). Thera (2014) further explains that this feature of mindfulness, called *bare attention*, involves registering the facts that are only observed by the five senses and the mind itself. In other words, this characteristic highlights accurate and objective observation with minimal interference by previous knowledge and experience.

The second characteristic of mindfulness is present-moment awareness. For example, one is encouraged to simply notice and observe internal and extern phenomena (e.g., a sad feeling) as they arise in the here and now and to focus on their moment-by-moment change (Gunaratana 2011). Present-moment awareness involves sustaining focused attention without drifting away into the past and future while minimizing judgmental reactions to the experience. Thus, the individual is able to keep the mind in a receptive mode and to maintain attention to the object of the mind.

Third, certain attitudes toward experience are either encouraged or discouraged in mindfulness practice. In Buddhist tradition, attachment is viewed as a cause of suffering. Thus, a decentered, impartial perspective without self-reference is presented as an antidote to attachment (Walshe 1995). All objects of mindfulness are viewed as transient mental events, and meditators are taught to maintain a detached attitude toward their experiences without clinging or resisting to them (Thera 2014). When someone clings to a mental phenomenon (e.g., infatuation) instead of letting it go, such mental state disrupts their ability to be mindfully and objectively aware of their experience. Likewise, when someone has strong aversive reactions to experience and resists seeing the experience as it is, their mind becomes divided and biased so that they will have trouble maintaining full awareness of their experience. For these reasons, mindfulness is described as a mental state where the mind is free from mental commentary, judgment, and pre-occupation (Thera 2014).

Finally, mindfulness reflects a clear awareness of where the mind is dwelling on each moment. This helps discern the mind state from its object, and the object of the mind (e.g., a feeling of sadness experienced in the present moment) from what gives rise to the object (e.g., loss of a loved one in the past). In other words, mindfulness reflects the meta-awareness of the state of the mind, which is linked to the third foundation of mindfulness: Mindfulness of the Mind (Thera 2014). Through honest but thorough self-examination, one can increase knowledge about the self, which in turn helps guide appropriate behavior in a given context.

We have so far discussed how mindfulness is characterized in the East Buddhist tradition. These characteristics include having a clear observation of mental phenomena including perception, a present-focused awareness, a decentered, accepting, and non-judgmental attitude toward experience, and a meta-awareness of the mind. However, mindfulness is generally considered a non-conceptual process in Buddhist tradition (Gunaratana 2011). Thus, there might be some remaining features that are integral to mindfulness but are not explicitly described in Buddhist texts.

While Eastern mindfulness practice has long been maintained under cultural and religious influence as a way of being and attaining personal enlightenment, the clinical utility and applications of mindfulness have been more appreciated in the West. Since Kabat-Zinn developed the MBSR to treat patients with chronic pain in the 1970s (Kabat-Zinn 1982), new MBIs have emerged: MBCT (Segal et al. 2002) for relapse prevention of depression, DBT (Linehan 1993) for treatment of borderline personality disorder and high risk behaviors (e.g., suicidality and self-harm), and ACT (Hayes et al. 1999) for individuals who are "experientially avoidant." As MBIs grew a clinical evidence base and popularity in clinical practice, researchers began to investigate into mindfulness in a deeper level.

Although efforts have been made to conceptualize and operationalize mindfulness, there is little consensual agreement on the definition of mindfulness among mindfulness researchers (Bishop et al. 2004). For instance, Kabat-Zinn defines mindfulness as "paying attention in a particular way: on purpose, in the present moment, non-judgmentally" (Kabat-Zinn 1994, p. 4). His definition emphasizes the importance of paying attention to whatever experience (e.g., bodily sensations, thought, images, and memories) unfolds and noticing the experience as it is without any judgments or evaluations. Likewise, Bishop et al. (2004) proposed a two-component model of mindfulness consisting of self-regulation of attention and orientation to experience (e.g., curiosity and acceptance). The former element is similar to Kabat-Zinn's conceptualization that places emphasis on maintaining attention to one's current experience, switching attention back to the object of mindfulness when one gets distracted, and abstaining from elaborative or evaluative processing (e.g., rumination). However, Bishop et al. (2004) incorporated additional attitudinal components such as curiosity and acceptance. To foster mindfulness, they argue that people need to be able to stay interested in their present-moment experience (curiosity) and to become experientially open to their experience without making any attempt to change it (acceptance). While Kabat-Zinn and Bishop et al. proposed multi-facets conceptualizations of mindfulness, Brown and Ryan (2003) considered mindfulness as a unidimensional construct characterized by open receptivity to the present-moment experiences while discounting any attitudinal components. Their argument is that although attitudinal and motivational attributes (e.g., acceptance, patience) are conducive to development of mindfulness, they are not an integral part of mindfulness. Finally, additional components have been suggested: decentered perspective that is devoid of self-focus or self-absorption (Lau et al. 2006), non-reactivity or non-habitual responding to one's experience and the ability to describe one's experience in words (Baer et al. 2006), and non-identification with one's own experiences and insightful understanding (Bergomi et al. 2013). In sum, there is clear evidence that most mindfulness researchers acknowledge attention to present-moment experience as a key component of mindfulness. However, significant conceptual divergence in additional components exists in the literature.

As noted earlier, there are considerable conceptual differences in the conceptualizations of mindfulness among researchers, and this conceptual divergence is derived from two primary sources. First, investigators themselves are not familiar with mindfulness practice. Grossman (2008) criticized that some investigators lack in-depth knowledge of Buddhist psychology and personal experience with meditation practice. It is possible that some Western scholars only reviewed contemporary literature on mindfulness, mostly written by the developers of MBIs, and understood mindfulness in a superficial way while neglecting its deep connection to Buddhist philosophy. Moreover, continuous meditation practice over time is considered necessary to cultivate mindfulness (Gunaratana 2011), but scholars' own mindfulness practice may be relatively short in time, which limits their understanding of this non-discursive but experiential process. Such a limited understanding and experience on the part of Western scholars may have contributed to the neglect of integral features and the inclusion of irrelevant aspects in their conceptualizations of mindfulness, thus increasing conceptual divergence.

Second, there exists a diverse form of mindfulness practices in Buddhist traditions. Buddhism originated in India and spread across Asia over 2500 years. When Buddhism was introduced to different cultures, each culture adopted Buddhism in a unique way, which contributed to various forms of meditation practices (e.g., Zen mediation in Korea and Japan, Vipassana meditation in Sri Lanka, Cambodia, Thailand, Laos, and Burma, and Tibetan mediation in Tibet). As a result, one type of mindfulness practice has its unique characteristics that differ from those of others. For example, focused attention meditation presets an object of meditation such as a mantra or external object while open monitoring meditation emphasizes keeping the mind in a receptive state that ongoing moment-by-moment experience becomes the object of mediation. This cross-cultural diversity in mindfulness practice is not a problem per se. Rather, such diversity reflects the richness of this Buddhist tradition. However, this clearly poses a problem for operationalizing and measuring mindfulness using self-report measurement because the heterogeneity of mindfulness traditions makes it hard to establish an objective criterion.

Methodologically, such conceptual divergence hinders the operationalization of mindfulness and hampers scale development. When a construct is poorly conceptualized, the subsequent scale becomes prone to measurement error, indicative of low construct validity. Thus, what can be inferred from collected data may significantly differ depending on the selection of mindfulness scales. Considering that mindfulness is still a burgeoning filed, further research on its conceptualizations and measurements is needed.

Existing Mindfulness Scales

This section will encompass a review of eleven existing mindfulness scales. In our review, we will primarily focus on their major features (e.g., theoretical sources and response options), psychometric properties, strengths, and limitations. As later mindfulness scales were often devised in an effort to improve limitations of early scales, the scales are generally arranged in chronological order. The overview of the eleven mindfulness measures reviewed here is presented in Table 1.

Mindfulness Attention Awareness Scale (MAAS)

The MAAS (Brown and Ryan 2003) is the most commonly used mindfulness questionnaire that

Table 1 Overview of 11 validated measures of mindfulness

	Validation study	# of facets	Facets	# of items	Response options	Validation sample	Trait or state	Assessment target	Internal consistency
MAAS	Brown and Ryan (2003)	1	Present awareness	15	6-point Likert	College students, non-college adults, and clinical sample	Trait	Meditators and non-meditators	0.82–0.87
KIMS	Baer et al. (2004)	4	Observing Describing Acting With Awareness Accepting without judgment	39	5-point Likert	College students and clinical sample	Trait	Meditators and non-meditators	0.76–0.91
FMI	Walach et al. (2006)	2	Presence Acceptance	8 or 14	4-point Likert	Meditating, clinical, and general community samples	Trait	Meditators and non-meditators	0.79–0.86
TMS	Lau et al. (2006)	2	Decentering Curiosity	13	5-point Likert	Community sample with various levels of meditation experience	State and trait	Meditators	0.91–93
CAMS-R	Feldman et al. (2007)	4	Attention Present focus Awareness acceptance	10 or 12	4-point Likert	College students	Trait	Meditators and non-meditators	0.74–0.77
SMQ	Chadwick et al. (2008)	1	Mindfulness awareness of distressing thoughts and images	16	7-point Likert	Both meditating and non-meditating community and clinical samples	Trait	Meditators and non-meditators	0.82–0.89
FFMQ	Baer et al. (2006)	5	Observing Describing Acting With Awareness Non-reactivity to Internal experience Non-judging of Experience	39	5-point Likert	College students and meditating and non-meditating adults	Trait	Meditators and non-meditators	0.75–0.91
DMS	Solloway and Fisher (2007)	1	Open awareness to the present Non-judgmental stance toward experience	30	8-point Likert	College students	Trait	Meditators and non-meditators	0.88–0.99
PHLMS	Cardaciotto et al. (2008)	2	Present-moment awareness Acceptance	20	5-point Likert	College students and clinical adults	Trait	Non-meditators only	0.75–0.90
EOM	Reavley and Pallant (2009)	2	Experiences during meditation Effects of meditation in everyday life	64	6-point Likert	Community sample with meditation experience	State and trait	Meditators	0.68–0.87
MMS	Haigh et al. (2011)	1	Mindfulness	9	7-point Likert	College students	Trait	Non-meditators only	0.76–0.85

assesses how frequently one is *not* paying attention to their thoughts, feelings, physical sensations, and tasks at hand (Sauer et al. 2013). The MAAS items were pooled mainly from literature on mindfulness and related conscious states (e.g., objective self-awareness) as well as the authors' personal experience. This brief instrument consists of 15 items that are rated on a 6-point Likert scale ranging from 1 (*almost always*) to 6 (*almost never*) with high scores representing heightened levels of mindfulness. A single factor of present awareness was extracted from a series of exploratory and confirmatory factor analyses using both college and non-college adult and clinical samples (Brown and Ryan 2003; Carlson and Brown 2005). The internal consistency is adequate (Cronbach's alpha = 0.82–0.87), and test–retest reliability was acceptable (intraclass correlation coefficient [*ICC*] = 0.81). Sample items include "I find it difficult to stay focused on what's happening in the present," "It seems I am 'running on automatic' without much awareness of what I'm doing," and "I find myself preoccupied with the future or the past."

Although the MAAS is the most widely used measure of mindfulness (Sauer et al. 2013), it has been criticized on several grounds. First, all MAAS items were developed to reflect *absence of mindfulness* because, according to the authors, people can better recall instances of mindlessness and may incorrectly endorse items reflecting mindfulness, thus yielding markedly skewed distributions. However, Grossman (2011) argued that the scale measures everyday inattentiveness which is not consistent with the original Buddhist conceptualization of mindfulness. Second, the MAAS does not directly assess attitudinal components (e.g., acceptance and non-judgment) that are considered integral to conceptualizations of mindfulness (Baer et al. 2006; Bishop et al. 2004; Kabat-Zinn 1994). Although the developers of the MAAS argued that the attitudinal components are subsumed under the present-moment awareness component, the issue is debatable and needs further investigation because a two-factor solution including non-judgmental acceptance as a distinct factor has been identified in the validation study of the Toronto Mindfulness Scale (Walach et al. 2006). Third, some MAAS items fail to reliably discriminate different trait levels. Van Dam et al. (2010) evaluated the MAAS items by applying item response theory and found that only five items carried the majority of the information about mindfulness while the rest poorly represented the latent trait mindfulness.

Despite these limitations, the MAAS demonstrated sound psychometric properties, and its solid unidimensional factor structure was replicated by an independent research group (MacKillop and Anderson 2007). There is also evidence for measurement invariance, suggesting that the underlying factor structure is stable across different populations (Carlson and Brown 2005). This brief 15-item scale is suitable for a concise measurement of mindfulness in individuals with and without mindfulness experience.

Kentucky Inventory of Mindfulness Skills (KIMS)

Influenced by the conceptualization of Dialectical Behavior Therapy (DBT; Linehan 1993), the KIMS (Baer et al. 2004) was designed to measure the general tendency to be mindful in daily life across four areas: observing, describing, Acting With Awareness, and Accepting Without Judgment. The KIMS consists of 39 items that are rated on a 5-point Liker scale ranging from 1 (*never or very rarely true*) to 5 (*almost always or always true*). The scale was validated college student and clinical samples who were diagnosed with borderline personality disorder, major depression, and post-traumatic stress disorder (Baer et al. 2004; Baum et al. 2010). Both Cronbach's alphas and test–retest reliability coefficients for the four facets were found to be adequate ranging between 0.76 and 0.91 for the former and between 0.65 and 0.86 for the latter (Baer et al. 2004). Participants who received the MBCT showed changes in their subscale scores suggesting its sensitivity to MBIs (Baum et al. 2010).

It is worth noting two issues regarding the KIMS. First, Baer et al. (2004) reported that three

Observe items (i.e., "I intentionally stay aware of my feelings," "I pay attention to how my emotions affect my thoughts and behaviors," and "I notice when my moods begin to change") were moderately but negatively loaded on the Accepting Without Judgment factor. Not surprisingly, the Observe factor was negatively correlated with the Accepting Without Judgment factor ($r = -0.14$, $p < 0.01$) and uncorrelated with the Acting With Awareness factor ($r = 0.09$, $p > 0.05$). Baer et al. (2004) argued that the three Observe items were retained for thorough coverage of this facet. However, these negative relationships are not consistent with how these facets are theorized to relate to one another (Gunaratana 2011). The authors also suggested that the Observe factor may differentially relate to the Accepting Without Judgment factor depending on levels of mindfulness, thus requiring further validation using a meditator sample. Additionally, Baum et al. (2010) a conducted factor analysis among clinical samples, and no second-order factor of mindfulness emerged (Baum et al. 2010). Regardless of how this issue is resolved, such negative factor correlation may discourage the use of total scores derived from the KIMS, and its factor structure needs to be re-evaluated without those three Observe items.

Second, there is a debate whether the Describe factor is an essential component of mindfulness. Simple labeling of observed experience may provide practical advantage, especially for novice meditators, and when MBIs are applied to individuals with severe psychological problems such as BPD (Linehan 1993; Segal et al. 2002). This labeling technique may foster a decentered perspective of ongoing experience and a meta-awareness of where the mind is dwelling on in a given moment. Such awareness may help one bring their attention back to the object of meditation, if mind wandering occurs. However, Buddhist texts have no mention about labeling, and it is rather discouraged (Gunaratana 2011). Labeling may disrupt focusing on ongoing experience because those labels intervene between the observer and the object of observation. In other words, even simple labeling such as "thinking" requires putting experience into a category and may filter out the experience that does not match the chosen category, thus preventing one from attending to the full spectrum of unfolding experience. Furthermore, when labeling is inappropriately used, unnecessary attention may be diverted to the label and subsequent reactions (e.g., "emotion makes me feel insecure"). Although labeling technique may carry practical utility, it is questionable whether it should be considered a key component of mindfulness.

To sum up, the KIMS items are anchored in mindfulness-specific, observable behavior and are written in a language that is understandable to individuals with no prior meditation experience. The scale has also demonstrated robust psychometric properties. However, the KIMS may contain a non-essential aspect of mindfulness (describing). Furthermore, development of the Five Facets Mindfulness Questionnaire (FFMQ), its upgrade version by the same developers, may render the KIMS obsolete.

Freiburg Mindfulness Inventory (FMI-14)

The item pool of the original 30-item FMI (Walach et al. 2006) was drawn from Buddhist scripts and writings by Buddhist scholars and meditation teachers. The authors note that a substantial body of selected literature pertains to insight mediation among different types of meditation practices (Buchheld et al. 2001). The items are rated on a 4-point Likert scale ranging from 1 (*rarely*) to 4 (*almost always*). The early 30-item version was validated in a sample of meditation retreat participants. Using the FMI-30, four factors (i.e., Mindful Presence, Non-judgmental Acceptance, Openness to Experiences, and Insight) were identified, but the factor structure was found to be unstable (Buchheld et al. 2001). Walach et al. (2006) conducted subsequent validation studies using meditation, clinical, and general samples and reported that some of the original 30 items did not show acceptable psychometric characteristics across samples, thus suggesting the use of a 14-item short form (FMI-14).

In addition to the reduction in item number, the FMI-14 has undergone two additional changes. First, items that are only familiar to meditators (e.g., "When I notice an absence of mind, I gently return to the experience of the here and now") were excluded in order to render the scale applicable to broader, non-meditating population. Second, the psychometric analysis indicated a unidimensional factor structure due to high factor loadings on the common factor and high cross-loadings of the items (Walach et al. 2006). The scale was found to have acceptable internal consistency (Cronbach's alpha = 0.79 for the general sample and 0.86 for the clinical sample). Sample items of the short form include "I am open to the experience of the present moment," "I see my mistakes and difficulties without judging them," and "I watch my feelings without getting lost in them."

It is noteworthy that some researchers disagree on the unidimensionality of the FMI-14. Ströhle et al. (2006) studied psychometric characteristics and proposed a two-factor solution. However, the developers (Kohls et al. 2009) later examined the factor structure with a mix of meditating and non-meditating samples using structural equation modeling (SEM), and they found that both one- and two-factor solutions did not yield acceptable fit indices. Therefore, they performed an exploratory factor analysis using the same sample. After removing six items that highly loaded onto both factors, a two-factor structure model (FMI-8) was identified that consists of "Presence" and "Acceptance" factors. Because no confirmatory factor analysis (CFA) has been performed on the FMI-8 with an independent sample, further investigation on this later version is needed. Furthermore, Belzer et al. (2013) examined the semantic understanding of the FMI-14 and found that participants with no mindfulness experience poorly understood the items. This comprehension problem is concerning because non-meditators are likely to misunderstand the FMI-14 items and provide inaccurate responses, thus reducing construct validity of the instrument.

The FMI encapsulates the most Buddhist conceptualizations of mindfulness among the self-report questionnaires reviewed here. Although the developers of the FMI excluded items that are difficult for non-meditators to understand, the FMI may be more suitable for individuals who have meditation experience. Furthermore, the new two-factor structure of the scale needs replication in an independent sample.

Toronto Mindfulness Scale (TMS)

The TMS (Lau et al. 2006) was developed based on the conceptualization of mindfulness by Bishop et al. (2004). While most mindfulness questionnaires assess a trait-like quality of mindfulness, the TMS offers both trait and state versions, and the state version is administered immediately following a meditation session. The TMS items concern how much one maintains an attitude of curiosity and a decentered perspective toward various mental events (e.g., thoughts and feelings) during a meditation session. For this reason, the scale is suitable only to individuals with meditation experience. This 13-item instrument is rated on a 5-point scale from 0 (*not at all*) to 4 (*very much*). Sample items include "I was curious about my reactions to things," "I was curious about what I might learn about myself by just taking notice of what my attention gets drawn to," and "I approached each experience by trying to accept it, no matter whether it was pleasant or unpleasant."

Lau et al. (2006) conducted a validation study using an adult sample with and without mindfulness experience and proposed a two-factor solution consisting of Curiosity and Decentering factors. However, a subsequent CFA found that data fit was inadequate, which the authors attributed to two cross-loading items, and they removed those items from the item pool (Lau et al. 2006). Although this change improved model fit, an additional confirmatory factor analysis in an independent sample is warranted because the cross-loadings were found only in the CFA sample, but not in the EFA sample (factor loadings for TMS20 and TMS29 = 0.10

and 0.08, respectively). The TMS demonstrated excellent internal consistency (Cronbach's alpha = 0.93 and 0.91 for Curiosity and Decentering factors, respectively) and low factor correlation ($r = 0.26$ and 0.42). TMS scores are related to theoretically related constructs (e.g., internal state awareness, reflective self-awareness, and psychological mindedness) in an expected way, suggestive of good convergent and divergent validity (Lau et al. 2006).

One thing to note here is that the TMS lacks a present-moment awareness factor, which almost all other mindfulness measures include. The authors argued that regulation of attention is not separable from the quality of attention (e.g., curiosity and acceptance) and some of the TMS items reflect present-moment awareness. However, there exist at least five mindfulness questionnaires (e.g., KIMS, FFMQ, FMI, CAMS-R, and PHLMS) that distinguish the two components (Baer et al. 2004, 2006; Cardaciotto et al. 2008; Feldman et al. 2007; Walach et al. 2006). Therefore, further research is needed to re-evaluate the factor structure of the TMS and its construct validity.

In summary, the TMS measures two unique facets of mindfulness (Curiosity and Decentering) that are not explicitly assessed by other mindfulness scales. Moreover, the TMS is one of the two questionnaires that are currently available to assess the state level of mindfulness. Considering the inclusion of two unique facets, the TMS can be used in a complementary way to broaden the coverage of mindfulness measurement.

Cognitive and Affective Mindfulness Scale Revised (CAMS-R)

The CAMS-R (Feldman et al. 2007) assesses four facets of mindfulness: self-regulation of attention, orientation to present-moment experience, awareness of experience, and accepting or non-judging attitude toward experience. Theoretically, the four facets were derived from the conceptualizations of Kabat-Zinn (1994) and Bishop et al. (2004). The items were rated on a 4-point Likert scale ranging from 1 (*rarely/not at all*) to 4 (*almost always*) with higher scores indicating higher levels of mindfulness. In a validation study of the early CAMS, low internal consistency and construct validity were observed, and the four factors that were extracted from an EFA were not replicated across samples (Feldman et al. 2005). Feldman et al. (2007) later combined 18 CAMS items and 17 new items into an item pool and conducted a factor analysis in a college sample. The final hierarchical model with a second-order factor of general mindfulness produced good model fit, $\chi^2(50) = 110.58$, $p < 0.001$, RMSEA = 0.064, SRMR = 0.052, CFI = 0.92 (Feldman et al. 2007). The CAMS-R demonstrated acceptable internal consistency for the total items (Cronbach's alpha = 0.74–0.77) and convergent validity. Sample items include "It is easy for me to concentrate on what I am doing," "I am able to focus on the present moment," and "I can tolerate emotional pain."

The CAMS-R offers broad conceptual coverage of four distinct mindfulness facets. However, the factor loadings of three items (i.e., Items 2, 3, and 5) were found to be low, which may inflate measurement error. The authors argued that they retained the items that had low factor loadings as low as 0.32 because these items supplement the model with broad conceptual coverage. However, using such a low cutoff may not be justifiable because a minimum factor loading cutoff of 0.40 or above is generally recommended (Steves 1992; Tabachnick and Fidell 2013). Furthermore, a follow-up analysis by the developers documented that two CAMS-R items with low factor loadings ("I am preoccupied by the future" and "I am preoccupied by the past") significantly confounded with the measures of worry and rumination, respectively. Additionally, these items did not correlate with other mindfulness measures (i.e., FMI and MAAS), suggesting that the two items have closer conceptual connection to worry and rumination than to mindfulness (Feldman et al. 2007). Thus, revision of these items and a subsequent factor analysis are warranted.

The CAMS-R is a brief measure that offers a broad coverage of mindfulness components. The

CAMS-R items are written in an everyday language that people with little meditation experience can understand. However, two CAMS-R items have questionable item content and low factor loadings. After these items were removed, Feldman et al. (2007) found that the scale related to criterion variables (e.g., distress and wellness) in a similar manner as the full 12-item scale. Thus, the 10-item version that excludes the two items with low content validity is recommended for use. Furthermore, the proposed factor structure of the CAMS-R has not been tested in a CFA, especially using a meditating sample, which warrants further validation of the scale.

Southampton Mindfulness Questionnaire (SMQ)

The SMQ (Chadwick et al. 2008) was developed to assess mindfulness awareness in response to distressing thoughts and images. Items were selected to reflect four facets of mindfulness: decentered awareness, staying open to difficult experience, non-judgmental acceptance, and seeing difficult cognitions as transient mental events without reacting to them. The SMQ consists of 16 items that are scored on a 7-point Likert scale ranging between 0 (*strongly disagree*) and 6 (*strongly agree*). The scale has been validated in both clinical and non-clinical community samples with and without mediation experience. The authors reported that the SMQ demonstrated good internal consistency (e.g., Cronbach's alpha = 0.82–0.89) and discrimination power among meditators, non-meditators, and individuals with psychosis. Sample items include "I'm able just to notice them without reacting," "I judge the thought/image as good or bad," and "I lose myself in the thoughts/images."

Two points are noteworthy regarding theoretical and practical aspects of the scale. First, although the authors originally conceptualized mindfulness as a multidimensional construct, a subsequent factor analysis provided only partial support for this proposition. Three factors whose eigenvalues were greater than one were identified in the principal components factor analysis with each factor accounting for significant amounts of variance. However, the authors noted that the three factors were not distinctly interpretable. One possible explanation is that compared to the 39-item FFMQ, the 16-item SMQ did not contain enough items that represent the full coverage of each facet, thus limiting its power to differentiate among the facets. Second, the SMQ items are framed to respond to how mindfully one related to distressing thoughts and images. Since MBIs are often administered in clinical settings, narrowing the focus of assessment to how an individual has dealt with disturbing experience may have clinical utility. However, it is unknown whether those who can stay mindful with regard to distressing thoughts and images are equally mindful in response to positive or neutral experience, or whether the same mindfulness skills can be translated into the dealings with feelings and bodily sensations.

The SMQ incorporated four mindfulness facets into a unidimensional self-report instrument. The scale demonstrated excellent psychometric properties and was validated in various samples although the scale needs further validation of the factor structure. Its narrow focus on unpleasant thoughts and images offers clinical utility of the scale but, at the same time, limits its general use.

Five Facets Mindfulness Questionnaire (FFMQ)

The FFMQ (Baer et al. 2006) was created by factor analyzing a 112-item pool derived from five validated mindfulness questionnaires including Mindfulness Attention Awareness Scale (MAAS; Brown and Ryan 2003), Kentucky Inventory of Mindfulness Skills (KIMS; Baer et al. 2004), Freiburg Mindfulness Inventory (FMI; Walach et al. 2006), Cognitive and Affective Mindfulness Scale (CAMS; Hayes and Feldman 2004), and an early version of the Southampton Mindfulness Questionnaire (SMQ; Chadwick et al. 2008). The scale consists of one emerging factor (Non-reactivity to Internal Experience) and the four factors that were already identified in the KIMS (Observing, Describing, Acting with Awareness, and Non-judging of Experience). The 39 items of the FFMQ are rated on a 5-point Likert scale ranging from 1 (*never or very rarely true*) to 5 (*very often or always true*). The scale showed acceptable psychometric properties, such as internal consistency (Cronbach's alpha for the subscales = 0.75–0.91), convergent and discriminant validity, and incremental validity in the prediction of general mental health (Baer et al. 2006; Curtiss and Klemanski 2014). Sample items include "I pay attention to how my emotions affect my thoughts and behavior," "I'm good at finding words to describe my feelings," "I am easily distracted," and "I criticize myself for having irrational or inappropriate emotions."

Two issues with the FFMQ are worth considering here. First, factor correlations involving the Observe factor may need further justification with theoretical support. As found in the validation study of the KIMS (Baer et al. 2004), the Observe factor weakly correlated with the Act With Awareness factor ($r = 0.15$, $p < 0.01$) and the Non-reactivity to Internal Experience factor ($r = 0.16$, $p < 0.01$), and it was uncorrelated with the Non-judging Of Experience factor ($r = -0.07$, *n.s.*). Since observing present-moment experience is considered a central feature of mindfulness (Bishop et al. 2004), the weak to negative correlations between the Observe facet and other subsidiary facets is puzzling. One possible explanation is that some of those individuals who rate high on the Observe items may have a heightened sensitivity to certain stimulus types (e.g., emotions and bodily sensations) but may be low in overall mindfulness. For example, anxiety-prone individuals may stay vigilant for any change in their emotional and bodily states or other signs of threat, thus providing high ratings of their observing skill. However, these individuals are probably low in mindfulness facets because they ignore important goal-relevant contextual information, which indicates a failure in self-regulation of attention. On a similar note, Baer (2016) suggests that a subset of individuals with little mindfulness practice may be attentive to present-moment experience, but in a reactive and judgmental way.

Second and related, there is evidence that the identified factor structure of the FFMQ differs between meditation-naïve and meditator groups. When two hierarchical models with and without the Observe facet were tested in the total sample with both meditating and non-meditating individuals, overall model fit was better for the four-factor model (Baer et al. 2006). However, when the factor structure was examined separately for each group, support was found for the five-factor hierarchical model in a meditating sample (Baer et al. 2006). Van Dam et al. (2009) reported that 18 of the FFMQ's 39 items favored either meditators or non-meditators suggesting differential item functioning (DIF) of these items. However, this finding was not replicated in the study using a demographically matched control sample (Baer et al. 2010). Although the FFMQ items showed minimal DIF in Baer et al. (2010) study, its factor structure still varied depending on respondents' meditation experience. Thus, it is recommended to use facet-specific subscale scores instead of a total score.

The FFMQ is one of the most popular mindfulness questionnaires with good psychometric characteristics, and its biggest strength lies in its coverage of five distinct mindfulness facets. However, the FFMQ items were mostly drawn from the KIMS and its factor structure was specified by a data-driven statistical approach without thorough examination of the items and their theoretical linkage. Furthermore, the DIF of some FFMQ items and lack of empirical support for the relation between the Observe factor and the other mindfulness factors warrant caution, and thus, the use of a total score is discouraged in a non-meditating sample.

Developmental Mindfulness Survey (DMS)

The DMS (Solloway and Fisher 2007) measures a unidimensional construct of non-judgmental observation of present-moment experience. The theoretical source for development of the DMS includes literature on mindfulness and journal responses to mindfulness practice by novice practitioners. Built upon item response theory, this 30-item questionnaire is rated on an 8-point scale ranging from 1 (*Absolutely disagree*) to 8 (*Absolutely agree*). During scale development, items were selected based on endorsement rates and other item properties to maximize discrimination power, and response options were grouped into three categories: disagree, agree, and strongly agree. These items were then transformed to produce a rescaled range between zero and one hundred. Sample items include "Mindfulness heightens my sense of smell," "I notice things about myself I never knew before," and "Mindfulness makes me a more attentive listener."

Three potential issues using the DMS are noted as follows. First, some items appear to lack content validity. For example, Item 16 ("Mindfulness can be learned") and Item 25 ("Mindfulness is harder than I first thought it would be") concern one's thought or feeling about mindfulness practice which is not synonymous with mindfulness level per se. Furthermore, the authors reported a discrepancy between their original conceptualization of item ordering and data-driven item difficulty, suggesting theory-data divergence and thus the need for subsequent re-evaluation of the scale. Second, measures based on Rasch analysis assume unidimensionality of the construct under investigation (Glas and Verhelst 1995). Individual items in a Rasch model are constructed to have discrimination power along the unidimensional continuum of mindfulness (Glas and Verhelst 1995). However, it is debatable whether the factor structure of mindfulness is unidimensional or multidimensional (Baer et al. 2006; Brown and Ryan 2003; Lau et al. 2006). If the underlying factor structure of mindfulness is multidimensional, items that assess a certain facet of mindfulness no longer retain similar discrimination power for items that belong to different subscales, especially when factor correlations are low. Third, it is important in scale development and validation to recruit samples that represent the whole spectrum of mindfulness skills including experienced meditators. However, the DMS was developed based on a sample of education students, most of whom are likely to have minimal exposure to mindfulness practice. Because the DMS items were calibrated to this restrictive sample, these items may function differentially toward individuals with higher degrees of meditation experience.

The DMS was developed using a unique approach to the measurement of mindfulness. The scale based on Rasch analysis offers higher discriminatory power to assess individuals with varying mindfulness skills. Despite this methodological advantage, the DMS contains items that lack theoretical support, and the scale was validated in a convenient sample with limited meditation experience. Thus, further validation of the scale is needed in individuals with varying levels of mindfulness skills.

Philadelphia Mindfulness Scale (PHLMS)

The PHLMS (Cardaciotto et al. 2008) was developed to measure two facets of mindfulness: present-moment awareness and acceptance. Inspired by conceptualizations of Kabat-Zinn (1994) and Bishop et al. (2004), the authors proposed two key elements of mindfulness defined as, "the tendency to be highly aware of one's internal and external experiences in the context of an accepting, nonjudgmental stance toward those experiences" (Cardaciotto et al. 2008). Using a 5-point Likert scale from 0 (*never*) to 4 (*very often*), the 20-item PHLMS asks respondents to rate the frequency of mindfulness-specific behaviors over the past week. The scale has been validated in clinical and non-clinical student samples while it may need further validation in people with extensive mindfulness practice (Cardaciotto et al. 2008). Subscale internal consistency across samples was within an acceptable range (Cronbach's alpha = 0.75–0.90), and convergent and discriminant validity was adequate when the relationships between the PHLMS subscales and measures of theoretically related constructs (e.g., mindful awareness, experiential avoidance, rumination, and suppression) were examined, except for the scale's non-significant correlation with psychopathology.

Although a CFA provides support for a two-factor model, the two subscales of Awareness and Acceptance were almost unrelated ($r = -0.10$, $p = 0.025$) in the student sample (Cardaciotto et al. 2008). Furthermore, the correlation between the MASS and PHLMS Awareness subscales was found to be low ($r = 0.21$, $p < 001$). The authors argued that acceptance and awareness are separate facets of mindfulness and can be measured independently. However, this orthogonality between the two factors is not consistent with the theory that suggests the intercorrelations among mindfulness facets (Baer et al. 2006; Gunaratana 2011). From a methodological standpoint, subfactors in a multidimensional scale are supposed to correlate with a higher order construct of mindfulness (Kline 2011). Thus, item content in the PHLMS subscales may need revision, and a subsequent factor analysis is necessary.

Effects of Meditation Scale (EOM)

The EOM (Reavley and Pallant 2009) consists of two subscales that assess the effects of meditation during meditation practice (EOM-DM) and in everyday life (EOM-EL). The 29-item EOM-DM subscale assesses five types of meditation effects: cognitive effects, emotional effects, mystical experiences, relaxation, and physical discomfort. The 35 items of the EOM-EL represent four types of meditation effects in everyday life: physical effects, expanded consciousness, emotional effects, and cognitive/behavioral effects. The cognitive and behavioral effects factor is further broken down into four subfactors including social, cognitive, and behavioral effects, and non-judgmental acceptance. All items are rated on a 6-point Likert scale ranging from 1 (*almost never*) to 6 (*almost always*). Internal consistency for the subscales was within an acceptable range with Cronbach's alpha values ranging between 0.68 and 0.87. Sample items include "I observe without judgment any negative thoughts or emotions that arise" (EOM-DM), "I feel a sense of physical wellbeing," (EOL-EL-Physical), and "I am less affected by habits such as biting nails, teeth grinding etc." (EOM-EL-Behavior).

Three limitations of the EOM are noteworthy. First, some EOM items may have questionable content validity because of the potential for multiple interpretations. For example, EOM-DM Item 49 ("I experience feelings of sadness and depression") and Item 15 ("I am aware of physical discomfort") may be intended to assess increased awareness of negative feelings or physical discomfort as a result of meditation practice. However, these items are possibly endorsed by individuals who are either undergoing a stressful situation or highly sensitive to negative information (i.e., depressed individuals) regardless of their mindfulness level. Likewise, items such as, "I have what I describe as a mystical experience" and "I observe inner colors, sounds, or visions" are not behavior-specific and lack any clear reference to what these terms mean. Second, some factors may lack concurrent validity. The authors noted that investigation into the effects of mindfulness practice is important because mindfulness effects link mindfulness practice with psychological outcomes (e.g., psychological problems or well-being). However, the emotional effects and relaxation factors of the EOM-DM were found to be mostly unrelated to weekly practice time, the degree of benefits in everyday life, and mediation experience (Reavley and Pallant 2009). These results are contrary to the generally accepted notion that mindfulness practice promotes emotion regulation and relaxation (Bishop et al. 2004). Third, a later validation study (Skipper et al. 2015) confirmed its five-factor structure of the 29-item EOM-DM. However, the seven-factor structure of the EOM-EL was not replicated. Thus, the EOM-EL's factor structure needs re-examination and if necessary respecification in the future.

While most mindfulness questionnaires concern the assessment of mindfulness skills, the EOM focuses on assessing one's experiences after mindfulness practice and the impact of mindfulness practice on everyday life. Since the scale presupposes that respondents have previous meditation experience, it is not suitable for non-meditating people. Additionally, the use of a total score is discouraged due to weak subscale correlations.

Mindfulness Mindlessness Scale (MMS)

The MSS (Bodner and Langer 2001; Haigh et al. 2011) was built on Langer's theory of mindfulness, described as "a general style or mode of functioning through which the individual actively engages in reconstructing environment through creating new categories or distinctions, thus directing attention to new contextual cues that may be consciously controlled or manipulated as appropriate" (Langer 1989, p. 4). The MSS consists of 21 items that assess four factors of mindfulness: Novelty Seeking, Engagement, Flexibility, and Novelty Producing. Items are rated on a 7-point Likert scale ranging from 1 (*strongly disagree*) to 7 (*strongly agree*). A CFA was conducted in student and community samples indicating adequate fit of a four-factor solution (goodness-of-fit index = 0.97; root mean square of approximation = 0.057). However, the developers reported that internal consistency for the Engagement and Flexibility factors was low (Cronbach's alpha = 0.63 and 0.54, respectively). Haigh et al. (2011) pursued further validation of the scale in undergraduate samples and found that the four-factor model proposed by Bodner and Langer (2001) yielded a poor fit to the data and failed to be replicated. Thus, Haigh et al. (2011) re-evaluated the factor structure of the MMS and suggested a single-factor solution that consists of nine out of the original 21 items. Internal consistency for the Mindfulness factor ranged between 0.76 and 0.85 across samples. Sample items for the 9-item version include "I like to investigate things," "I am always open to new ways of doing things," and "I 'get involved' in almost everything I do."

Two issues with the MMS are briefly mentioned here. First, Langer's conceptualization of mindfulness has the weakest connection to traditional Buddhist conceptualizations. Based on information processing theory, Langer and Moldoveanu (2000) argued that "drawing novel distinctions" and "creating new categories for structuring perception" are key aspects of mindfulness. However, such notions of mindfulness contradict with non-analytical and non-discursive quality of mindfulness suggested by Buddhist scholars and mindfulness teachers (Gunaratana, 2011). Second, some MMS items lack content validity. For example, Item 10 ("I am very creative"), Item 14 ("I try to think of new ways of doing things"), and Item 17 ("I like to be challenged intellectually") may tap one's creativity and preference of intellectual challenge but may not have much relevance to mindfulness.

In sum, the MMS represents the most Westernized conceptualization of mindfulness among the reviewed scales. Strongly influenced by information processing theory, the MMS items do not adequately capture the key aspects of mindfulness as they originate in Buddhist tradition. Re-evaluation of item content may be needed in a future validation study.

Open Issues and Research Implications

Can Mindfulness Be Assessed Using Self-reports?

This section seeks to explore two open issues regarding the measurement of mindfulness. The first issue relates to the adequacy and utility of self-report questionnaires in measuring mindfulness. The chapter so far discussed eleven existing self-report measures of mindfulness and their characteristics under the assumption that, despite some weaknesses and the needs of further validation, these measures are generally deemed to assess mindfulness accurately and reliably. However, there exists a group of researchers and mindfulness teachers that disagree with this premise.

According to Buddhist tradition, practicing mindfulness involves becoming a detached observer and staying fully engrossed in the observing process without engaging in any analytical and interpretative activity (Bodhi 1984). When a researcher attempts to assess the degree to which people engage in their experience mindfully, individuals who are not mindful or attentive may not be able to provide a valid report. This concern is consistent with the well-known phenomenon, called the Dunning–Kruger effect (Kruger and Dunning 1999), where low-ability individuals overestimate their ability in question and fail to recognize their inadequacy. Even if respondents are attentive to their mindfulness experience, their self-estimated experience may significantly differ from their actual mindfulness state considering that mindfulness consists of multiple preverbal facets (Grossman 2008). Moreover, mindfulness is often discussed in relationship to the other elements of the Noble Eightfold Path rather than in isolation. For example, staying mindful (Right Mindfulness) requires the proper amount of effort (Right Effort) and concentration (Right Concentration). The relationships among these elements and within mindfulness facets are characterized as interdependent, transactional, and nonlinear (Buddhadāsa and Santikaro 1988). However, the available mindfulness research seldom assesses the other seven elements of the Noble Eightfold Path.

Some empirical support against the use of mindfulness questionnaires is found in a study by Christopher et al. (2009). These researchers administered two popular questionnaires of mindfulness (MAAS and FFMQ) to Thai monks and students from Thai and American universities. As expected, the mean scores of the MAAS were higher for the Thai monks than for the two student groups. However, the American students scored higher on Observing and Accepting Without Judgment of the KIMS than the Thai monks and students. The American students also provided higher ratings on KIMS Describing compared to the Thai monks. Although these results do not confer direct evidence that mindfulness is not measurable using self-reports, the significant group difference in self-reported mindfulness between American and Thai samples indicates a considerable discrepancy between Eastern and Western conceptualizations, and the existing self-report questionnaires developed by Western scholars may have limitations in assessing levels of mindfulness among people outside the West.

The debate may continue as to whether self-reports are a valid method of assessing mindfulness, and we need more conclusive evidence in order to settle this issue. In addition to further validation of existing measures, research efforts are needed to examine whether the self-assessed mindfulness relates to other theoretically relevant constructs in a treatment outcome or longitudinal study. In fact, validation studies exist that investigate convergent and divergent validity by evaluating constructs that are supposed to either positively (e.g., well-being and self-awareness) or negatively (e.g., psychological problems and neuroticism) correlate with mindfulness (Baer et al. 2006; Lau et al. 2006). Although these correlational studies provide partial support for mindfulness questionnaires, more solid evidence will be found in a mediation study demonstrating that treatment type (e.g., MBI vs. control) and practice time predict pre/post-treatment scores of a mindfulness scale, which in turn are associated with outcome measures. It is also important to simultaneously assess other plausible constructs such as attention and emotional regulation and examine whether mindfulness accounts for the variance in treatment outcome above and beyond what may be predicted by the competing constructs.

Is Mindfulness a State or Trait?

Mindfulness is often used interchangeably even when the term refers to three different types of mindfulness. First, mindfulness is generally considered a trait that is stable over time and less susceptible to situational changes (Davidson 2010; Lau et al. 2006). In this view, individuals with high dispositional mindfulness are expected to live mindfully (e.g., having a clear awareness of what is happening in the present moment and accepting their experience without any negative judgment) in most of their life domains compared with those with low dispositional mindfulness. Their proneness to be mindful is kept relatively stable across time and place, and most mindfulness questionnaires such as the MAAS and FFMQ are purported to measure this stable quality of mindfulness. Such stability allows for the comparison of individual differences in relation to various psychological and biological processes that are presumed to co-vary with mindfulness such as brain functions and cognitive ability.

The second type of mindfulness resembles a trait-like quality but is amenable to treatment such as mindfulness training. For example, a self-report questionnaire used in a treatment outcome study is assumed to respond to changes in overall mindfulness levels, but not to short-lived fluctuations in mindfulness state. However, there is little empirical data showing the sensitivity of mindfulness questionnaires. Since mindfulness is a hypothetical construct that is not directly accessible, it is difficult to see how a change in scores of a mindfulness questionnaire corresponds to the "true" change in the amount of mindfulness. One can argue that if no difference in pre/post-treatment scores is found, this result could not be only because the selected MBI is not effective, but also because the self-report measure fails to respond to a "true" change in mindfulness. To determine the sensitivity and stability of a mindfulness questionnaire, a long-term longitudinal study is needed that tracks changes in self-report scores, the amount of intervention and individual practice, and other cognitive and neurophysiological measures that are known to be stable over time, and then evaluates the temporal relationship among these measures.

Third, mindfulness is also viewed as a state that varies depending on time and context (Lau et al. 2006). Currently, there are two questionnaires (i.e., TMS and EOM) that assess the state quality of mindfulness. A state mindfulness measure is useful when one needs to examine immediate effects of daily mindfulness practice and effectiveness of a brief (e.g., 30 min) MBI. Since brief mindfulness training may be limited in terms of the magnitude and scope of treatment effect, questionnaire items need to be specific rather than general and to correspond to the mindfulness facets that the MBI or individual practice promotes. To capture the full spectrum of the short-term impact of mindfulness training, it is also recommended to concurrently measure physiological and emotional processes as well as behavioral performance.

I have so far reviewed three types of mindfulness. It is all critical to understand individual differences in dispositional mindfulness, both short-term and long-term effects of MBIs, and fluctuations in mindfulness state. Compared to other mindfulness measures, the FFMQ and MAAS have been used in a large number of studies using correlational, experimental, and longitudinal study designs. Thus, these studies provide preliminary evidence showing how these two scales respond to different types of mindfulness. Overall, research evidence is not sufficient to determine the adequacy of current mindfulness questionnaires in relation to mindfulness type.

Implications for Future Research

The current review of the existing mindfulness questionnaires highlights some implications for future research. First, further investigations into identified facets are encouraged, as there is no clear consensus in the current literature on the dimensionality of mindfulness. As seen in the questionnaires reviewed here, some mindfulness scales contain items that are weak in content validity, and questionnaires vary in terms of the number of facets and the existence of the higher order mindfulness factor. In addition, the relationship among mindfulness facets needs to be explicitly theorized and empirically tested. To conduct statistical analysis and infer overall levels of mindfulness, researchers often use total scores of a mindfulness questionnaire with multiple subscales. This practice is potentially problematic unless we know how mindfulness facets relate to each other. There is evidence that the relationship among mindfulness facets differs depending on levels of mindfulness. Baer et al.

(2004) suggested that people with limited mindfulness practice may have a strong tendency to attend to their experience, but often in a judgmental way while those with experienced meditators are more likely to attend to experience and accept it without judgment. This is consistent with neuropsychological findings showing an inverse U-shaped relationship between meditation experience and brain activity (Brefczynski-Lewis et al. 2007). Thus, further research effort is needed to identify mindfulness facets and their relationship.

Second, although continued effort is needed to increase validity and reduce measurement divergence among mindfulness scales, the inherent heterogeneity in Eastern mindfulness tradition and the complexity of factor relationship make it difficult to develop a valid and coherent measure of mindfulness. Thus, I propose that research should focus on selecting mindfulness facets that are of investigators' interest and studying the relationship between these facets and other variables until such validity issue regarding mindfulness questionnaires is reasonably addressed.

The facet-focused approach provides a practical advantage compared to the approach to assessing overall levels of mindfulness. As noted above, Western investigation into mindfulness has primarily focuses on the clinical applications of MBIs. Researchers are curious about the underlying mechanisms through which MBIs work and which facets of mindfulness lead to particular clinical outcomes because such knowledge allows for the modification of MBIs and thus an increase in their effectiveness. Moreover, when a MBI is delivered to diverse clients, facet-level changes may differ depending on various factors (e.g., clients' meditation experience and presenting problems, and characteristics of the MBI). It is possible that such nuanced but clinically important information is obscured if a researcher aggregates data across facets and examines only overall levels of mindfulness using the total score of a mindfulness questionnaire. For example, most MBIs begin with attending to breathing and, as treatment progresses, the object of mindfulness is extended to other internal events (e.g., thoughts and feelings) that may evoke more strong emotional reactions. Since the early-stage mindfulness practice involves focusing attention on a relatively benign stimulus (e.g., breathing), the development of attitudinal components (e.g., non-judgmental acceptance) may be delayed until a later time. Although the attainment of such low-level mindfulness skills may not be strong enough to change the total score of a mindfulness scale, this small change can still carry a significant clinical importance and still have a measurable impact on clinical outcomes (e.g., improvement in focused attention).

Third, a multimethod approach using alternative methods is encouraged in future research. Currently, there exists no established referent of mindfulness that self-report questionnaires can be tested against. For this reason, Baer (2003) pointed that some mindfulness questionnaires overlook essential components of mindfulness and as a result possess weak construct validity. The multimethod triangulation across various modalities (e.g., self-report, behavioral tasks, and biological activities) can address this pitfall because convergence among different assessment methods undergirds construct validity of the measures in use and thus increases internal validity in research findings (Kopinak 1999). When the construct validity of a mindfulness questionnaire is in question, an additional assessment tool can provide a robust safeguard against the measurement drift. For example, a researcher can choose one mindfulness facet such as the ability to maintain attention to present-moment experience among others. This demands sustained attention while resisting distraction so that those who are high on the present-moment awareness facet are expected to demonstrate superior performance in a sustained attention task. A high correlation between self-reported ability to sustain attention and task performance will strengthen the confidence in this questionnaire. In addition, a meta-analysis on sustained visual attention reports increased neural activities in the right-lateralized areas such as anterior insula, mid-lateral prefrontal cortex (PFC), posterior ventrolateral PFC, and intraparietal sulcus (IPS) (Langner and Eickhoff 2013), thus predicting a positive correlation between self-reported present-moment awareness and the magnitudes of the activities in these area. Although these alternative measures need to be shown to have appropriate characteristics as a measurement tool (e.g., linearity of the scale), converging evidence among these methods will increase confidence in self-reported data and contribute to the modification of the existing questionnaires.

Conclusion

Despite over 20 years of rapid research growth, the field of mindfulness is in a relatively early developmental stage. No consensual agreement on the definition of mindfulness has emerged among researchers, and the underlying mechanisms of MBIs mostly remain unknown. Moreover, there exists a view that mindfulness can hardly be captured via a self-report instrument because mindfulness involves direct experience with thoughts, feelings, and bodily sensations without engaging any discursive and analytical processes. When one reports on a mindfulness questionnaire, responses may reflect cognitively filtered self-knowledge, not necessarily how truly they are aware of and relate to various experiences.

To date, eleven mindfulness questionnaires have been developed by researchers from various backgrounds. As these instruments differ in terms of conceptualizations of mindfulness, theoretical sources, the number of included facets, methods of scale development, and validation samples, each instrument provides unique measurement advantages over the others. However, such a large divergence among the instruments also reflects the misspecification of mindfulness facets and the inadequate psychometric properties of the instruments, mainly due to lack of a criterion measure of mindfulness. For this reason, when selection of a mindfulness questionnaire is considered, a careful examination of the scale is warranted in order to match the research goals.

It is also noteworthy that most mindfulness questionnaires need further validation of their factor structure and other psychometric properties, especially in both meditating and non-meditating samples, to ensure that the broad distribution of mindfulness skills is captured. Despite these limitations, there has certainly been continued effort to verify and improve mindfulness scales. In addition to subjective reports, biological and behavioral data have accumulated and are available for the cross-validation and improvement of self-report measures. It will be exciting to see how far the field of mindfulness advances in the future.

References

Baer, R. (2016). Assessment of mindfulness and closely related constructs: Introduction to the special issue. *Psychological Assessment*.

Baer, R. A. (2003). Mindfulness training as a clinical intervention: A conceptual and empirical review. *Clinical Psychology: Science and Practice, 10*(2), 125–143.

Baer, R. A., Samuel, D. B., & Lykins, E. L. (2010). Differential item functioning on the Five Facet Mindfulness Questionnaire is minimal in demographically matched meditators and nonmeditators. *Assessment*, 1073191110392498.

Baer, R. A., Smith, G. T., & Allen, K. B. (2004). Assessment of mindfulness by self-report the Kentucky inventory of mindfulness skills. *Assessment, 11* (3), 191–206.

Baer, R. A., Smith, G. T., Hopkins, J., Krietemeyer, J., & Toney, L. (2006). Using self-report assessment methods to explore facets of mindfulness. *Assessment, 13* (1), 27–45. doi:10.1177/1073191105283504.

Baron, R. M., & Kenny, D. A. (1986). The moderator–mediator variable distinction in social psychological research: Conceptual, strategic, and statistical considerations. *Journal of Personality and Social Psychology, 51*(6), 1173.

Baum, C., Kuyken, W., Bohus, M., Heidenreich, T., Michalak, J., & Steil, R. (2010). The psychometric properties of the Kentucky Inventory of Mindfulness Skills in clinical populations. *Assessment, 17*(2), 220–229.

Belzer, F., Schmidt, S., Lucius-Hoene, G., Schneider, J. F., Orellana-Rios, C. L., & Sauer, S. (2013). Challenging the construct validity of mindfulness assessment—A cognitive interview study of the Freiburg mindfulness inventory. *Mindfulness, 4*(1), 33–44.

Bergomi, C., Tschacher, W., & Kupper, Z. (2013). Measuring mindfulness: First steps towards the development of a comprehensive mindfulness scale. *Mindfulness, 4*(1), 18–32.

Biegel, G. M., Brown, K. W., Shapiro, S. L., & Schubert, C. M. (2009). Mindfulness-based stress reduction for the treatment of adolescent psychiatric outpatients: A randomized clinical trial. *Journal of Consulting and Clinical Psychology, 77*(5), 855.

Bishop, S. R., Lau, M., Shapiro, S., Carlson, L., Anderson, N. D., Carmody, J., et al. (2004). Mindfulness: A proposed operational definition. *Clinical Psychology: Science and Practice, 11*(3), 230–241.

Bodhi, B. (1984). *The noble eightfold path—The way to the end of suffering*. The Wheel Publication.

Bodhi, B. (2010). *The noble eightfold path: The way to the end of suffering*. Kandy: Buddhist Publication Society.

Bodner, T. E., & Langer, E. J. (2001). *Individual differences in mindfulness: The Mindfulness/Mindlessness Scale*. Paper presented at the 13th annual American Psychological Society Conference, Toronto, Ontario, Canada.

Brefczynski-Lewis, J. A., Lutz, A., Schaefer, H., Levinson, D., & Davidson, R. (2007). Neural correlates of attentional expertise in long-term meditation practitioners. *Proceedings of the National Academy of Sciences, 104*(27), 11483–11488.

Brown, K. W., & Ryan, R. M. (2003). The benefits of being present: Mindfulness and its role in psychological well-being. *Journal of Personality and Social Psychology, 84*(4), 822.

Buchheld, N., Grossman, P., & Walach, H. (2001). Measuring mindfulness in insight meditation (Vipassana) and meditation-based psychotherapy: The development of the Freiburg Mindfulness Inventory (FMI). *Journal for Meditation and Meditation Research, 1*(1), 11–34.

Buddhadāsa, B., & Santikaro, B. (1988). *Ānāpānasati: Mindfulness with Breathing; Unveiling the Secrets of Life; a Manual for Serious Beginners*. Dhamma Study-Practice Group.

Cardaciotto, L., Herbert, J. D., Forman, E. M., Moitra, E., & Farrow, V. (2008). The assessment of present-moment awareness and acceptance the Philadelphia mindfulness scale. *Assessment, 15*(2), 204–223.

Carlson, L. E., & Brown, K. W. (2005). Validation of the Mindful Attention Awareness Scale in a cancer population. *Journal of Psychosomatic Research, 58* (1), 29–33.

Chadwick, P., Hember, M., Symes, J., Peters, E., Kuipers, E., & Dagnan, D. (2008). Responding mindfully to unpleasant thoughts and images: Reliability and validity of the Southampton mindfulness questionnaire (SMQ). *British Journal of Clinical Psychology, 47*(4), 451–455.

Christopher, M. S., Christopher, V., & Charoensuk, S. (2009). Assessing "Western" mindfulness among Thai Theravāda Buddhist Monks. *Mental Health, Religion and Culture, 12*(3), 303–314.

Creswell, J. D., Irwin, M. R., Burklund, L. J., Lieberman, M. D., Arevalo, J. M., Ma, J., et al. (2012). Mindfulness-based stress reduction training reduces loneliness and pro-inflammatory gene expression in older adults: a small randomized controlled trial. *Brain, Behavior, and Immunity, 26*(7), 1095–1101.

Curtiss, J., & Klemanski, D. H. (2014). Factor analysis of the five facet mindfulness questionnaire in a heterogeneous clinical sample. *Journal of Psychopathology and Behavioral Assessment, 36*(4), 683–694.

Davidson, R. J. (2010). Empirical explorations of mindfulness: Conceptual and methodological conundrums.

Feldman, G., Hayes, A., Kumar, S., Greeson, J., & Laurenceau, J.-P. (2007). Mindfulness and emotion regulation: The development and initial validation of the Cognitive and Affective Mindfulness Scale-Revised (CAMS-R). *Journal of Psychopathology and Behavioral Assessment, 29*(3), 177–190.

Feldman, G., Hayes, A. M., Kumar, S. M., Kamholz, B., Greeson, J. M., & Laurenceau, J. P. (2005). *Assessing mindfulness in the context of emotion regulation: The revised cognitive and affective mindfulness scale (CAMS-R)*. Paper presented at the annual convention of the Association for Behavioral and Cognitive Therapies, Washington, DC.

Glas, C. A., & Verhelst, N. D. (1995). *Testing the Rasch models* (pp. 69–95).Berlin: Springer.

Grossman, P. (2008). On measuring mindfulness in psychosomatic and psychological research. *Journal of Psychosomatic Research, 64*(4), 405–408.

Grossman, P. (2011). Defining mindfulness by how poorly I think I pay attention during everyday awareness and other intractable problems for psychology's (re) invention of mindfulness: Comment on Brown et al. (2011).

Gunaratana, B. (2011). *Mindfulness in plain English*. New York: Simon and Schuster.

Haigh, E. A., Moore, M. T., Kashdan, T. B., & Fresco, D. M. (2011). Examination of the factor structure and concurrent validity of the Langer Mindfulness/Mindlessness Scale. *Assessment, 18*(1), 11–26.

Hayes, A. M., & Feldman, G. (2004). Clarifying the construct of mindfulness in the context of emotion regulation and the process of change in therapy. *Clinical Psychology: Science and Practice, 11*(3), 255–262.

Hayes, S. C., Strosahl, K. D., & Wilson, K. G. (1999). *Acceptance and commitment therapy*. New York: Guilford Press.

Kabat-Zinn, J. (1982). An outpatient program in behavioral medicine for chronic pain patients based on the practice of mindfulness meditation: Theoretical considerations and preliminary results. *General Hospital Psychiatry, 4*(1), 33–47.

Kabat-Zinn, J. (1994). *Wherever you go, there you are: Mindfulness meditation in everyday life*. New York, NY: Hyperion.

Keng, S.-L., Smoski, M. J., & Robins, C. J. (2011). Effects of mindfulness on psychological health: A review of empirical studies. *Clinical Psychology Review, 31*(6), 1041–1056.

Khoury, B., Lecomte, T., Fortin, G., Masse, M., Therien, P., Bouchard, V., et al. (2013). Mindfulness-based therapy: A comprehensive meta-analysis. *Clinical Psychology Review, 33*(6), 763–771.

Kline, R. B. (2011). *Principles and practice of structural equation modeling* (3rd ed.). New York, NY: Guilford Publications.

Kohls, N., Sauer, S., & Walach, H. (2009). Facets of mindfulness—Results of an online study investigating the Freiburg mindfulness inventory. *Personality and Individual Differences, 46*(2), 224–230.

Kopinak, J. K. (1999). The use of triangulation in a study of refugee well-being. *Quality & Quantity, 33*(2), 169–183.

Kruger, J., & Dunning, D. (1999). Unskilled and unaware of it: how difficulties in recognizing one's own incompetence lead to inflated self-assessments. *Journal of Personality and Social Psychology, 77*(6), 1121.

Langer, E. J. (1989). *Mindfulness*. Addison-Wesley/ Addison Wesley Longman.

Langer, E. J., & Moldoveanu, M. (2000). The construct of mindfulness. *Journal of Social Issues, 56*(1), 1–9.

Langner, R., & Eickhoff, S. B. (2013). Sustaining attention to simple tasks: A meta-analytic review of the neural mechanisms of vigilant attention. *Psychological Bulletin, 139*(4), 870.

Lau, M. A., Bishop, S. R., Segal, Z. V., Buis, T., Anderson, N. D., Carlson, L., et al. (2006). The Toronto mindfulness scale: Development and validation. *Journal of Clinical Psychology, 62*(12), 1445–1467.

Linehan, M. (1993). *Cognitive-behavioral treatment of borderline personality disorder*. New York: Guilford press.

MacKillop, J., & Anderson, E. J. (2007). Further psychometric validation of the mindful attention awareness scale (MAAS). *Journal of Psychopathology and Behavioral Assessment, 29*(4), 289–293.

Reavley, N., & Pallant, J. F. (2009). Development of a scale to assess the meditation experience. *Personality and Individual Differences, 47*(6), 547–552.

Regehr, C., Glancy, D., & Pitts, A. (2013). Interventions to reduce stress in university students: A review and meta-analysis. *Journal of Affective Disorders, 148*(1), 1–11.

Sauer, S., Walach, H., Schmidt, S., Hinterberger, T., Lynch, S., Büssing, A., et al. (2013). Assessment of mindfulness: Review on state of the art. *Mindfulness, 4*(1), 3–17.

Segal, Z. V., Williams, J., & Teasdale, J. D. (2002). Mindfulness-based cognitive therapy for depression: A new approach to relapse prevention: New York: Guilford Press.

Skipper, T., O'Donovan, A., Conlon, E., & Clough, B. (2015). An examination of the factor structure of the Effects of Meditation scale. *Personality and Individual Differences, 86*, 57–62.

Solloway, S. G., & Fisher, W. P. (2007). Mindfulness practice: A Rasch variable construct innovation. *Journal of Applied Measurement, 8*(4), 359.

Steves, J. (1992). *Applied multivariate statistics for the social science*. New Jersey: Hillsdale.

Ströhle, G., Heidenreich, T., Michalak, J., & Nachtigall, C. (2006). *Empirische Erfassung der Achtsamkeit* (Unpublished master's thesis). Universität Jena, Jena.

Tabachnick, B. G., & Fidell, L. S. (2013). *Using multivariate statistics* (6th ed.). New Jersey: Pearson.

Thera, N. (2014). *The heart of Buddhist meditation: The Buddha's way of mindfulness*: Weiser Books.

Van Dam, N. T., Earleywine, M., & Borders, A. (2010). Measuring mindfulness? An item response theory analysis of the Mindful Attention Awareness Scale. *Personality and Individual Differences, 49*(7), 805–810.

Van Dam, N. T., Earleywine, M., & Danoff-Burg, S. (2009). Differential item function across meditators and non-meditators on the Five Facet Mindfulness Questionnaire. *Personality and Individual Differences, 47*(5), 516–521.

Walach, H., Buchheld, N., Buttenmüller, V., Kleinknecht, N., & Schmidt, S. (2006). Measuring mindfulness—The Freiburg mindfulness inventory (FMI). *Personality and Individual Differences, 40*(8), 1543–1555.

Walshe, M. (1995). *The long discourses of the Buddha: A translation of the Digha Nikaya (teachings of the Buddha)*. Boston, USA: Wisdom Publications.

Remembering-and-Receiving: Mindfulness and Acceptance in Zen

Josh Bartok and Lizabeth Roemer

Keywords
Mindfulness · Acceptance · Zen · Buddhism · Behavioral health

Stay with that just as that
Stay with this just as this.
—*Hongzhi Zhengjue (Leighton 2000, p. 31)*

The concepts of mindfulness and acceptance have become ubiquitous in behavioral health intervention and prevention efforts (e.g., Hayes et al. 2011; Kabat-Zinn 2013; Linehan 1993; Roemer and Orsillo 2009; Segal et al. 2013), and these approaches have demonstrated efficacy in addressing a wide range of psychological disorders and psychological symptoms associated with medical issues (e.g., A-Tjak et al. 2015; Gotink et al. 2015). Generally speaking, mindfulness-based approaches incorporate meditation practices (often formal sitting practices as well as others) to help people to bring their awareness back, again and again, to this moment in order to be choicefully present in their lives. Acceptance-based practices help people open to, allow, and recognize experiences as they are, rather than engaging in futile efforts to avoid, ignore, suppress or change these experiences—all of which ultimately further increase distress. The practices of mindfulness are intended to cultivate this accepting way of relating to experiences.

Both mindfulness and practices to enhance acceptance can be found in Buddhism, including within the Zen Buddhist tradition. Modern psychological interventions vary in their grounding within these spiritual traditions.

This is a jointly written chapter. We write this chapter as a Zen teacher—in a Buddhist tradition (Boundless Way Zen) that includes lineages of both Soto and Rinzai Zen, who is also an editor of Dharma books and a Buddhist pastoral counselor (JB), and a clinical psychologist, grounded in the behavioral tradition, who has co-developed an acceptance-based behavioral therapy for anxiety disorders (LR). The authors also happen to be married to one another—and have come to

J. Bartok (✉)
Greater Boston Zen Center, Boundless Way Zen, Cambridge, USA
e-mail: jbartok@gmail.com

L. Roemer
University of Massachusetts Boston, Boston, USA
e-mail: Lizabeth.Roemer@umb.edu

A. Masuda and W.T. O'Donohue (eds.), *Handbook of Zen, Mindfulness, and Behavioral Health*, Mindfulness in Behavioral Health, DOI 10.1007/978-3-319-54595-0_18

deeply influence one another. From these positions, we have a respect for the value of distinguishing spiritual, religious practice from provision of behavioral health services and encourage (and engage in) secular adaptations of mindfulness-based approaches that draw from evidence-based practice and psychological theory. At the same time, we appreciate the ways that the depth of Zen tradition can inform these adaptations and our own ability to flexibly implement them with attention to the complexity of the lived experience of acceptance and its relationship to suffering in its many forms. Toward that end, we endeavor to provide here an illustration of the Zen teachings that inform our understanding of acceptance and how it can promote freedom amid suffering. The bulk of this chapter presents these teachings in the voice of a Zen teacher (JB), with the psychologist adding some psychological interpretation periodically.

Defining Acceptance and Mindfulness

Acceptance has long been incorporated into psychological perspectives (see Hayes and Pankey 2003, for a brief overview of this history), with Rogers (1961) particularly emphasizing the central role of acceptance in psychological and behavioral health and well-being. Our work is particularly influenced by behavioral perspectives on acceptance. The common emphasis on strategies to promote change within this tradition has been balanced by attention to promotion of acceptance over the past two decades (e.g., Hayes et al. 2011; Linehan 1993), with a specific emphasis on experiential acceptance, or acceptance of internal thoughts, feelings, sensations, and memories. In his review of these approaches, Cordova (2001, p. 215) defines acceptance as "allowing, tolerating, embracing, experiencing, or making contact with, a source of stimulation that previously evoked escape, avoidance, or aggression" and "a change in the behavior evoked by a stimulus from that functioning to avoid, escape, or destroy, to behavior functioning to maintain or pursue contact." He notes that this does not mean attempting to increase (or decrease) the frequency of these experiences, only an end to trying to avoid or struggle with them. In essence then, acceptance is learning to respond differently to internal experiences. A metaphor from acceptance and commitment therapy (Hayes et al. 2011) helps to illustrate the concept of acceptance: rather than engaging a futile tug-of-war with thoughts, feelings and sensations, acceptance is "dropping the rope." Acceptance is distinguished from resignation in that acceptance means accepting what is already present; not condoning it or refraining from efforts to make situations different. For instance, Linehan (1993) describes the related concept of willingness as acceptance of what is, as well as responding to what is, effectively and appropriately.

We would like to offer a definition of acceptance from a Zen perspective—which will also provide an opportunity to explore Zen's relationship to seeming paradox and to language, which we will do immediately below. From a Zen perspective, we might define acceptance as turning toward, making space for, and *receiving* this moment of this one thing that is self-and-the-universe-together just as it is. We receive what is and simultaneously entrust ourselves to what is. We entrust ourselves-and-the-universe to ourselves-and-the-universe. This is a subtle inward gesture of contact that, though in one sense is so small as to be almost trivial, also represents a radically transformed relationship to all that arises, inwardly and outwardly. Acceptance reveals, affirms, and honors the reality that this moment—inclusive even of present suffering—rests on an unconditioned, unconditional ground of *okayness* and *enoughness*—a wholeness that does not require any element of experience be obtained nor any element of experience be expunged.

This Zen definition of acceptance points to a key characteristic and function of meditation in the Zen tradition: it enlarges our heart's capacity to hold both sides of a seeming paradox, to make space for simultaneous and non-identical truths. This is in itself a profoundly liberating capacity. The text at the very core of the Zen tradition, the Heart Sutra, offers a particularly succinct and dramatic example of this: "form is exactly emptiness; emptiness, exactly form."[1] A thorough exploration of form and emptiness is beyond the scope of this chapter but is alluded to in the compound term coined above: "self-and-the-universe-together." This term points to an element of the Zen perspective that regards "me" not only as a discrete entity, but also as *essenceless* and fundamentally inextricable from the vast interconnected whole of the universe. In a sense "I" (and "my experience") is not separate from "the universe"—but rather I-and-my-experience is what the *universe* is *doing* right here. It is our enlarged capacity to hold truths that precisely allows us to express (and be liberated by) the fact that "everything is a mess, yet all is well" (Bayda and Bartok 2005, p. 28).

Zen's relationship to paradox informs and transforms its relationship to language and its characteristic modes of expression. In an important way, Zen specializes in using *seeming* paradox as well as artful, poetic language to express what is fundamentally inexpressible. In this way, the language of Zen—especially as it unfolds over years of practice and study—can be radiant to the heart even though it may also be dark to the mind. Zen language can be met as a kind of verbal art in the way one meets an abstract expressionist's painting: it evokes rather than explains; it points directly to an aspect of the human heart rather than being "about" something else. And yet even so, after years of study and practice, one comes to see that, in fact, the language of Zen is also direct, succinct, and clear.

Within the behavioral health literature, mindfulness strategies are typically introduced as a way to cultivate acceptance and to relate differently to one's internal experiences. Mindfulness is commonly defined as "paying attention in a particular way, on purpose, in the present moment, and nonjudgmentally" (Kabat-Zinn 1994, p. 4), or "open or receptive attention to and awareness of ongoing events and experience" (Brown and Ryan 2004, p. 245). Another, related, often-cited definition is "the awareness that arises through intentionally attending in an open, kind, and discerning way" (Shapiro and Carson 2009, p. 15). Most interventions incorporate *formal* practices, or time set aside to develop the skills of mindfulness, for instance by sitting and returning attention to the breath, again and again. *Informal* practices involve applying this awareness within daily life, for instance while washing dishes or folding clothes or even in more stressful contexts. Often formal practices become synonymous with mindfulness-based treatments; however, informal practices are equally, if not more, important. It is easy to fall into the trap of regarding formal meditation as some kind of sacred or "real" practice and informal practice as its vastly inferior stand-in in the mundane world—but this misunderstands both. From a Zen perspective, Dogen Zenji (the peerless master who was the founder of the Japanese Soto School of Zen) says, "Those who think that worldly tasks hinder Buddhism know only that there is no Buddhism in the world; they do not know that there is nothing that can be set apart as worldly tasks in Buddhism" (this translation is from Masunaga 1958; also translated by Leighton 2011).

Although terms such as *mindfulness, acceptance,* and even *Zen* do have precise, expansive definitions in the behavioral health field, they have become so common in the behavioral health literature, culture of self-help, and everyday life that they are easily oversimplified or misunderstood. For instance, the word *mindfulness* often evokes focusing in on paying attention, slowly and narrowly and perhaps somehow preciously, often with an intention to focus the mind. Similarly, the word *Zen* has entered the popular lexicon as a synonym for a kind of chilled-out, it's-all-good almost tranquilized equanimity. And *acceptance* often has a connotation of passivity or resignation, rather than being an important step in promoting effective, meaningful action. From a Zen perspective, acceptance is at the very heart of what enables us to be choicefully present in our lives, continually reorienting ourselves to harmonious action in alignment with our values. Truly noticing and accepting things as they are,

[1]All presentations of Zen liturgy are drawn from the *Boundless Way Zen Sutra Book* (Boundless Way Zen 2015).

including injustices and inequities, can even be a catalyst for the awakening that leads to empowerment and social action (e.g., Williams 2002; Manuel 2015).

The Pali word that is commonly translated as mindfulness is *sati*—and this word could also be translated as "remembering." This points to an aspect that can be easily overlooked. Within Zen, an important part of Dharma practice is the practice remembering—remembering our values, our intentions, and our aspirations—and remembering to show up to the big mess of our lives and the big mess of our selves.

Zazen, meditation practice in the Zen tradition, is Zen's formal practice of mindfulness-and-acceptance (hyphenated because this refers to a single unitary practice, not two practices done in succession). We could also call zazen "accepting-and-entrusting" or "remembering-and-receiving."

The Practice of Zazen

Awareness of What Is—Zazen Highlights the Nature of Our Minds

Okumura (2010, p. 64) says of zazen that it "goes beyond and yet includes complete acceptance and complete rejection of thoughts."

What we are practicing in zazen is beginning to free ourselves from the shackles of our own minds. In zazen, we are being intimately present to the arising of grasping, aversion, and delusive certainties that claim to us that they are true. In other words, we are familiarizing ourselves with all of the ways in which we are constantly, moment after moment, pushing away, grabbing on, and telling ourselves a story. When we first start to sit in zazen, this becomes vividly apparent as we see our monkey mind jump from narrative to narrative, reactive impulse to reactive impulse—and seeing this is actually a very good thing, a positive development. It can be easy to feel that you are doing meditation completely wrong or that somehow meditation is making your mind worse, because, now that you've started meditating you see how vividly and ceaselessly this grasping, aversion, and these stories, arise. In truth though, such ceaseless arising is not a new development within your mind—it has actually been going on since time immemorial. Your mind has always been doing that—it is just that now we have finally gotten around to noticing.

The Zen-influenced writer Tollifson (2012, p. 112) points to the power of this awareness itself: "part of waking up is becoming sensitive to how we become discouraged, how we close down, and where we go for false comfort. To wake up is to become aware of the tendency to judge ourselves, to take our failures personally, to fall into despair, self-pity, depression, frustration, anger, or wherever we tend to go when we believe the story that we are a loser who cannot do it right. Seeing all of this is enough. Awareness is its own action. We do not need to analyze it mentally or try to impose changes willfully based on our ideas of what 'should' be happening, and in fact, that rarely works. Just being awake to the present moment, as it is, and seeing clearly what is happening—not what we think is happening—this is transformative." When we start to settle down and practice opening the hand of thought—bringing some awareness and attention—we start to *see* our mind's conditioned nature. When we start to see it, we are laying the groundwork for working flexibly with the arising of these impulses in the rest of our lives.

In the simplified experimental container of formal meditation practice, we begin to develop and cultivate a skill—unhooking from thoughts, opening the hand of thought, receiving what is—and then in the messy conditions of our lives, we gradually gain a capacity to apply that skill.

Acceptance and Not-knowing—Zazen Illuminates a New Way of Responding to Arisings in Our Minds

Zazen is not about trying to still the mind, quiet the mind, or empty the mind. It is not about trying to feel calm or trying to feel relaxed or trying to feel any way and not some other way. The practice of zazen is actually the most simplified form that remembering-and-receiving can take. It is the easiest way to cultivate and train this capacity—quite literally *practice*—as hard as it may feel. In a stripped-down fashion, it allows us to begin to get familiar with the way our minds amplify and create suffering, in ourselves and around us. We are practicing the skills we need to be able to live from a place of freedom in our lives, to have freedom amid suffering—which is very different from freedom *from* suffering. *Freedom amid* takes place simultaneously with the arising of a suffering and distress, of all arising thoughts and feelings, whereas striving for *freedom from* is a manifestation of both aversion and grasping: aversion to this moment as it is, and an impulsive reaction that tries to make this moment different. *Freedom from* is an imagined state (a narrative) in which we are somehow beyond our ordinary humanness. *Freedom amid* embraces the full scope of our humanity.

As humans, we naturally have reactions to distress and discomfort—and in accordance with our conditioning, we try to relieve it. One place we engage with this dynamic in zazen is in regard to maintaining complete stillness. People new to zazen may conclude that those old hands who sit so still do so because it is easy for them —effortless and completely comfortable. Comparing our insides to other people's outsides, we may imagine the impulse to shift, or scratch, or flee never arises for the type of people we see sitting so still. Yet this is not so. Even Zen masters sit zazen in human bodies. The posture of zazen, whether on a cushion, a bench, or a chair allows us to sit in a way that is *moderately* comfortable—but it is generally not a position of optimal, perfect comfort. With our very stillness itself, we are enacting and embodying a practice of acceptance—this is the great gift of stillness.

Our conditioning, our habit energy, our *karma* (about which, more below) is such that sensations of discomfort may arise—as indeed will the whole gamut of mental formations—and our conditioned response to these arisings is to automatically try to push away the unpleasant ones. This impulse of aversion arises so instantaneously on the heels of the original sensation that we conflate those elements as being one and the same. Sensations themselves are *all* fundamentally neutral, but we become conditioned to believe that the certain sensations themselves, certain arisings themselves, are a problem, are inherently bad. In fact, though, sensations are just sensations, so too with mental formations—the larger category that includes sensations, emotions, perceptions, impulses, thoughts, and beliefs. They are just a manifestation of the universe arising right here, right now. We need not endorse an interpretation of their arising as an objective problem, or our impulse to push away as a command to act. Each mental formation is not a truth, and not a problem. All that arises: not a truth, not a problem. Our practice of zazen is meeting all arisings equally. A famous classical Chinese Zen poem "Trust in Mind" *(Xinxinming)* describes this practice as immediately affirming "not-two" (Soeng 2004, p. 16).

We use the external container of physical stillness as a place to explore this—the not-a-truth-and-not-a-problem quality of mental formations. By remaining still when the impulse to move or scratch an itch arises screamingly, we demonstrate to ourselves a flexible way of interacting with our mental formations. Sitting upright and unmoving in the midst of those things arising is demonstrating and actualizing reality that your thoughts and your opinions do not and need not define the situation; they need not carry the force of truth. We need not believe everything we think.

Part of the nature of the delusive stories we tell ourselves is that they seem to fill the whole frame of our experience, or we might say that our experience narrows to be no larger than this small thought. Each time we return our attention back to the breath, come back to the physicality of sitting, we expand our awareness to be more inclusive. We are practicing sitting in a spacious awareness, which may include the breath, which may include mental formations, which may include physical formations, but is not limited to any of those things. In this way, zazen is not fundamentally a concentration practice. Expanded awareness allows us to meet our thoughts as *just thoughts* without infusing them with the force of truth.

Another name for believing our thoughts, taking our thoughts as truth or impulses as requirements, is *delusive certainty*. And each time we see a thought as a thought rather than a truth, a story as a story, a sensation as a sensation, we are actualizing the antidote to delusive certainty. We are also cultivating a capacity to simply be with not-knowing, without needing to replace not-knowing with some knowing. This too is part of the great liberating value of zazen.

And this, in turn, allows us to enlarge our capacity to be with the reality of uncertainty. We have stories of certainty, we have stories about the certainty for the future, but as true as these stories may claim to be to us, they are in the end just stories—whose main function is to create an illusion of certainty, and illusion of knowing. Part of zazen is befriending, becoming familiar, and keeping company with this reality of not-knowing—and this is actually quite radical, quite flexible, and profoundly useful.

Formal-and-Informal Practice

When I (JB) meet with people individually in *dokusan*—formal guidance in Zen meditation—frequently people say to me, "I haven't been practicing." When they say that, what they often mean is, "I haven't been sitting in formal meditation." To be sure, a certain amount of formal practice is essential—but it is not the whole of the endeavor, or the only way to practice. When people tell me they have not been practicing, I encourage them to not mistakenly identify *practice* with formal meditation on the cushion. Practice is your life, and practice is available continually throughout the whole your life. This is *informal* practice—and it cannot be overvalued. Some amount of formal practice supports our ability to do informal practice—it orients us to the nature of the work to be done—but there is not a dose-related response with regard to the amount of formal practice. It is not the case that more formal practice is better than less; what is true is that more *formal-and-informal* practice is better than less formal-and-informal practice. Informal practice is simply noticing (whenever, and wherever we can) the arising of grasping, aversion, and delusive certainty, unhooking from those karmically conditioned automatic action tendencies, and being choicefully present in our lives. This lets us at least slightly more often make a choice for a valued action rather than a conditioned response.

Torei Enji, a disciple of the great Rinzai Zen Master Hakuin in the eighteenth century, offers a frame for appreciating our noticing the arising of attachments, aversions, and stories: "This is the Buddha appearing to us, finding ways to free us from our own attachments—the very ones that have made us suffer, again and again and again."

When anxiety arises, when difficulties arise, when some problem arises, if we accept that as an opportunity to practice the fundamental essence of Zen—accepting-and-entrusting, remembering-and-receiving—this is the Buddha appearing to us, inviting us to meet directly with the arising of our own suffering-causing mental formations. In this way, the arising of a difficulty can itself remind us to practice—whether formally or informally. A fearful thought, a rageful thought, can thus become like a big neon arrow saying, "Right here in this moment is an opportunity for you practice." Our very suffering reminds us to practice.

When fear arises or when anger arises, rather than getting caught up in the energy of fear, and hiding or turning away from what matters to us, or rather than just reacting angrily and creating more harm and suffering for ourselves and others in the world, we start to have a little moment of choice. We start to notice a choice-point, a moment in which we can "stand behind" our grasping and aversion—believing it, endorsing it, and acting from it—or see through it and instead choose an action that has a potential to be useful, skillful, and kind.

The Subtleties and Complexities of Practicing Acceptance on and off the Cushion

Although zazen and the practice of acceptance can seem simple, the experience of turning toward, noticing, and allowing our experience raises endless complexities. Below, we highlight CBT-resonant Zen practices that address these subtleties and challenges.

"Inviting Demons"—The Mess of Being Human

Naming has, in many cultures, actually been a magical power: the power of naming demons gives you power over those demons. In our daily lives on and off the cushion, demons are these struggles that we continually come up against. Many of them become quite familiar to us, easily recognizable: the demon of inadequacy, the demon of fear, the demon of black mood, the demon who tells me I'm an imposter. One way we can work with the arising of these demons is to name them and welcome them—remember and receive them—inviting them to join us and keep us company as we engage in our valued action. "Here's the demon of anxiety—glad you could make it. Right now we're sitting zazen. There's a spot for you right here." "Ah, here's my old friend—the demon of not-good-enough. Welcome. Right now we're writing a chapter."

Inviting is a form of acceptance. Awareness and naming, combined with inviting, is a powerful practice. Sometimes, the demon who drops by is the one who screams: *No! I will not welcome a demon!* And we can welcome *that* demon, the demon of unwillingness, as well. This is welcoming not-welcoming: "Ah, my old friend non-acceptance has dropped by. Welcome." Any problematic moment, any piece of what's arising, including aversion, including avoidance, is our demon in that moment—and every moment can be invited in. Any moment in which we stop pushing, we experience a release. Even allowing unwillingness is an allowing, a dropping the rope of the struggle.

Zazen allows us to start to really see and become intimately familiar with our experience. There is a liberating value in being able to say to ourselves, "Oh right! This thing where it feels like *this*, this is anxiety." "Oh right, this is the thing where my thoughts just continue to do *this thing*. It's anxiety." Eventually, we become able to say, "Ah yes, this is anxiety." When we're able to do that, we also have the possibility of remembering that that anxiety, that struggle, is honestly come by. That in itself actually begins to open up a kind of space and a kind of possibility.

In a way, this practice of noticing and naming demons, and thereby diminishing their power, has its roots in the Pali canon, the oldest of the Buddhist scriptures: When Shakyamuni Buddha sat down under a tree and resolved to not get up until he penetrated through the root of suffering, he met the King of All Demon's, Mara. Mara is the personification of all suffering-causing energy; he is also known as Mara the Deceiver. As Shakyamuni sat in meditation, Mara took the form of a charging elephant, trying to frighten the Buddha away from his seat. And the Buddha saw the demon and said, "I see you, Mara." And the scriptures say, charmingly, that "sad and disappointed" Mara disappears. Then, Mara comes back as a huge snake, a hail of boulders, sensually provocative dancers, and an old man challenging the Buddha's integrity. Each time, Buddha recognizes and names the demon—"I see you, Mara"—and each time, "sad and disappointed," Mara disappears.

A Zen Catechism of Impermanence

Everything changes—this is the teaching of impermanence, a cornerstone of Buddhist teaching. Connecting to this reality can be tremendously helpful in times of distress—severe anxiety, catastrophic thinking, overwhelmedness, black depressions. One way that I (JB) have found helpful is with the following script, which I have come to think of as a kind of catechism of impermanence.

My answers to myself appear in parentheses:

Beginning state: I feel devastatedly terrible, utterly overwhelmed with anxiety and fear, or in black pit of depression.

- *Is the first time I have felt this way? (No.)*
- *Was it permanent last time? (No—but this time it definitely feels permanent, so it is surely different.)*
- *Is the first time I have been sure* this time *is different? (No.)*
- *Was it permanent when I felt that way before? (No—but this one may be The Big One.)*
- *Is this the first time I have thought* that*?...*

This catechism can be applied with infinite recursion—yet ultimately what using this practice does is enlarge our capacity to be patiently present to what is. The value of it is twofold: (1) it grounds us in the truth of impermanence *as seen in our own direct experience*; and (2) it can allow us access to more patience, more courage, and a greater ability to entrust ourselves to what is—in short, to practice acceptance. At some point we stop recursing, and we have to practice acceptance of the fact that although there is absolutely no precedent whatsoever in our experience or in history of the universe, *this might actually be The Big One, The One That Is Permanent.*

In this practice, ultimately we *do* in fact have to accept at least provisionally that our current state might be permanent, and that is of course difficult and scary—but this catechism can enhance our ability to patiently and unpanickingly be present with the pain and fear that that provisional acceptance may bring with it. Moreover, provisional acceptance of something that our own experience shows has absolutely no precedence of being true is much easier than trying to force ourselves to *deny* something that, from the perspective of being caught in the web of our own delusive certainty, we are absolutely sure is Definitely True. And having cultivated, through Zen practice, a capacity to be present to not-knowing, having befriended uncertainty, is of great value here too.

This catechism allows us to call ourselves to this moment, to call ourselves to notice our stories of delusive certainty—to notice our predictions of a certain and permanent future, to notice our stories simply as stories. This is the practice of waking up, this is the practice of not being deceived by Mara, even when he arises inside our own thoughts.

Accepting suffering diminishes suffering—but it must be genuine, complete, acceptance, which is itself a form of surrendering to the moment. To access the full power of acceptance, Hongzhi Zhengjue (an influential twelfth-century Chinese Zen master; Leighton 2000, p. 36) writes that we must "straightforwardly abandon strategems"—that is to say we must directly give up all our attempts to fix and all our techniques for improvement. If we accept suffering *instrumentally,* in order to, in this moment, make suffering go away—this is not genuine acceptance, but rather is aversion masquerading as acceptance. That never works to diminish suffering—and ultimately functions to maintain it. Hongzhi holds up the alternative to such instrumental acceptance: we must "contact phenomena with total sincerity, not a single atom of dust outside yourself."

In the context of this catechism, true acceptance involves accepting that, universal truth of impermanence notwithstanding, there is the possibility that this suffering *might be permanent* —we have to accept that wholly and fully. And when we do that, then we open up space for change—but we cannot actually skip the step of really, fully, unconditionally accepting, including unconditionally accepting even our inability to unconditionally accept.

This truth—that acceptance can, and often does, reduce suffering, and yet if we do it for that purpose, it is likely to backfire—is particularly challenging within behavioral health contexts. In those contexts, clients seek treatment expressly to reduce their suffering—they want strategies that will reduce their anxiety, promote relaxation, reduce their worry, or improve their mood—and indeed, we do know that mindfulness- and acceptance-based strategies can, in fact, help with all of this. And yet, to some extent, we also know that the more we do not want some experience, the more we have it. In such contexts, being explicit about this paradox is helpful. We might tell clients that we do know that being aware, in the moment, and allowing what arises to arise often does, in time, lead to distress not lingering quite as long and perhaps not being as intense—and we know it does not always have this effect, particularly immediately. Also, we might tell that them, that the diminution of suffering really only happens when we are open to what is actually happening for us in the moment, and not attached to an outcome of reducing distress immediately. Usually clients have their own experiences of this truth to draw from, so this information is validating—even if somewhat disappointing because people naturally want to reduce their distress reliably and instantly. At such times, we might communicate to clients that if they respond differently to their internal experiences, they can have much more agency and choice in what they actually do in their lives. This is where the more reliable capacity for change lies.

Accepting Our Unwillingness to Accept

Sometimes acceptance of some element of our experience seems (or in fact is) impossible. Again, zazen is the practice of unhooking from our preferences, our stories of certainty about what we need, what want, what we cannot stand. One translation of the beginning of "Trust in Mind" is, "The Great Way is not difficult for those who do not pick and choose"… and we can well imagine that this might be so for such people—but what about for those who *do* pick and choose, how can we engage the Great Way? We may find ourselves grasping at being someone who does not pick and choose, or telling ourselves stories about how we are causing our own suffering.

Similarly, the American Soto Zen teacher Reb Anderson (2005, p. 12) says, "Zazen does not prefer success to failure, or enlightenment to delusion. If we are enlightened, we sit still in the middle of enlightenment with no preference for it. If we are deluded, we sit still in the middle of delusion with no aversion to it." This seems to be quite a tall order! What about when we do have preferences for enlightenment, or for feelings of calmness and spaciousness and clarity? And what about when we are sitting with aversion to our anxiety, our agitation, our physical, emotional, or psychic pain?

In fact, there is a beautiful quality of recursion to the practice of Zen, one that is always accessible—and one that honors the fact that ultimately, we cannot control or otherwise suppress the natural, human, inevitable arising of preferences, of picking and choosing. If we cannot control the arising of aversion (which we could call A_1), we can practice acceptance in the presence of that aversion rather than continuing to mentally reinforce our aversion with another form of aversion (A_2); we can practice acceptance of the arising of preferences (P_1), rather than continuing to cultivate preferences (P_2) for our preferences. And if we cannot do that, if we have aversion to our aversion to our aversion (A_3), we can practice acceptance of our aversion to our aversion to our aversion, rather than endorsing A_4. And the really remarkable thing is that acceptance breaks the cycle wherever it is practiced; peeling back one layer of the onion is actually the whole of the endeavor. It truly does not matter whether we accept A_1, A_2, or $A_{1,000,007}$. Ultimately, accepting $A_{1,000,007}$ rather than endorsing it and moving on to $A_{1,000,008}$ is the essence of the practice. In Zen, each iteration is called a "mind-moment"—and each mind-moment, though also different, is always the same. We always work with *exactly just this*. *Just this* is It.

Letting Be Versus Letting Go

There is a way that the language of "let go" has permeated into Buddhist discourse, popular psychology, and the self-help literature—though this language is sometime useful, and we may even occasionally use it ourselves, it is also problematic. Telling ourselves or another to "let go" can so easily become another way of trying to get our experience to go away, to be other than it is. More useful language is *letting be*. Here is an image for the difference: imagine whatever experience we are having that we are supposed to be letting go of as a butterfly in our closed hands. Letting go suggests we are trying to get the butterfly to *go away now—begone!* Letting be, the fundamental gesture of acceptance, is actually a much more spacious practice. Letting be is opening our hands and letting the butterfly stay as long as it stays, and leave when it leaves.

In this way, zazen is described as "opening the hand of thought" (Uchiyama 2004). Zazen is not about removing thoughts or experiences from us, and it is not about trying to have or keep some specific experience or state of mind.

Modern Soto Zen teacher Okumura (2010, p. 64) uses the language of "letting go" in a way that fully evokes the aspect of *letting be:* "Letting go is on the one hand the complete rejection of any thought based on our limited karmic experiences. Yet, on the other hand, letting go is the acceptance of all thoughts as mere secretions of the mind…We just let thoughts come up, and we just let them go away. We neither negate nor affirm anything in zazen."

Zazen is the practice of letting come all that comes, letting be all that is, and letting go all that goes.

Other Zen Principles and Practices that Cultivate Acceptance

In this section, we will provide a brief overview of a few other aspects of Zen practice that inform our understanding of how people can cultivate a complex, multifaceted experience of acceptance that allows them to engage meaningfully in their lives even in the face of inevitable pain, suffering, and discomfort.

Understanding the Karma of Suffering

The word *karma* essentially points to actions-and-their-consequences, all of which is conditioned by causes and conditions. In the realm of psychology, this is a person's learning history. Let us consider the example of the arising of fear.

There are a lot of good reasons for fear to develop—fear is an adaptive response. In our personal learning history, our personal karma, we may have had challenging experiences in the past that taught us some circumstances are dangerous. With regard to our familial karma, we may have seen fear modeled and taught within our family —and similar dynamics take place on a societal scale as well, cultural karma. And then, there is our evolutionary karma: as a species we are hard-wired to enact fear as a survival response. This is the karma that we have inherited and it can be helpful to acknowledge it because doing so gives rise to a little bit of space for compassion for ourselves when fear arises.

With this perspective, when we notice anxiety arising for us, we may have a feeling of "Why is this happening?" One aspect of the Zen perspective is simply this: the answer to *why* is always going to be "because of causes and conditions." It is not actually essential to identify *which* causes and conditions—and ultimately that is impossible anyhow, because there are infinite vectors of causes and conditions impinging on this moment, and the sum total of them give rise to my experience of fear—to this moment, just as it is. Though not specific, in some obvious sense, recalling that things arise because of causes and conditions is nonetheless psychologically valuable. This perspective allows us to appreciate that all of our difficulty, all of our fear, all of this karma, is honestly come by—it is not an indication of brokenness; it is not an indication of moral or spiritual failure; it is not an indication of weakness. It is simply the universe of causes and conditions arising *thus*, arising right here in this form. This in turn allows our relation to our internal experience to shift from, "Why, why am I like this? What is wrong with me?" to simply, "Ah, yes. This is what's here and now."

Fear is in a certain way indelible. Part of what that means is that we are unlikely to become a person for whom fear does not arise—because that is actually the karma of millennia and hundreds and thousands of years as a species. So it is important to distinguish between fear arising ("Ah yes, here's some fear") and fear taking control of our actions and putting us on automatic pilot of choiceless action. As we have said above, fear is one psychological term for a part of what the dharma calls aversion. "That thing over there I need it to go away, I need to avoid that, I need to avoid this." All of this *pushing away* is one of the main modes through which we create internal suffering for ourselves—and that impulse to push away, that impulse to turn away to run away to avoid, is honestly come by. It is part of the machinery of being human, of having a family, of having hearts and minds and relationships. This is what it means to be an actual human being. And all of this practice from the psychological perspective, from the Zen perspective, is about helping us fully unfold into the full being of humanness with compassion and awareness and a capacity to move toward what matters to us.

Within Zen practice, the principle of karma is taught in dharma talks, and then is clarified in zazen practice, and in life, as causes and consequences are observed, again and again. "Ah, this thought that I'm not good enough is followed, again, by the urge to find faults in others." "That knot in my stomach arises after thoughts of my family." Behavioral health practice may use psychoeducation as a way to introduce causes and conditions. Various awareness practices (formal mindfulness practices, informal practices, self-monitoring) can promote observation of these patterns, and cultivate self-and other-compassion for the way these patterns unfold so quickly.

Zen Liturgy that Cultivates/Embodies Acceptance

In the Boundless Way Zen tradition, we recite a teaching called the Five Remembrances at the beginning of our liturgical service. That recitation goes like this:

> I am of the nature to grow old; there is no way to escape growing old.
> I am of the nature to have ill health; there is no way to escape having ill health.
> I am of the nature to die; there is no way to escape death.
> All that is dear to me and everyone I love are of the nature of change; there is no way to escape being separated from them.
> My deeds are my closest companions. I am the beneficiary of my deeds; my deeds are the ground on which I stand.

Part of the value of this practice is that it functions, in a way, to help us "pre-accept" these conditions in advance of their coming to the fore in our lives. This practice is a countercultural foregrounding of the realities of old age, sickness, death, loss, and change—and responsibility. The value of this practice of pre-accepting is that when these circumstances do materialize for us, rather than being shocked by their arising or seeing their presence as, somehow, a defect in the universe or ourselves, we are able to recall that these things are in fact part of our very nature. The power of practicing *turning toward* rather than turning away from these elements of human existence helps diminish our suffering when these circumstances inevitably arise.

This points to something important about the power, value, and aim of Zen practice as distinct from the approaches taken in certain forms of psychotherapy: Zen does not aim to *fix* problems but to change our relationship to them—and to examine that "problems" may not be quite what we always imagined them to be. We are not trying to be liberated *from* our life but liberated *into* it. Rather than seeking freedom *from* suffering, we cultivate a perspective that allows to find freedom *amid* suffering—right in the center of it.

Dogen points to life that includes death rather than a life that is somehow free of it or negated by it. He says "this birth and death is the life of Buddha, if you try to exclude it, you will lose the life of Buddha, if you try to cling to it in me or in you, trying to remain in it, you will also lose the life of Buddha." (Tanahashi 1985, p. 75).

Another element of Zen liturgical practice that has a direct relationship with acceptance is the practice of *atonement*. In my tradition, each period of liturgy includes the Gatha of Atonement (a *gatha* is a short verse to be used as a point of practice). The Gatha of Atonement goes like this:

> All evil karma ever committed by me since of old,
> Because of my beginningless greed, anger, and ignorance,
> Born of my body, mouth, and thought,
> Now I atone for it all.

For our purposes, here we can hear the word *evil* as a synonym for "suffering-engendering" or "harm-causing." We say "beginningless" to acknowledge the vast web of causes and conditions that extends infinitely far into the past—this refers to our karma and karmic conditioning, our personal, familial, cultural, and evolutionary learning history, all of which is manifest in this moment. "Greed, anger, and ignorance" points to the three fundamental energies of mind—collectively known as the *three poisons*—that, according to the Dharma tradition, are ultimately at the root of all harm-causing, all suffering-causing. Those three energies can also be translated and usefully thought of as the energies of grasping, aversion, and delusive certainty—the mind gets trapped in stories and takes its stories as truth.

In the Mahayana tradition of which Zen is part, we do not hold as a goal somehow purifying ourselves into a permanent state in which grasping, aversion, and delusion do not arise; we acknowledge that their arising is, in fact, part of what it means to be human. What is essential, however, is being able to see such arisings, and work with them—to take choiceful, values-consistent actions even amid their arisings. And yet, even so, sometimes we fail—sometimes our automatic, conditioned, reactive minds get triggered and we cause harm, we create suffering with our body, mouth, or mind—our actions, words, or thoughts. Because this is an inevitable part of being human, it is of utmost importance that we be able to find our ways back to the possibility of reorienting to our values, aspirations, and intentions and starting in this moment afresh. This is the practice of *atonement*, sometimes referred to by the more Christian-sounding term *repentance*.

Etymologically, the word *atonement* is "at-one-*ment*"—and thus to *atone* means to be "at one with" this moment, the whole big mess of ourselves-and-the-universe. Atonement is fundamentally a practice of acceptance, acceptance of the consequences and impact of our actions, acceptance of ourselves as an imperfect human being who sometimes causes harm to ourselves or others. Accepting ourselves as imperfect, as having caused harm, we are then able to reorient ourselves to our values, and do what is within our limited power to redress the situation.

While atonement may seem to be more in the domain of spiritual than behavioral health contexts, the concept of human imperfection and the inevitability of causing harm has ramifications in the behavioral health spheres as well. Recognition that the continual repetition of habits makes it challenging to develop new habits, so that we will inevitably *lapse* into old behavior patterns is an essential part of avoiding *relapse* into ongoing patterns we are trying to change (Marlatt and Donovan 2005). Understanding and having compassion for ourselves as these lapses occur, coupled with awareness of how the patterns evolved so that we can try to change them in the future, helps with long-term change. Also, guilt and self-blame often interferes with our ability to face situations when we have harmed others; acceptance and atonement can free us up to find corrective actions on an interpersonal level (e.g., making amends with a loved one) and a societal one (e.g., taking action for social justice in response to recognizing our own experiences of privilege and unearned advantage).

The Liberation of Vulnerability

In a certain sense, many of us come to meditation, to spiritual practice, from some desire to have better and thicker armor that can more effectively keep the world at bay. We want to be better able to withstand and just knock away the arrows of suffering that come so constantly at us. And the first great bait-and-switch of spiritual practice is this: rather than getting thicker more impermeable armor, we find we are called upon to take off even the limited armor we have, to disburden ourselves of the fear-driven need to protect ourselves from the world. This is actually the real, true, and genuinely valuable functioning of liberation—but it is not the thing that, in the beginning, anyone thinks they want. Rather than being more able to reject suffering—to prevent pain and difficulty from arising—Zen offers liberation through expansive acceptance. Unarmored, we have the profound opportunity to see that we can actually *let in* (or let be) even tremendous suffering and be *undestroyed* by it. This opens the possibility of a profound kind of fearlessness that is fully inclusive of the arising of fear. Removing our limited and limiting armor is part of the practice of becoming fully human, fully accepting even our vulnerabilities. And it is precisely these vulnerabilities, our cracked and broke-open heart, that let us connect as humans to other humans—and to ourselves.

In this way, what can feel like our greatest moments of weakness are actually our greatest moments of strength. We may find ourselves unable to hide our cracks, our vulnerabilities anymore—and in that moment we may choose to accept them, receive them, and perhaps even share them. This can be due to great courage, or sometimes just due to not knowing what else to do. And yet, if we pay attention in those moments, we may see that that vulnerability and sharing is actually what helps give our lives meaning—and our doing that can be helpful to other people as well.

My (LR) own experience taught me the truth of this teaching. When I started giving talks on how to help people with anxiety disorders, I experienced tremendous public speaking anxiety. My voice would drop so people had trouble hearing me, and my hand would shake (to this day, I still do not use a laser pointer). I gave talks anyway, because the work we were doing was important to me and I wanted to share it and that was what I was trying to teach. So I started to explicitly model *speaking while anxious*, referring in my talks to my own experiences of anxiety in front of rooms of strangers who could see how anxious I was. I did not do this because I was brave or courageous. I literally did not know what else to do because I could not make the anxiety go away, and I did not want to not give the talk. And then, I discovered something surprising—people really responded to the vulnerability I shared. They told me that it made them feel they could share their perspectives with groups of people, or go out on dates, or do whatever they feared, even if their voices trembled or their thinking was not as clear as they wished. And I experienced more meaning and satisfaction in what I was doing than I had imagined possible. I used to wish I was like those people who either do not experience anxiety when speaking or do not show it the way I do—now I'm grateful for being exactly the way I am because of the connectedness to others being this way has brought to me.

We can only practice as ourselves. We can only meet this moment with the self (or the self-and-the-universe) we in fact have—not the one we would have if only everything were different: if only we had more sleep, if only we had a different family, if only we had a better set of reactions, if only we had more tools, or if only we had some other culture, society, and planet. We must accept the constraints of circumstances to be free of them. Zazen holds out the possibility of absolute freedom—and this includes the freedom to fail when we fail, to struggle when we struggle, and to die when we die. Complete freedom includes the freedom to be bound when we are bound.

This practice releases us into this life of ourselves-and-the-universe-together, into this life not of just joy or just pain but of joy-and-pain; into this existence not of just life or just death but of life-and-death; into this life not just of self but of self-and-universe-arising-together.

And this is indeed something of consequence.

References

Anderson, R. (2005). *Warm smiles from cold mountains: Dharma talks on Zen meditation*. San Francisco, CA: San Francisco Zen Center.

A-Tjak, J. G. L., Davis, M. L., Morina, N., Powers, M. B., Smits, J. A. J., & Emmelkamp, P. M. G. (2015). A meta-analysis of the efficacy of acceptance and commitment therapy for clinically relevant mental and physical health problems. *Psychotherapy and Psychosomatics, 84*, 30–36.

Bartok, J. (Ed.). (2015). *Boundless Way Zen Sutra book* (3rd ed.). Worcester, MA: Boundless Way Zen.

Bayda, E., & Bartok, J. (2005). *Saying yes to life (Even the hard parts)*. Somerville, MA: Wisdom Publications.

Brown, K. W., & Ryan, R. M. (2004). Perils and promise in defining and measuring mindfulness: Observations from experience. *Clinical Psychology: Science & Practice, 11,* 242–248.

Cordova, J. V. (2001). Acceptance in behavior therapy: Understanding the process of change. *The Behavior Analyst, 24,* 213–226.

Gotink, R. A., Chu, P., Busschbach, J. J. V., Benson, H., Fricchione, G. L., & Myriam Hunink, M. G. M. (2015). Standardised mindfulness-based interventions in healthcare—An overview systematic reviews and meta-analyses of RCTs. *PLoS ONE, 10,* 1–17.

Hayes, S. C., & Pankey, J. (2003). Psychological acceptance. In W. T. O'Donohue, J. E. Fisher, & S. C. Hayes (Eds.), *Empirically supported techniques of cognitive behavior therapy: A step by step guide for clinicians*. New York: Wiley.

Hayes, S. C., Strosahl, K. D., & Wilson, K. G. (2011). *Acceptance and commitment therapy, 2nd edition: The process and practice of mindful change.* New York: The Guilford Press.

Kabat-Zinn, J. (1994). *Wherever you go, there you are: Mindfulness meditation in everyday life.* New York: Hyperion.

Kabat-Zinn, J. (2013). *Full Catastrophe Living (Revised Edition): Using the wisdom of your body and mind to face stress, pain, and illness.* New York: Bantam Books.

Leighton, T. D. (2000). *Cultivating the empty field: The silent illumination of Zen master Hongzhi.* Clarendon, VT: Tuttle Publishing.

Leighton, T. D. (2011). *The Wholehearted Way: A translation of Eihei Dogen's Bendowa, with commentary by Kosho Uchiyama Roshi.* Clarendon, VT: Tuttle Publishing.

Linehan, M. M. (1993). *Cognitive-behavioral treatment of borderline personality disorder.* New York: The Guilford Press.

Manuel, Z. E. (2015). *The way of tenderness: Awakening through race, sexuality and gender.* Somerville, MA: Wisdom Publications.

Marlatt, G. A., & Donovan, D. M. (2005). *Relapse prevention: Maintenance strategies in the treatment of addictive behaviors.* New York: Guilford Press.

Masunaga, R. (1958). *The Soto approach to Zen.* Tokyo: Layman Buddhist Society Press.

Okumura, S. (2010). *Realizing Genjokoan: The key to Dogen's Shobogenzo.* Somerville, MA: Wisdom Publications.

Roemer, L., & Orsillo, S. M. (2009). *Mindfulness and acceptance-based behavioral therapies in practice.* New York: The Guilford Press.

Rogers, C. R. (1961). *On becoming a person: A therapist's view of psychotherapy.* Boston: Houghton Mifflin.

Segal, Z. V., Williams, J. M. G., & Teasdale, J. D. (2013). *Mindfulness-based cognitive therapy for depression* (2nd ed.). New York: The Guilford Press.

Shapiro, S. L., & Carlson, L. E. (2009). *The art and science of mindfulness: Integrating mindfulness into psychology and the helping professions.* Washington, DC: American Psychological Association.

Soeng, M. (2004). *Trust in mind: The rebellion of Chinese Zen.* Somerville, MA: Wisdom Publications.

Tanahashi, K. (1985). *Moon in a dewdrop: Writings of Zen master Dogen.* New York: North Point Press.

Tollifson, J. (2012). *Nothing to grasp.* Salisbury, UK: Nonduality Press.

Uchiyama, K. (2004). *Opening the hand of thought: Foundations of Zen Buddhist practice.* Somerville, MA: Wisdom Publications.

Williams, A. K. (2002). *Being Black: Zen and the art of living with fearlessness and grace.* New York: Penguin Books.

Brief Thoughts on Zen and Behavior Therapy

Marsha Linehan and Kayla Sargent

Keywords
Zen · Religion · Buddhism · Behavior therapy · Behavioral health

As a girl who was raised in the heart of Catholicism, it is hard to believe that my journey led me into the development of behavior therapies that incorporate Zen and mindfulness as a core component of treatment. Even more surprising is that I went on to become an actual Zen master (e.g., a Roshi) who is simultaneously a dyed-in-the-wool behavior therapist. I am certain now that the Catholic priest who was my spiritual director when I was a graduate student at a Catholic University many years ago would faint if he knew this. Although these identities appear upon first glance to be mutually exclusive—Zen versus Catholic or Behaviorist versus Roshi—the two Zen teachers that have guided me most in Zen were, in fact, Catholic priests. When I first became a Zen teacher, many of my students struggled with the perceived distinctions they had internalized about these "conflicting" identities, but as you can see, they can coexist. In this chapter, I will paint a picture of Zen and Behavior therapy and present what I see as two processes with much in common. Although differences are also present, my hope is that after reading this chapter you will gain and understanding of the similarities between Zen and Behavior Therapy.

People who are raised and socialized in what we consider Western countries tend to see Eastern practices within the framework of their own cultures. Thus, it is common for Zen to be referred to as a religion. Zen is not a religion; instead, it is a practice, one that includes individuals with a wide range of spiritual practices from atheism to Islam. To put it in the words of my teacher Willigis Jaeger:

> Zen is Zen and will always be Zen, irrespective of whether it is taught and practiced in the East or the West. The core of Zen is always the same, aimed at experiencing reality as it is. To do this, Zen points to an inner experiential existence transcending our rational capabilities.

The aim of Zen is for the individual to experience what is called *Satori*, a difficult concept to articulate in translation. In essence, satori is a Japanese term for awakening to awareness of one's own comprehension and understanding of one's own true nature. It is also known as *kenshō*

Edited by Kayla Sargent

M. Linehan (✉)
University of Washington, Seattle, USA
e-mail: linehan@uw.edu; efranks@uw.edu

K. Sargent
University of Hawaii at Manoa, Honolulu, USA
e-mail: kaylansargent@gmail.com

A. Masuda and W.T. O'Donohue (eds.), *Handbook of Zen, Mindfulness, and Behavioral Health*, Mindfulness in Behavioral Health, DOI 10.1007/978-3-319-54595-0_19

(*ken* meaning "seeing" and *shō* meaning "essence"), which is derived from the Japanese verb *satoru* which means "to know or understand." In the Zen Buddhist tradition, satori refers to the experience of *kenshō*, the experience of seeing into one's true nature or true essence. The experience is similar to what could be described as a mystical experience in a Christian practice. Both radiate an experience of oneness that almost always leads to an experience of ecstatic joy. It is important to recognize that such experiences are experienced by people with a variety of spiritual beliefs and practices; many are not practicing Zen or on a specific spiritual path at all. Of the clients in my own skills training program, over half endorse having had at least one experience of "oneness." I respond to my clients who endorse these experiences with wonder, charging them to hold the experiences closely. Without a teacher to help us understand the importance of such events, it can be difficult to keep them in mind.

Behavior Therapy, on the other hand, is a process rooted in empiricism. The focus of behaviorism is on reducing problematic behavioral patterns by observing and changing factors that are immediately present. These current factors are ones that cause and maintain problematic behaviors. In addressing current patterns, it is possible to teach new, more functional, or more helpful behaviors. Behavior from a behavioral perspective is defined as anything that changes, including thoughts, feelings, or actions. Behavior itself includes a range of actions and mannerisms made by individuals (including organisms, systems, or artificial entities) in conjunction with themselves or their environment (including other systems, organisms, and physical environments). Behavior is a response to various stimuli: internal or external, conscious or unconscious, overt or covert, voluntary or involuntary. In this sense, Zen and Behaviorism have the common goal of understanding and living in the present moment, of having a firm grasp upon reality.

Zen teachers and behavior therapists both have regular individual meetings with their students and clients. When done well, both have the capacity to bring about positive therapeutic outcomes, although the two differ in that the goal of Behavior Therapy is to create these positive outcomes, whereas no such goal exists in Zen. The focus of these meetings is another difference between the two. In Zen, the teacher listens and talks with students about their Zen practice, giving advice on how to solve problems they are having in their practice, offering acceptance, and encouraging them to persist in their practice. The teacher's aim is to help the student stay in his or her Zen practice instead of getting stuck in their current patterns of behavior. In contrast to Behavior Therapy, where the goal is to reduce symptoms of mental disorders, the goal of Zen is to help the student experience their ultimate reality, all things as one.

Both Zen and behavior therapy focus on the present. From a Zen perspective, the present is all there is. Zen meditation practice, zazen, which makes up much of Zen practice is a silent focus on the present moment. Behavior therapists also focus on client's current difficulties and goals. They may conduct a clinical analysis of the present and the past to determine the variables that control the problem behaviors, but ultimately these efforts contribute directly to their understanding of the present factors that are maintaining a specified problem. Their work, after this analysis has been conducted, is to help the client change the causal factors maintaining problem behaviors in the present. Behavioral change, ultimately, can only happen in the service of present moment awareness.

Although Zen and behaviorists have different ways of talking about the self, both recognize a sense of "no self" or a sense of the self as a matter of perspective. That is, from a Zen perspective there is no independent self because all is one. The belief in an independent self is viewed as a delusion that all humans carry with them. Zen practice is aimed at experiencing the wonder of the oneness of all beings. Behavior therapists also do not hold on to an idea of an independent "self" within the individual that influences action. Although the role of genes is not discounted, Behaviorist is more likely to focus on learning experiences and environmental events, no matter how small or large. Individuals, as well as their behaviors, are seen as products of contexts, relationships, and environments; thus, an individual can never actually be seen as a separate entity. In this sense, Zen and behavior therapy both recognize unity. As noted above, the focus of Zen is on experiencing the unity of all things. Similarly, behaviorists view behavior and context as connected and behavior cannot be understood outside of its context. In other words, there is always a unity between context and behavior.

At the same time, both practices have a way of honoring and respecting individual preferences and personalities. That is, the sense of "no self" does not extend to imply that all people are inherently the same; on the contrary, people, systems, and the cultures they grow out of are diverse *and* interconnected. Both Zen and Behavior therapy maintain these individual, diverse threads. Both the Zen teacher and the behavior therapist tailor what they say and do to the unique needs of the individual person they are working with.

Nonjudgment is a core theme of Zen and Behavior Therapy. Although Zen does have a set of precepts that guide a Zen students' moral behavior, the concepts of "good" versus "bad" are not present. As my Zen teacher, (Do you know his/her name? insert here), used to say, "Shit and gold are the same. They are one." From a Zen perspective, "good" and "bad" are in the minds of the observers and are incompatible with oneness. From a behavioral perspective, all behavior is caused and therefore all behavior should be as it is given the causes. Changing behavior requires changing causes. Both Zen teachers and Behavior therapists offer corrective feedback while also interacting with their students and clients with kindness and compassion.

Practice, or behavioral activation, are integral components of behavioral therapy and Zen. Training in Zen can last for years. Instructions from Zen teachers consistently include the prescription of maintaining a practice of meditation —daily at best—and as often as possible otherwise. Students are also encouraged to attend Zen retreats once a year or as often as possible. In a similar strategy, behavior therapy includes teaching a new behaviors and such behavior includes practice. Both Zen and behavior therapy often focus on practicing new behaviors with a firm footing in the present moment. In many ways, they voice similar prescriptions and proscriptions to those they work with. For example, Robert Aitken Roshi, who founded the Zen Diamond Sangha, in one of his many books on Zen said the following:

> The first truth is that life is suffering. Avoidance of suffering leads to worse stuffing.

Such a sentiment could easily be expressed by any modern behavior therapist, as their work focuses on helping clients face rather than avoid the difficult issues in their lives. Exposure interventions in particular focus on a client's coordinated and careful practice of confronting painful cues in real time while simultaneously blocking avoidance and escape patterns.

Pat Hawk Roshi said to "practice these things, wisdom, compassion, freedom as if you already have," and Bob Aitken Roshi said to "act as if you always had compassion, and then you will find you always did." Although the belief that behaviors exist within us inherently is a Zen sentiment, the idea itself of practicing as if you can engage in effective behaviors could easily be suggested by a behavior therapist; this emphasis on altering cognitive self-statements is foundational to modern therapeutic techniques.

Zen practitioners and Behavior therapists arrived at a similar view of reality by similar paths based on validation of observations, or, mindful present moment awareness. Behavior therapy endorses treatments that have been scientifically found to be effective, and how is this achieved? Treatments have to be validated by clinical trials where outcomes are observed and evaluated by groups of scientists. Similarly, Zen is a practice where the experience of students must be verified by a Zen master. A Zen student who becomes a Zen teacher is also an outcome of observations over years by senior Zen masters. In fact, the average Zen student, at some point, is sent by his or her teacher to another teacher for confirmation of their experience and competency to teach.

Among these similarities between Behavior Therapy and Zen, differences also exist. The primary difference is that behavior therapy focuses on what can be observed through the senses, and Zen focuses on what can be observed in the center of one's self. Basically, Zen as a practice rooted in spirituality (not to be confused with religion), proposes that there is more than can be observed through the senses. From that perspective, Zen is in line with mystical traditions whereas behavior therapy is in line with science. The two coexist nicely when one remembers what many astronomers have posited: scientists who the study the universe ultimately become mystics themselves.

Zen, Mindfulness, and Cognitive-Behavior Therapy

Holly Hazlett-Stevens

Keywords
Zen · Mindfulness · Cognitive-Behavior therapy · Behavioral health · Buddhism

Introduction

Approximately 2600 years ago, a young prince named Siddhartha Gautama left his luxurious life to wander the Indian subcontinent in search of freedom from mental suffering. After six years of intensive practice in various meditation traditions, he discovered the clarity of mind he originally sought, became known as the Buddha ("the awakened one"), and spent the rest of his life teaching his methods to others (see Smith and Novak 2003). After his death, his teachings spread throughout Asia, divided into three prominent traditions (Theravada, Mahayana, and Vajrayana) and accumulated a wide variety of religious rituals, ceremonies, and cultural trappings.

However, the Buddha also might be considered a brilliant early psychologist, whose observations about the nature of the human condition and the workings of the human mind are consistent with modern scientific research findings and effective clinical interventions later developed in the West. As His Holiness the Dalai Lama once said, "Buddhist teachings are not a religion, they are a science of mind" (Kornfield 2008, p. xi). In the early 1900s, American psychologist William James famously stopped his lecture at Harvard when he recognized an Asian Buddhist monk in the audience, saying "Take my chair. You are better equipped to lecture on psychology than I. This is the psychology everybody will be studying twenty-five years from now." (Epstein 1995, pp. 1–2). Likewise, former Buddhist monk and American psychologist Jack Kornfield considers Buddhists the first cognitive-behavior therapists (Kornfield 2008). From his perspective, both Buddhism and cognitive-behavior therapy (CBT) have identified how automatic patterns of thought outside of awareness can lead to maladaptive emotion and behavior. Furthermore, both approaches teach methods designed to increase present-moment awareness of thoughts for the purpose of challenging underlying assumptions and beliefs, resulting in more skillful behavior. Thus, authorities from both Buddhist and Western psychological backgrounds have long acknowledged

H. Hazlett-Stevens (✉)
University of Nevada, Reno, USA
e-mail: hhazlett@unr.edu

A. Masuda and W.T. O'Donohue (eds.), *Handbook of Zen, Mindfulness, and Behavioral Health*, Mindfulness in Behavioral Health, DOI 10.1007/978-3-319-54595-0_20

the value of Buddhist insights to alleviate human mental suffering.

In the twentieth century, Buddhism spread to the Western Hemisphere. Although Theravada Buddhism already was under study in Great Britain, Buddhism first came to America in the form of Zen—a form stemming from the Mahayana sect—when American Buddhist enthusiast Paul Carus brought Japanese Zen Master D.T. Suzuki to America to translate classic texts (Smith and Novak 2003). By the 1970s, Theravada Buddhist practices known as *vipassana*—a meditation approach practiced to increase insight into the nature of the mind and reality directly—also arrived in the USA. In 1979, Indian vipassana teacher S.N. Goenka began teaching abroad, leading to the development of retreat centers across America. In addition, Americans including Joseph Goldstein, Jack Kornfield, and Sharon Salzberg returned from extensive monastery practice in Southeast Asia (including India, Burma, and Thailand), seeking to bring the core teachings of Buddhism to Americans without dividing the teachings into different traditions or sects. Goldstein, Kornfield, Salzberg, and other Buddhist meditation teachers returning from extensive study in Asia founded the Insight Meditation Society (IMS) in 1975. They opened a meditation retreat center in Barre, Massachusetts to teach a vipassana-based method termed *insight meditation* in the local community and to provide intensive meditation instruction within a residential retreat setting.

In 1979, one particular insight meditation practitioner named Jon Kabat-Zinn, a medical researcher with a Ph.D. in molecular biology, brought these teachings and practices into the American medical setting. Kabat-Zinn opened a stress reduction clinic at the University of Massachusetts (UMass) Medical School to teach *mindfulness*, the essence of insight meditation practice, to medical patients suffering from chronic pain and other conditions. Kabat-Zinn later defined mindfulness in the scholarly literature as "the awareness that emerges through paying attention on purpose, in the present moment, and nonjudgmentally to the unfolding of experience moment to moment" (Kabat-Zinn 2003, p. 145). His intensive eight-week curriculum taught the Buddhist meditation practices of the insight meditation tradition, but were free from traditional Buddhist cultural rituals and Asian language terms, deliberately presented in a fashion acceptable to the average American medical patient. Given its emphasis on cultivating mindfulness, the qualities of attention considered essential to Buddhist meditation, this secular stress reduction program eventually became known as "mindfulness-based." Eventually, the clinical benefits of this mindfulness-based stress reduction (MBSR) program and its mindfulness meditation approach became known throughout the UMass Medical School hospital; physicians and other healthcare professionals themselves began to attend the UMass Medical School MBSR program to alleviate their own stress. Early research demonstrating the effectiveness of MBSR from the original UMass stress reduction clinic led to exponential growth, both in terms of implementation and further research. An extensive Campbell Systematic Review (de Vibe et al. 2012) including 26 randomized controlled trials of MBSR (1456 participants) reported post-intervention Hedges' *g* effect sizes of 0.53 for anxiety, 0.54 for depression, and 0.56 for stress/distress. MBSR is listed in the Substance Abuse and Mental Health Services Administration (SAMHSA) National Registry of Evidence-based Programs and Practices (NREPP) as an intervention evaluated in comparative effectiveness research studies, and hundreds of MBSR programs have been implemented in medical settings worldwide.

Since the 1970s, Western psychologists have incorporated Buddhist practices and principles into their clinical work as well. Long-time mindfulness meditation practitioners Phillip Aranow, Christopher Germer, and Ronald Siegel, along with Zen Buddhist Paul Fulton, formed the Institute for Meditation and Psychotherapy (IMP) in the mid-1990s. These American clinical psychologists have led a growing professional discourse about how meditating therapists might best integrate mindfulness into the practice of psychotherapy. Around this same time, Zen Buddhist and American clinical psychologist

Marsha Linehan drew heavily from traditional Zen mindfulness practices as well as other sources as she developed dialectical behavior therapy (DBT) for chronic self-harm and suicidal behavior (Linehan 1993). In addition, clinical psychologist Alan Marlatt developed a relapse prevention approach for substance use disorders largely informed by his own long-time vipassana meditation experience (Witkiewitz and Marlatt 2004). He and his colleagues also implemented a traditional 10-day silent vipassana meditation retreat intervention into a prison setting within the state of Washington. Compared to an inmate-matched control group, inmates attending the 10-day meditation retreat reported greater improvement on measures of impulse control, drug use, drug abuse severity, and drinking-related locus of control, as well as reduced thought suppression and increased optimism (Marlatt et al. 2004).

During the 1990s, Western clinical psychologists without meditation backgrounds began to take note of this trend, leading to further psychotherapies that teach mindfulness in some form to patients. Many of these psychologists practiced psychotherapy from a cognitive-behavioral perspective and found a natural compatibility between mindfulness meditation principles and cognitive-behavior therapy (CBT). Indeed, CBT is predicated on the notion that emotional distress often stems from distorted mental perceptions as well as cognitive and behavioral habits, all learned under earlier conditions yet no longer serve the individual. Therapy procedures therefore teach patients to identify and then to objectively evaluate their thoughts as they occur, thereby promoting adaptive behavior change.

One leading example of how mindfulness became integrated into CBT is mindfulness-based cognitive therapy for depression (MBCT; Segal et al. 2013) developed by cognitive therapy researchers Zindel Segal, Mark Williams, and John Teasdale. In 1993, they visited Jon Kabat-Zinn's stress reduction clinic and eventually came to practice mindfulness meditation themselves. Over the following several years, they adapted the original MBSR protocol to develop a maintenance form of therapy to prevent future relapse specifically for patients with a history of recurrent major depressive episodes. While much of the curriculum structure and mindfulness meditation practice schedule of MBSR was maintained, MBCT sessions incorporate psychoeducation specific to the nature of depression. For example, didactic material is presented and discussed throughout the curricu lum regarding: (1) how on "automatic pilot," ruminative thought patterns are more likely to lead to depression, (2) the role of negative interpretive bias in emotion, (3) the self-referential nature of thoughts (i.e., most thoughts involve content so close to an individual's sense of self and/or personal values, they are difficult to recognize as mere mental events in the mind), and (4) how mood can influence thoughts and behavior. MBCT participants learn to meet difficult emotions such as sadness with acceptance and practice allowing such unpleasant affective experiences rather than trying to eliminate or to fix them. Subsequent research showed that MBCT significantly reduced the risk of depressive relapse by 35%, with this rate increasing to 44% for patients with three or more past episodes (Piet and Hougaard 2011).

Other adaptations of MBSR emerged in the field as well, including mindfulness-based eating awareness therapy (MB-EAT; Kristeller et al. 2006), mindfulness-based childbirth and parenting (MBCP; Duncan and Bardacke 2010), mindfulness-based relationship enhancement (MBRE; Carson et al. 2004), mindfulness-based therapy for insomnia (MBT-I; Heidenreich et al. 2006), mindfulness-based mind fitness training for military troops, police officers, and firefighters (MMFT; Stanley et al. 2011), and mindful self-compassion (MSC; Neff and Germer 2013). Furthermore, Western psychologists adapted other behavioral and cognitive-behavioral therapies by incorporating mindfulness into existing treatment protocols. For example, Steven Hayes adapted his original behavior therapy acceptance and commitment therapy (ACT; Hayes et al. 1999) by incorporating mindfulness principles into ACT as it developed into its current form (Hayes et al. 2012). Lizabeth Roemer and Susan Orsillo integrated components of CBT with

MBSR, MBCT, DBT, and ACT methods to develop an evidence-based therapy protocol for generalized anxiety and worry (Roemer et al. 2008). As such mindfulness-oriented psychotherapies developed, subsequent research and scholarly articles followed. Indeed, only 365 peer-reviewed articles on mindfulness could be identified using the PsycINFO database in 2005; this number grew to over 2200 by 2013 (Germer 2013). A comprehensive meta-analysis including 209 studies enrolling over 12,000 participants (Khoury et al. 2013) reported moderate effect sizes for mindfulness-based therapies in pre-post comparisons (Hedge's $g = 0.55$), when compared to waitlist controls (Hedge's $g = 0.53$), and when compared with other active treatments (Hedge's $g = 0.33$).

This chapter will explore the common ground between key fundamental Buddhist teachings, mindfulness-based interventions informed by Buddhism, and Western CBT approaches. General Buddhist principles found throughout Buddhism's different sects as well as specific ways of teaching these principles within the Zen tradition will be included. The term "mindfulness meditation" typically is associated with vipassana meditation methods from the Theravada tradition, and "mindfulness-based" secular interventions were largely based on this approach. However, mindfulness is considered essential to all forms of Buddhist meditation, including Zen. Each principle, beginning with mindfulness, will be described first from its Buddhist roots, followed by the discussion of how this principle is presented in mindfulness-based clinical interventions and how it corresponds to CBT theory and procedures. Specific ways that cognitive-behavioral clinicians might integrate Buddhist and Zen principles, including mindfulness, into their CBT practice will be offered. Potential pitfalls that sometimes arise have been identified as well.

Common Principles

MBSR and related mindfulness-based interventions are based directly upon several axioms of Buddhism. Since the 1960s, the Western psychotherapy approach of CBT also has addressed the complex interaction between thoughts, emotional reactions, physical sensations, and behavior, largely independent of Buddhist influences. As this evidence-based orientation to psychotherapy has evolved over the past 50+ years, many CBT observations and practices share a striking similarity with Buddhism. While certainly not exhaustive, the following list reviews core Buddhist principles, how these principles are taught in mindfulness-based interventions, and ways in which they share similar principles and practices of Western CBT.

Mindfulness

The term mindfulness captures the quality of awareness required for effective investigation of first-hand direct experience. The importance of mindfulness to Buddhist practice can be found throughout the different sects of Buddhism. Theravada Buddhist Nyanaponika Thera referred to mindfulness as the "heart" of Buddhist meditation, describing it as a form of "bare attention" and "the clear and single-minded awareness of what actually happens to us and in us, at the successive moments of perception" (1965, p. 30). Thich Nhat Hanh, the well-known Vietnamese Zen Buddhist monk, defined mindfulness as "keeping one's consciousness alive to the present reality" (Hanh 1976, p. 11). Buddhist monk and scholar Bhante Gunaratana described mindfulness as a "special mode of perception" that involves a "special way of seeing life" that contrasts with our usual tendency to "see life through a screen of thoughts and concepts, and we mistake those mental objects for reality" (Gunaratana 1992, p. 37). After reviewing many discussions of mindfulness across Western clinical and Buddhist literatures, Germer (2005) concluded that most definitions of mindfulness contain three basic elements: (1) awareness, (2) of present experience, (3) with acceptance.

The word mindfulness first entered the English language when the word *sati* was translated from Pali, the original language of the Buddha. Buddhist teachings about the qualities of awareness known as sati appear throughout many Buddhist discourse documents, including both the *Anapanasati* and the *Satipatthana Sutras* (Thera 1965). Many Buddhist meditation practices are specifically intended to cultivate *sati* to provide a necessary foundation for subsequent practice. A set of Buddhist teachings known as the *Four Foundations of Mindfulness* guide meditation practitioners to cultivate mindfulness of the body, mindfulness of feelings (pleasant, unpleasant, or neutral), mindfulness of mind (memories and thoughts), and mindfulness of phenomena, including mental reactions to experience and the nature of experiential phenomena itself (Gunaratana 2012).

Jon Kabat-Zinn also acknowledged the importance of mindfulness to meditation, making mindfulness the central focus of his stress reduction program. In both MBSR and MBCT curricula, the teaching of mindfulness begins with the first foundation of mindfulness, mindfulness of the body. Naturally occurring body sensations are experienced directly in formal practice beginning with mindfulness of breathing. Participants also learn to cultivate mindfulness of other sensations in the body in a formal practice known as the body scan, in which attention is systematically directed throughout all areas of the body. During the body scan, participants are instructed to allow themselves simply to feel whatever sensations are present in each area of the body, corresponding to the Buddhist first foundation of mindfulness. After the first week of this formal practice, participants are further encouraged to notice whether sensations are pleasant, unpleasant, or neutral (corresponding to the second foundation of mindfulness), and the mind's habitual reaction to push away unpleasant experience, to try to create or hold onto pleasant experience, and to ignore or become bored with neutral experience. Eventually participants learn to investigate mental states, such as boredom, restlessness, and irritation, as well as thoughts and emotional reactivity that arise during formal practices (corresponding to the third and fourth foundations of mindfulness). Formal sitting meditation instructions expand beyond focus on the breath to a series of other objects of attention, including body sensations, sounds, thoughts, and emotions, and eventually "choiceless awareness," in which the constantly changing flow of experiential phenomena itself is perceived (corresponding to the fourth foundation of mindfulness). In both MBSR and MBCT, the process of thinking is examined in meditation directly and then discussed in group dialogue, revealing the "storytelling" nature of the mind which creates and reifies personal narratives about experience and then confuses these thoughts with reality (Kornfield 2008). In addition to formal meditation practice, formal mindfulness practice assignments promote mindfulness in daily activities and in stressful situations. As participants gain experience in formal meditation and applying mindfulness in daily life, they discover how the interplay of these different types of phenomena can unfold in an ephemeral and impersonal way. As a result, participants become more able to respond deliberately after reflection, even in challenging real-life situations, rather than follow habitual patterns of stress reactivity which are likely to be unskillful and to intensify negative affect and depression.

Although not rooted in Buddhism, CBT relaxation training procedures were developed to calm the body and settle the nervous system with focused attention to direct somatic experience in the body. Consistent with a component of the first foundation of mindfulness in Buddhism known as "calming the bodily function" (Thera 1965, p. 110), Western psychologists also discovered clinical value in directing present-moment attention to felt experience in the body. Diaphragmatic breathing techniques teach patients to focus attention on breathing sensations for the purpose of slowing and deepening the breath, maximizing physical and mental relaxation. Likewise, progressive muscle relaxation methods teach directed attention to sensation in muscle groups as patients learn to discriminate between subtle unnecessary muscle tension and complete muscle relaxation (Hazlett-Stevens 2008). In addition, increased awareness of habitual thought patterns, narratives, and core beliefs is a foundation of cognitive therapy. Standard CBT procedures incorporate self-monitoring of thoughts, feelings, and behaviors in between therapy sessions, so that patients can identify automatic thoughts and respond to such thoughts with skepticism rather than adopting as truth. Therapists work with patients in session further to identify underlying narratives and core beliefs, subjecting long-held cherished beliefs about oneself, the outside world, and the future to the same standards of empirical examination as any other thought. As patients become increasingly aware of habitual thought patterns when they arise, patients become better able to see thoughts are mere conjecture, become less emotionally reactive, and deploy adaptive behavioral responses, all of which can interrupt habitual cycles of thoughts, sensations, emotions, and behavior (Hazlett-Stevens 2008).

Empirical Emphasis

Buddhism including Zen Buddhism has been described as a first-person empirical approach (Wallace 2007), in which the careful and systematic observation of one's own direct experience is valued over any assumptions, beliefs, judgments, or opinions. Others' claims and even Buddhist teachings are not to be taken as truth without careful investigation within one's own awareness. As Zen priest Steve Hagen described, Buddhism is "about examining the world clearly and carefully, about testing everything and every idea" (1997, p. 8). He also repeated a famous Buddhist teaching in which the original Buddha invited his students to test him, saying "Don't believe me because you see me as your teacher. Don't believe me because others do. Don't rely on mere logic, or inference, or appearances, or speculation" (p. 8). Instead, the Buddha encouraged his students to see for themselves what was true, while suspending judgment and criticism in the meantime. Buddhist empiricism is encouraged by the well-known Zen phrase "beginner's mind." As Suzuki-roshi famously exclaimed, "In the beginner's mind there are many possibilities, but in the expert's there are few." (Suzuki 1970, p. 21). The beginner's mind is open to any occurrence, perceiving each experience as if for the first time. In addition to freedom from expectations, the open mind is also free from opinions and judgments. The Third Great Ancestor of Zen in China promoted empiricism in the following way: "If you wish to see the truth then hold no opinions for or against anything. To set up what you like against what you dislike is the disease of the mind." (Goldstein and Kornfield 1987, p. 197).

This same value of first-person empiricism is the cornerstone of mindfulness-based interventions. In the first session of MBSR and MBCT, the instructor passes out raisins and invites each participant to bring an open and curious attention to their immediate and direct sensory experience while slowly eating the raisin. This approach is contrasted with getting caught up in mental reactions and eating the raisin quickly without awareness (Kabat-Zinn 2013). When discussing expectations about the program itself, participants are asked to suspend any beliefs that MBSR will or will not be helpful to them. Although research from third-person observations of Western science has shown MBSR to benefit many people with similar conditions, each person enters the program not knowing if the program indeed will help them personally. Instead, instructors invite participants to treat the next eight weeks as a "personal experiment." Only after dedicated practice and session attendance with an open mind will they be able to determine for themselves whether or not the program helped. This approach, of course, does not prevent instructors or therapists from carefully monitoring week to week progress and providing other clinical services when needed in accordance with clinical standards of care.

When participants share their experiences with the practice in session, instructors are careful to direct inquiry toward what actually happened within the practice, teasing the original direct experience (such as an uncomfortable sensation) apart from any beliefs, judgments, or emotions that arose in reaction. As an example, the instructor might accomplish this by asking a participant reporting pain to describe only what was felt in the body at first: Exactly where in the body was the sensation felt? Where were its boundaries with tissue in which the sensation was not felt? How might the participant describe the sensation of pain in terms of quality: burning, dull, sharp, aching, pulling? Was there any change in intensity, location, or quality of the sensation over time? After such inquiry into the original direct experience of a body sensation, the instructor then might ask about other experiences, including any thoughts or emotions, also noticed in reaction to the physical sensation. As the participant voices any emotions, such as frustration or fear, or any thoughts, such as worrying about future consequences of the pain, the instructor points out how such experiences were mental reactions to the original direct experience of physical sensation.

CBT has been considered an empirical approach to psychotherapy since its inception in the 1960s and 1970s. Cognitive therapy emphasizes cognition as habits of subjective perception —a series of assumptions, beliefs, and expectations, which may closely reflect or grossly distort external reality. Thoughts are viewed as conditioned habits of mind; mere products of the mind that often do not reflect external reality without some degree of misperception, inference, or distortion. However, because thoughts originate within one's own mind, they are typically experienced as compelling truths. CBT therapists therefore educate patients of this nature of thoughts, often using the well-known cognitive therapy adage "a thought is just a thought." Patients are then assigned self-monitoring of thoughts at home, increasing awareness when particularly troublesome thoughts are perceived and responding with cognitive therapy strategies such as examining evidence that counters the underlying belief. Therapy sessions explore the veracity of the mind's claims with direct personal experience as evidence, often leading therapist and patient to construct personal experiments in which the patient can test the assumption as a hypothesis out in the real world. Thus, the therapeutic relationship is described as "collaborative empiricism," in which all thoughts can be examined objectively and tested. CBT also emphasizes the third-person empiricism of Western science, as these therapy approaches and its underlying theory developed from systematic scientific investigation and continue to receive empirical research support.

Emphasis on Direct Experience

Since its beginning, Buddhism has emphasized direct experience as the primary means of knowing. One Buddhist teaching traced back to the original Buddha says, "In seeing there is just what is seen. In hearing there is just what is heard." (Goldstein and Kornfield 1987, p. 191). Zen Buddhism, famous for its use of incomprehensible riddles, paradoxes, and dialogues, exposes the serious limitations of language based in conceptual thought. Instead, practitioners are encouraged to experience reality in its natural non-conceptual way without confusing the experience itself with any words used to describe it, often likened not to mistaking the menu for the meal itself (Smith and Novak 2003). Experienced vipassana insight meditation teacher Phillip Moffitt described how direct experience can deepen with practice according to the *Three Insights*. In the *First Insight*, an existential truth, such as the truth of suffering, is examined critically with discursive thought and understood only as a concept that is generally true in life. In the *Second Insight*, direct personal experience of the truth is gained in the context of one's own moment-to-moment actual life experience. For example, a woman grieving the recent death of her beloved husband might move from an intellectualized knowledge that life involves suffering (i.e., the First Insight) to direct knowledge of this truth (i.e., the Second Insight) when she allows herself to feel emotions of sadness and longing within her body and mind as these experiences naturally arise over time. Eventually, the *Third Insight* can develop, allowing this embodied knowledge to be integrated into daily life as a profound experiential understanding (Moffitt 2008). The woman in the previous example might develop the Third Insight once her own personal direct experience with grief allows her to feel a social connection to others suffering, motivating her to reach out to others with compassion while offering assistance and comfort. Moffitt also observed that many practitioners are tempted to skip the Second Insight step, thereby remaining stuck with only the superficial and intellectual knowledge characterized by the First Insight. Intensive formal and informal meditation practices are viewed as the means by which individuals can train the mind to attend to direct experience without the distractions and distortions of conceptual thought. Mindfulness-based interventions also emphasize direct experience over mental concepts and ideas about experiences. Consistent with the epistemology of humanistic psychology (Bakan 1967) as well as Buddhism, MBSR and MBCT participants are encouraged to attend to the direct experiences perceived in the mind and body. Formal and informal mindfulness meditation practices are designed to provide opportunities for experiencing sensations directly. When attention is fully focused on internal direct experience in formal meditation, participants learn how to identify its pleasant, unpleasant, or neutral tone, and become aware of subsequent reactions of wanting pleasant experience, not wanting unpleasant experience, ignoring neutral experience, and further thinking in reaction to the original experience. For this reason, meditation has been likened to a microscope, in which moment-to-moment experience and mental reactivity can be seen much more clearly than when one is engaged with activities of daily life. For example, a participant struggling with chronic pain may learn to disentangle an uncomfortable sensation in the body from the mental state of aversion and any following thoughts and emotions that arise in reaction to the initial sensation.

CBT also emphasizes direct experience as the primary form of evidence. When patients express strongly held beliefs about the way things are or about what will happen in the future, therapists typically respond by pointing out the patient's conjecture and exploring how the patient might seek direct experiences to know the truth for themselves. In addition to seeking direct experience as evidence, patients are encouraged to behave in ways that counter such beliefs to allow for new experiences and to promote new learning. One classic example involves exposure therapy for anxiety. Exposure to feared environmental situations or imagined scenarios for the purpose of eliciting anxiety in the context of actual safety has been the cornerstone of CBT for decades. Patients might be educated about the realities of low risks and learn to challenge assumptions of danger intellectually, but the direct experience of personal safety and specific feared outcomes not actually happening while confronting their fear remains a powerful therapeutic intervention. Relaxation techniques found in CBT approaches also emphasize direct experience of body sensations. Both diaphragmatic breathing and progressive muscle relaxation procedures require the patient to feel sensations of breath or muscle tension/release in the body, allowing the direct experience of nervous system relaxation to be learned non-conceptually.

Non-striving Effort

Original Buddhist teachings detail how to implement the teachings into daily life with a series of instructions for both formal meditation and daily living practices known as the eightfold path. One component known as *right* or *wise effort* captures the inherent paradox of wanting a wholesome outcome, such as awakening or enlightenment, yet observing that too strong an emotional investment in attaining desired outcomes as soon as possible often proves counterproductive. Rather than straining, forcing, pushing, or trying to control factors beyond one's control, right effort teaches dedication to the path of practice itself with persistence and patience, trusting that this process will unfold naturally in its own time. This process of practice is not necessarily linear or always predictable, as profound learning and personal change can occur in the face of challenge or can follow apparent setbacks. Zen priest Steve Hagen (1997) recounts a famous story of a Zen master who was asked by an eager new student how long it would take for him to achieve enlightenment. "Ten years" was the master's initial response, but when the student persisted that he would really work at it, the master changed his response to "twenty years," and after another protestation, "thirty years." Right effort therefore teaches meditation practitioners to direct their efforts toward the practice itself with an earnest attitude of resolve and dedication. Such an attitude also fosters self-reliance, in which practitioners hold themselves responsible for their own efforts and the natural results of their behavior.

These same qualities of self-responsibility, persistence, and patience are deliberately cultivated in MBSR and other mindfulness-based interventions. In the initial MBSR session, the instructor explicitly acknowledges that participants enrolled to take an active role in their own health and well-being. Participants are encouraged to focus their efforts on attending sessions and completing daily home practices and assignments as faithfully and wholeheartedly as possible, rather than to approach the practice merely as a means to an immediate end. When participants voice discouragement that initial meditation practices were not pleasant or relaxing, the instructor might query to see if participants held a hidden agenda characterized by striving for immediate results and then might validate their efforts to follow the practice instructions earnestly. Instructors also might invite participants to investigate how such attachment to outcome affected the course of experience during the practice itself, guiding participants to discover for themselves how "trying too hard" actually backfired and produced experiences opposite those desired.

Likewise, CBT therapists readily discuss the essential paradox of relaxation training by inviting patients to remember times when they felt they must relax right away and the subsequent increase in tension that resulted. Lying awake in bed feeling pressured to relax in order to fall asleep is a common example of this phenomenon. Similarly, deploying cognitive therapy techniques to reduce immediate anxiety or depression without careful empirical examination of the evidence are likely to have little impact. Therapists also might educate patients about the "thought suppression" psychology experiments that began in the 1980s (e.g., Wegner et al. 1987) showing how the deliberate attempt not to think about something often leads to a paradoxical increase in the frequency of the suppressed thought. When CBT therapists suspect that patients are inadvertently circumventing the therapeutic learning process out of impatience or desperation, they encourage patients to redirect their efforts toward the therapeutic process itself. CBT therapists also promote a "take-charge attitude," in which patients take responsibility for participating actively in their own treatment. Accordingly, CBT therapists explicitly review the role of patient commitment, effort, and patience at the beginning of the therapy (Hazlett-Stevens 2008).

The Role of Perception

All Buddhist traditions address our human habits of subjective perception, which often prevent us from seeing reality clearly yet without awareness that this is the case. The Tibetan lama Kalu Rinpoche once said "You live in illusion and the appearance of things. There is a reality but you do not know this." (Kornfield 2008, p. 223). A well-known Zen Buddhist analogy describes a person who paints a picture of a tiger on the wall then cowers in fear from mistaking the painted tiger for a real live one (Suzuki 1949). Kornfield (2008) identified three primary forms of misunderstanding taught across various Buddhist traditions. The first, inattention, captures our tendency to live on "automatic pilot," engaging in activities without much awareness and constantly seeking distraction from present-moment direct experience. The second form, denial, refers to a failure or unwillingness to believe direct experience. Common examples include denial of past abuse or denial that a loved one is dying. The third form, misperception of reality, reflects deeply held assumptions, such as beliefs that material wealth will protect us from suffering or that change is not really inevitable.

MBSR, MBCT, and similar mindfulness-based interventions explicitly address the human tendency toward distracted attention and "automatic pilot," offering mindfulness meditation training as an antidote. In addition, MBSR emphasizes the role of perception in stress. In the second MBSR session, participants discuss their experiences with the "nine dots" problem, in which participants struggle to connect a square formation of nine dots on a piece of paper and cannot follow all given rules to accomplish this unless they see the problem from the broader view of the whole page. The potential impact of perception when encountering stressful life events is discussed in the context of stress resilience research findings, such as associations between stress-hardiness and tendencies to: (1) believe that an individual can exert an influence on their surroundings ("control"), (2) feel engaged and committed to life's activities ("commitment"), and (3) consider change and difficult life circumstances as challenges and opportunities for growth ("challenge") (Kobasa et al. 1982). Likewise, MBCT emphasizes the role of perception in depression. Distorted perceptions increase vulnerability for subsequent depression, and a currently depressed mood increases the likelihood of depressive thoughts. Awareness of this vicious cycle allows the individual to disengage from this habitual cognitive pattern and to respond differently (Segal et al. 2013).

CBT has emphasized the role of cognitive misperception in anxiety, depression, and other emotional difficulties since its inception. Much research has documented cognitive vulnerabilities among individuals prone to depression (Abramson et al. 1988), and a large body of cognitive research details how anxious individuals demonstrated both pre-attentive and interpretive biases toward threat (Eysenck 1992). From this perspective, certain individuals are prone to anxiety because they have learned to attend selectively to potential threats and to interpret ambiguous or neutral stimuli as threatening. As a result, they react to innocuous environmental circumstances as if they were truly in immediate danger, leading to heightened anxiety, worry, or panic. CBT strategies for anxiety therefore foster re-appraisals of misperceptions of threat as they occur, challenge underlying core beliefs that the outside world is inherently threatening and/or that the person is unable to cope, and promote behavior change that counter such beliefs (Hazlett-Stevens 2008).

Nature and Causes of Human Suffering

According to Buddhist accounts, the Buddha's first discourse addressed the topic of suffering directly in a series of teachings known as the *Four Noble Truths* (Smith and Novak 2003). From this perspective, suffering is considered inherent to the human condition. Although the original word used, *dukkha*, was often translated to the English word "suffering," this inevitable human experience is not limited to intense experience; suffering on a small scale involves the chronic dissatisfaction that results from the human mind wanting to experience something other than what actually exists in any given moment. Although much has been written about the nuances of meaning found in the Four Noble Truths, they consist of four main axioms: (1) human suffering is an inevitable aspect of human life, (2) suffering results when we try to obtain whatever object or experience we desire without fully accepting present-moment reality, (3) suffering naturally ceases when we relinquish the struggle against present-moment reality, and (4) practicing a specific way of life, the eightfold path, is the means to reduce such suffering (Moffitt 2008). Buddhist meditation practices therefore teach an experiential means of increased acceptance of three basic characteristics of human existence reflected in the Four Noble Truths: (1) the nature of suffering, (2) the temporary and ever-changing nature of life (i.e., "impermanence"), and (3) experiential phenomena are empty of a separate egoistic self (i.e., "selflessness") (Goldstein and Kornfield 1987).

In MBSR, MBCT, and similar clinical interventions, mindfulness meditation practices facilitate awareness of how habitual mental reactions of striving toward pleasant experience and of rejecting unpleasant experience increase a sense of dissatisfaction and suffering. As participants begin formal meditation practice with focused attention on the breath or other body sensations, their natural preferences to feel pleasant experience and to avoid unpleasant experience are known directly. Often with the guidance of the instructor, participants discover first-hand how resistance to present-moment experience actually increases negative affectivity and sometimes paradoxically increases the intensity of the unpleasant sensation itself. MBSR and MBCT curricula include the well-known poem by the Sufi poet Rumi entitled "The Guest House," in which readers are invited to treat each experience, whether sorrow, shame, malice, or joy, as a welcome guest who visits their home. Formal meditation instructions also direct awareness to the constantly changing nature of experience, pointing out the mind's tendency to create a solid, fixed, representation of the flow of experiential phenomena. The impersonal nature of experience is also highlighted to expose the mind's tendency to identify with passing experiences as if they reflected one's personal sense of self.

CBT therapists have long worked with patients to reveal the self-defeating paradox associated with trying to avoid unpleasant experience. In cases of fear and anxiety, patients often have developed elaborate or disabling behavioral limitations to avoid feeling the body's natural fight-or-flight physiological responses. Therapists educate patients about the physical safety of such responses as well as the need to allow oneself to feel them to counter cycles of fear and avoidance. Therapy procedures of exposure are carefully implemented to ensure that patients allow the experience of fear without a "hidden agenda" of getting through the exposure exercise with minimal discomfort. Subtle protective behaviors, attempts at immediate relaxation, or rehearsing false reassurances will prevent patients from learning to tolerate uncomfortable feelings. As patients successfully face feared situations, they learn first-hand how to allow themselves to feel the effects of the emotion without needing to try and change such feelings. Discoveries that such feelings naturally change over the course of time on their own and that experiences such as anxiety do not define a person's identity typically occur as well.

Incorporating Buddhism and Mindfulness into Cognitive-Behavioral Practice

As Buddhism and mindfulness-based interventions become increasingly popular in the West, clinicians are motivated to integrate these principles and practices into their clinical work. The following list identifies ways in which clinicians might modify instructions and procedures of common cognitive-behavioral techniques. Other practices from Buddhist meditation, MBSR, and MBCT that might be introduced to patients in a secular, culturally sensitive manner also are described. Finally, potential pitfalls that sometimes arise as clinicians attempt to integrate mindfulness into therapy are identified.

Breathing Practices

Meditation on the breath is the hallmark of formal Zen practice (Suzuki 1970) and considered the crucial starting point for Theravada vipassana meditation (Thera 1965). Not surprisingly, MBSR and MBCT begin with mindfulness of breathing as the initial formal meditation practice as well. Standard instructions encourage the individual to sit in a comfortable upright position, close the eyes, and simply allow attention to rest upon sensations of breathing. Attention may be directed toward one area of the body, such as the rising and falling of the belly. Individuals are instructed to maintain the focus on these sensations, "being with" each inbreath and each outbreath for their full duration. Each time the individual recognizes that attention has wandered away from the breath, the instruction is just to notice what was on the mind at that time and to bring attention back to the breath. This formal practice can be done daily for 10–15 min. in a secluded setting free from external distractions (Kabat-Zinn 2013). In mindfulness-based interventions, instructions emphasize feeling sensations of breath as they naturally occur in an open and receptive fashion, rather than encourage explicit attempts to change the rate or depth of breathing. In contrast, the CBT technique of diaphragmatic breathing is traditionally introduced to teach patients how to slow and deepen the breath deliberately for the purpose of promoting relaxation. CBT clinicians also typically explain the physiology of the diaphragm muscle and how breathing from this area of the body stimulates parasympathetic nervous system activity, thereby slowing down physiological arousal (Hazlett-Stevens 2008). When this practice is introduced in CBT, more mindfulness-oriented therapists still might explain the benefits of diaphragmatic breathing yet invite a receptive nature of attention as described above rather than aim for a certain rate or depth of breathing. Therapist instructions more similar to MBSR and MBCT interventions therefore could prevent unhelpful habits of striving, reducing the chance of paradoxical tension and frustration while lowering the risk of inadvertently sending a mixed message that patients need to relax immediately or to avoid unpleasant experience to benefit.

Mindfulness of breathing also can be applied as an informal practice in daily life. Traditional Buddhist meditation instructions often guide practitioners to bring awareness to the breath for brief moments in the course of daily life (Thera 1965). Likewise, Kabat-Zinn (2013) recommended frequently bringing awareness to feelings of breathing throughout the day for the duration of two whole breaths as part of his MBSR program. As attention collects around sensations of breathing, individuals also can bring awareness to any current thoughts, emotions, how they are seeing things and feeling about themselves; whether they are at all "caught" in their thoughts, emotions, or mental perceptions at the time. MBCT procedures teach applied breathing practice in a format known as the "3-minute breathing space" (Segal et al. 2013). Several times per day, participants "step out of automatic pilot mode" and bring awareness to any thoughts or feelings present, remembering that these experiences are only experiential phenomena. Next, participants collect attention on the breath and feel sensations of breathing, eventually expanding the field of attention to sense the body breathing as a whole. As with formal breathing practice, when instructing clients or patients to apply mindfulness of breathing in daily life, such instructions could emphasize increased mindfulness of the body rather than explicit attempts to change the depth or rate of breathing or to relax.

Relaxation Techniques

Even with CBT procedures designed to induce relaxation, therapist instructions for techniques such as progressive muscle relaxation can emphasize awareness of sensations in the body rather than striving toward immediate relaxation. Initial discussion with clients or patients can include warnings about the counterproductive nature of trying too hard to relax, and encouraging them instead to view relaxation practice as an opportunity to become more aware of direct experience. Whether or not practicing over time eventually increases relaxation can be treated as an empirical question worthy of testing. Alternatively, clinicians might choose to begin with body scan procedures, as used in MBSR and MBCT, instead of physical relaxation instructions. Beginning somatic practice with the body scan might help clients or patients reduce such striving efforts at first, eventually making relaxation more natural and possible to experience.

Self-monitoring Instructions

Most CBT protocols begin with daily self-monitoring of thoughts, emotions, body sensations, and behavior. Through this exercise, clients or patients come to see how states such as anxiety, depression, and stress actually reflect moment-to-moment processes, building over time as a series of reactions to reactions. Rather than more traditional CBT instructions which might focus on immediate reduction of difficult emotion when detected, mindfulness-oriented instructions might invite patients to investigate this process of habitual reactivity as it unfolds. Therapists can frame the purpose of self-monitoring to increase awareness of how these states develop from an empirical perspective with the aim of allowing direct experience of bodily sensations. Awareness of the breath and the body can serve as a "stress barometer" to cue clients that automatic reaction patterns might be occurring. One particular strategy from the MBSR literature presents the acronym STOP (Stahl and Goldstein 2010). Throughout the day or whenever stress is noticed, individuals are invited to work through four simple steps: "S" serves as a reminder to stop, pausing to turn attention inward; "T" reminds the individual to take a breath (mindfully); "O" stands for observe, inviting the individual to observe objectively whatever is occurring, externally as well as any thoughts, emotions, and sensations that are present; in the final step, "P" for proceed invites the individual to respond skillfully to the situation, including attending to one's own needs or reducing tension. This simple practice can be applied at predetermined times throughout the day or whenever stress, anxiety, depression, or tension are detected.

Exposure Practices

CBT therapists routinely assist their clients to approach and to face feared situations in the course of exposure therapy procedures. Consistent with mindfulness-based approaches, modern CBT therapists explain that the goal of such exposure exercises is to allow oneself to experience the fear reaction. Opening oneself up to feel the fear rather than resisting or fighting direct experience helps the patient learn that sensations of "fight-or-flight" are harmless and can be tolerated. In addition, therapists might point out how the experience of fear includes characteristics of impermanence and selflessness. Just like all experiential phenomena, sensations come and go naturally on their own, particularly when the mind is not fighting against reality. Rather than self-identifying with moments of anxiety, fear, or depression and viewing these experiences as an unchangeable aspect of one's identity, clients can remember that every human being has experienced such states at one time or another and such experiences are inherently "impersonal."

Mindfulness in Daily Activities

A common practice found across Buddhism, mindfulness-based interventions, and CBT involves bringing present-moment awareness to direct experience during routine activities of daily living. As an introduction to Buddhist meditation, Zen master Hanh (1976) described how washing dishes, washing clothes, housecleaning, making tea, eating, and walking all can be approached as mindfulness practice, cultivating full consciousness of bodily sensations, breathing, thoughts, and movements during the activity. Zen teacher Miller (2011) explained how engaging everyday chores, such as gardening, cooking, cleaning, and laundry, in this way can reveal the inherent value in living. In early MBSR sessions, instructors invite participants to expand applied mindfulness practice from eating to other routine activities, including brushing teeth, showering, washing hands, driving, reading to children, and folding laundry. Instructions are to approach the activity with the deliberate intention to experience any bodily sensations and movements associated with the activity in an open and accepting way, bringing attention back to direct experience in the body whenever the mind wanders in distraction. CBT expert Borkovec (2002) described how activities ranging from washing the dishes to writing grant proposals can be done while focusing on present-moment experience of the process itself instead of rushing through merely to achieve some extrinsic outcome. Borkovec outlined how orienting generalized anxiety clients toward direct experience in the present moment can facilitate letting go of attachment to outcome, thereby reducing worry and promoting natural experiences of pleasure and joy. Clinicians might introduce this simple informal mindfulness practice to clients or patients struggling with symptoms of stress, anxiety, or depression, encouraging them to self-monitor mood and associated symptoms on a daily basis once mindfulness of daily activities has become part of their routine. Therapists might query for a specific activity to be assigned for mindfulness practice (e.g., brushing teeth) to begin, adding more specific activities one at a time. Alternatively, clients may choose to remind themselves to engage in mindfulness each time they notice they are engaged in typical activities of daily living.

Pitfalls of Integrating Mindfulness into Clinical Practice

As behavioral health clinicians discover the value of Buddhist meditation and mindfulness practice in their own lives, the temptation to bring this knowledge into the therapy room naturally follows. The most fundamental way in which therapist mindfulness practice informs therapy is improving the attentive and compassionate presence of the therapist, regardless of the therapeutic approach. Buddhist ideals, such as beginner's mind, first-person empiricism, and an ability to focus the mind in the present, all can serve the assessment and therapy process. Clinicians easily might argue that a certain degree of therapist mindfulness and selflessness are required for empathy and development of a productive therapeutic alliance. While emerging research suggests a potential benefit for the clients of meditating therapists (Hick 2008), meditating therapists must remain humble in their efforts and recognize that at any moment mindfulness may lapse. In other words, having an established meditation practice does not insulate a therapist from all the distracting and destructive habits of mind elucidated in Buddhist teachings.

One particular pitfall of meditation has been identified for Western practitioners, including psychotherapists. Clinical psychologist Welwood (2000) described noticing in the 1970s that many Western practitioners were using spiritual practices to avoid dealing with unresolved personal or emotional issues. He coined the term "spiritual bypass" to denote this temptation to transcend basic human needs or developmental tasks prematurely, using spiritual practices to create a new yet dysfunctional "spiritual" identity. Meditating clinicians therefore might honestly examine their motivation for meditation practice, investigating whether they are using meditation to turn away from difficulties or to rationalize or reinforce old defensive habit patterns.

Other pitfalls can arise when clinicians attempt to teach mindfulness meditation practices to their clients or patients without sufficient experience with meditation themselves. Given that MBSR and MBCT interventions involve teaching formal mindfulness meditation, the professional training organizations associated with these interventions require instructors to have prior personal meditation experience. The developers of MBCT explained this requirement as follows: "Without such experience, the approach cannot be called mindfulness-based cognitive therapy; in fact, it is not mindfulness-based anything at all, since 'mindfulness-based' actually *means* teaching from the basis of your own mindfulness practice" (Segal et al. 2013, p. 79). Given the emphasis on non-conceptual direct experience as the only means of understanding mindfulness, clinicians who do not practice themselves may only understand mindfulness at an intellectual level. They also might fail to grasp the many challenges inherent in meditation practice, ranging from finding the time for formal practice to summoning the courage required to allow difficult experience. Furthermore, traditional psychotherapeutic training in which the therapist is viewed as the expert within a hierarchy can interfere with both the patient and the therapist fully acknowledging that the therapist is simply a fellow human being; this humanistic and egalitarian relationship is crucial to the skillful instruction of MBSR (McCown et al. 2010). As a general guideline, the developers of MBCT recommend that prospective MBCT instructors have an established daily formal mindfulness meditation practice in their own lives for at least one year before teaching it to clients or patients (Segal et al. 2013). In addition to an established meditation and mindful movement ongoing practice, the UMass Center for Mindfulness in Medicine, Health Care, and Society requires completion of one 5–10 day, silent, teacher-led mindfulness meditation residential retreat before enrollment in their foundational MBSR instructor training programs.

One final pitfall may arise when therapists first introduce mindfulness practices into the therapy session. Some clients or patients may be reluctant to try experiential practices associated with meditation out of concern that the Buddhist roots of such practices conflict with their personal religious beliefs. Others may fear that the therapist is teaching meditation out of desire to impose his or her Buddhist religious views onto the client. Therapists must be sensitive to these possible perceptions, responding to any client concerns with attention and care. In MBSR and MBCT interventions, mindfulness is described as a universal quality of human awareness. Although Buddhist meditation has been taught throughout human history as a way of cultivating mindfulness, secular mindfulness meditation can be practiced by anyone coming from any religious background, including atheism or a lack of religion. Mindfulness is presented simply as a way of paying attention: on purpose, in the present-moment, without judgment, and with acceptance. Therapists might increase client acceptance by describing how an everyday activity, such as eating or washing hands, can be done mindfully and then inviting the client to practice breathing mindfully in the same way. Therapists should be careful to avoid Buddhist terminology as much as possible, describing all aspects of mindfulness practice in the simplest common language available.

Summary and Conclusions

As Buddhism spread to the West, its wisdom eventually informed the work of clinicians in the fields of medicine and psychology. Resulting mindfulness-based interventions have received much research support over recent years, and mindfulness meditation training for clinicians has become increasingly popular. CBT developed within the area of Western psychology largely independent of these advancements, yet emphasized many of the same principles, including empiricism, emphasis on direct experience, non-striving effort, the importance of perception, the role of resisting experience in human suffering, and the benefits of an accepting present-moment attention. Clinicians can modify traditional CBT instructions and techniques in ways that are more consistent with Buddhist and mindfulness-based practices. Common pitfalls for meditating clinicians as well as for clinicians without a personal meditation practice hoping to teach mindfulness to their clients or patients require careful consideration.

References

Abramson, L. Y., Alloy, L. B., & Metalsky, G. I. (1988). The cognitive diathesis-stress theories of depression: Toward and adequate evaluation of the theories' validities. In L. B. Alloy (Ed.), *Cognitive processes in depression* (pp. 3–30). New York: Guilford.

Bakan, D. (1967). *On method: Toward a reconstruction of psychological investigation*. San Francisco, CA: Jossey-Bass Publishers.

Borkovec, T. D. (2002). Life in the future versus life in the present. *Clinical Psychology: Science and Practice, 9,* 76–80.

Carson, J. W., Carson, K. M., Gil, K. M., & Baucom, D. H. (2004). Mindfulness-based relationship enhancement. *Behavior Therapy, 35,* 471–494.

de Vibe, M., Bjørndal, A., Tipton, E., Hammerstrøm, K., & Kowalski, K. (2012). Mindfulness-based stress reduction (MBSR) for improving health, quality of life, and social functioning in adults. *Campbell Systematic Reviews* 3.

Duncan, L. G., & Bardacke, N. (2010). Mindfulness-based childbirth and parenting education: Promoting family mindfulness during the perinatal period. *Journal of Child and Family Studies, 19,* 190–202.

Epstein, M. (1995). *Thoughts without a thinker*. New York: Basic Books.

Eysenck, M. W. (1992). *Anxiety: The cognitive perspective*. Hove, UK: Lawrence Erlbaum Associates.

Germer, C. K. (2005). Mindfulness: What is it? What does it matter? In C. K. Germer, R. D. Siegel, & P. R. Fulton (Eds.), *Mindfulness and psychotherapy* (pp. 3–27). New York: Guilford Press.

Germer, C. K. (2013). Mindfulness: What is it? What does it matter? In C. K. Germer, R. D. Siegel, & P. R. Fulton (Eds.), *Mindfulness and psychotherapy* (2nd ed., pp. 3–35). New York: Guilford Press.

Goldstein, J., & Kornfield, J. (1987). *Seeking the heart of wisdom: The path of insight meditation*. Boston: Shambhala Publications.

Gunaratana, B. (1992). *Mindfulness in plain English, 20th* (Anniversary ed.). Boston: Wisdom Publications.

Gunaratana, B. (2012). *The four foundations of mindfulness in plain English*. Boston: Wisdom Publications.

Hagen, S. (1997). *Buddhism plain and simple*. New York: Broadway Books.

Hanh, T. N. (1976). *1976*. The miracle of mindfulness. Boston: Beacon Press.

Hayes, S. C., Strosahl, K., & Wilson, K. G. (1999). *Acceptance and commitment therapy: An experimental approach to behavior change*. New York: Guilford.

Hayes, S. C., Strosahl, K. D., & Wilson, K. G. (2012). *Acceptance and commitment therapy: The process and practice of mindful change* (2nd ed.). New York: Guilford.

Hazlett-Stevens, H. (2008). *Psychological approaches to generalized anxiety disorder: A clinician's guide to assessment and treatment*. New York: Springer.

Heidenreich, T., Tuin, I., Pflug, B., Michal, M., & Michalak, J. (2006). Mindfulness-based cognitive therapy for persistent insomnia: A pilot study. *Psychotherapy and Psychosomatics, 75,* 188–189.

Hick, S. F. (2008). Cultivating therapeutic relationships: The role of mindfulness. In S. F. Hick & T. Bien (Eds.), *Mindfulness and the therapeutic relationship* (pp. 3–18). New York: Guilford.

Kabat-Zinn, J. (2003). Mindfulness-based interventions in context: Past, present, and future. *Clinical Psychology: Science and Practice, 10,* 144–156.

Kabat-Zinn, J. (2013). *Full catastrophe living, Revised and updated edition*. New York: Bantam Books.

Khoury, B., Lecomte, T., Fortin, G., Masse, M., Therien, P., Bouchard, V., et al. (2013). Mindfulness-based therapy: A comprehensive meta-analysis. *Clinical Psychology Review, 33,* 763–771.

Kobasa, S. C., Maddi, S. R., & Kahn, S. (1982). Hardiness and health: A prospective study. *Journal of Personality and Social Psychology, 42,* 168–177.

Kornfield, J. (2008). *The wise heart: A guide to the universal teachings of Buddhist psychology*. New York: Bantam Books.

Kristeller, J. L., Baer, R. A., & Quillian-Wolever, R. (2006). Mindfulness-based approaches to eating disorders. In R. A. Baer (Ed.), *Mindfulness-based treatment approaches: Clinician's guide to evidence base and applications* (pp. 75–91). London: Academic Press.

Linehan, M. M. (1993). *Cognitive-behavioral treatment of borderline personality disorder*. New York: Guilford Press.

Marlatt, G. A., Witkiewitz, K., Dillworth, T. M., Bowen, S. W., & Parks, G. A. (2004). Vipassana meditation as a treatment for alcohol and drug use disorders. In S. C. Hayes, V. M. Follette, & M. M. Linehan (Eds.), *Mindfulness and acceptance: Expanding the cognitive-behavioral tradition* (pp. 261–287). New York: Guilford.

McCown, D., Reibel, D., & Micozzi, M. S. (2010). *Teaching mindfulness: A practical guide for clinicians and educators*. New York: Springer.

Miller, K. M. (2011). Do dishes, rake leaves. In B. Boyce (Ed.), *The mindfulness revolution* (pp. 68–72). Boston: Shambhala.

Moffitt, P. (2008). *Dancing with life: Buddhist insights for finding meaning and joy in the face of suffering*. New York: Rodale Inc.

Neff, K., & Germer, C. K. (2013). A pilot study and randomized controlled trial of the mindful self-compassion program. *Journal of Clinical Psychology, 69,* 28–44.

Piet, J., & Hougaard, E. (2011). The effect of mindfulness-based cognitive therapy for prevention of relapse in recurrent major depressive disorder: A systematic review and meta-analysis. *Clinical Psychology Review, 31,* 1032–1040.

Roemer, L., Orsillo, S. M., & Salters-Pedneault, K. (2008). Efficacy of an acceptance-based behavior therapy for generalized anxiety disorder: Evaluation in a randomized controlled trial. *Journal of Consulting and Clinical Psychology, 76,* 1083–1089.

Segal, Z. V., Williams, J. M. G., & Teasdale, J. D. (2013). *Mindfulness-based cognitive therapy for depression* (2nd ed.). New York: Guilford Press.

Smith, H., & Novak, P. (2003). *Buddhism: A concise introduction*. New York: HarperCollins.

Stahl, B., & Goldstein, E. (2010). *A mindfulness-based stress reduction workbook*. Oakland, CA: New Harbinger Publications.

Stanley, E. A., Schaldach, J. M., Kiyonaga, A., & Jha, A. P. (2011). Mindfulness-based mind fitness training: A case study of a high-stress predeployment military cohort. *Cognitive and Behavioral Practice, 18,* 566–576.

Suzuki, S. (1970). *Zen mind, beginner's mind*. New York: Weatherhill Inc.

Thera, N. (1965). *The heart of Buddhist meditation*. San Francisco, CA: Weiser Books.

Wallace, B. A. (2007). *Contemplative science*. New York: Columbia University Press.

Wegner, D. M., Schneider, D. J., Carter, S. R., & White, T. L. (1987). Paradoxical effects of thought suppression. *Journal of Personality and Social Psychology, 53,* 5–13.

Welwood, J. (2000). *Toward a psychology of awakening*. Boston: Shambhala.

Witkiewitz, K., & Marlatt, G. A. (2004). Relapse prevention for alcohol and drug problems: That was Zen, this is Tao. *American Psychologist, 59,* 224–235.

Acceptance and Commitment Therapy and Zen Buddhism

Kenneth Po-Lun Fung and Josephine Pui-Hing Wong

Keywords
Acceptance and commitment therapy · Zen buddhism · Third-wave behavior therapy · Acceptance · Mindfulness

Most people are afraid of suffering. But suffering is a kind of mud to help the lotus flower of happiness grow. There can be no lotus flower without the mud.

Thích Nhất Hạnh

Do not just look for what you want to see, that would be futile. Do not look for anything, but allow the insight to have a chance to come by itself. That insight will help liberate you.

Thích Nhất Hạnh

Introduction

For more than a century, many aspects of Buddhist teaching and practices have been recognized for its psychotherapeutic effects by Western scholars (Davids 1914). Psychotherapy and Buddhist practice share similar objectives in reducing human suffering associated with the mind and promoting humanity (Young-Eisendrath and Muramoto 2002). There is also increasing recognition of the potential mental health benefits of the practice of mindfulness in Buddhism, both in the mental health field and in the general public.

In recent years, a group of evidence-based psychotherapies have been noted to share in common the incorporation of the principles of acceptance and mindfulness, and they have been collectively termed "third-wave" behavioral interventions (Hayes et al. 2004). Acceptance and Commitment Therapy (ACT) is an exemplar of this family of psychotherapy. It has been used in many clinical and nonclinical populations, from the treatment of depression, anxiety, addictions, and psychosis, to improving patient outcomes with diabetes and epilepsy, to reducing stigma and burnout (Ruiz 2010). A recent meta-analysis of 39 randomized controlled trials on mental disorders and somatic health problems found that ACT outperformed control conditions and treatment as usual (A-Tjak et al. 2015).

K.P.-L. Fung (✉)
University of Toronto, Toronto, Canada
e-mail: kenneth.fung@utoronto.ca

J.P.-H. Wong
Ryerson University, Toronto, Canada
e-mail: jph.wong@ryerson.ca

A. Masuda and W.T. O'Donohue (eds.), *Handbook of Zen, Mindfulness, and Behavioral Health*, Mindfulness in Behavioral Health, DOI 10.1007/978-3-319-54595-0_21

Although ACT reflects many common tenets underlying Zen Buddhism, little has been written about the relationship between Zen Buddhism and ACT. A few researchers have highlighted the parallels between Zen Buddhism and ACT (Fung 2015; Hayes 2002), but writing about the plausible influences of Buddhism on the development of ACT is almost nonexistent. In this chapter, we provide a short account of the historical development of Western Buddhism in America and explore its influence on ACT; describe how ACT is similar to and different from Zen Buddhism; and propose a more explicit integration of Zen Buddhism into ACT to strengthen its practice.

Influence of Buddhism on Western Thought

While a comprehensive account of Buddhist influence on Western thought is beyond the scope of this chapter, reflecting on the historical development of Western Buddhism in America allows us to examine the cultural appropriation, diffusion, and hybridization of Buddhist philosophy in present day's field of psychology and the self-help industry in the West. While some researchers and practitioners like Tara Brach openly declare themselves as Buddhist psychologists, many others use or promote therapeutic approaches that resemble Buddhism without making any explicit reference to it. Non-Christian and non-Western approaches for mental well-being are often Westernized, and this norm to Westernize or appropriate foreign thoughts can be seen in Jon Kabat-Zinn's reflection on his ambivalence to accept an endorsement from a Buddhist Monk on his book, *Full Catastrophe Living*:

> … it would be disrespectful, having asked for it, not to use it. However, I did think twice about it. It precipitated something of a crisis in me for a time, because not only was Thich Nhat Hanh definitely a Buddhist authority, his brief endorsement used the very foreign word *dharma* not once, but four times… I wondered: 'Is this the right time for this? Would it be skillful to stretch the envelope at this point? Or would it in the end cause more harm than good?' In retrospect, these concerns now sound a bit silly to me. But at the time, they felt significant. (Kabat-Zinn 2011, pp. 282–283)

Kabat-Zinn's reticence to openly acknowledge the Buddhist foundation of his work in mindfulness-based stress reduction (MBSR) a decade after he had established his MBSR Clinic's work speaks to the power of the embedded Orientalist "Othering" and Anglo-Eurocentrism in American culture. Identifying this dynamic is important in understanding the development of Western Buddhism and the invisibility of Buddhist influence on modern and postmodern Western thoughts and therapeutic approaches.

European contact with Buddhist cultures started as early as the mid-thirteenth century when Franciscan pilgrims journeyed through Mongolia, China, and Japan. However, Western interest on the systematic study of Buddhism began only in the nineteenth century when transcendentalists rejected Christian puritanism and looked to Eastern religions for philosophical truths (Franklin 2008; Tamney 1992). Prior to the 1800s, Hinduism was an object of systematic study due to European political, commercial, and colonial interests on India. Thus, in the early days of intellectual encounters with Buddhism in the West, many transcendentalists, including Ralph Waldo Emerson, confused Buddhism with Hinduism; others understood Buddhism through an Orientalist lens and held the view of Buddhism as an atheistic religion grounded in pessimistic nihilism (Tamney 1992).

American transcendentalists were drawn to Buddhism for its emphasis on personal awakening instead of glorifying a deity. In his essay on transcendentalism, Emerson wrote:

> …if there is anything grand and daring in human thought or virtue, any reliance on the vast, the unknown. . . adopts it as most in nature. The oriental mind has always tended to this largeness. Buddhism is an expression of it. The Buddhist who thanks no man, who says, "do not flatter your benefactors," but who in his conviction that every good deed can by no possibility escape its reward, will not deceive the benefactor by pretending that he has done more than he should, is a Transcendentalist (Emerson and Myerson 2015, p. 168)

While Emerson resonated with the karmic suppositions in Buddhism, he was not a Buddhist. Like many others, his interest in Buddhism was more literary, whereas Henry David Thoreau's interest was more contemplative (Fields 1992).

In 1844, Thoreau published passages of the Lotus Sutra in the Ethnical Scripture section of the *Dial*, a journal on new spirituality established by Emerson, and it opened up discussions on Buddhism within the transcendentalist literacy circles. However, wider interest on Buddhism in America emerged around 1875 when the Theosophical Society was established in New York City and when Sir Arnold Edwin published his book *Light in Asia* in 1879. Its popularity, with eighty editions and sales between half a million to one million copies, was attributed to Edwin's ability to tell the story of Buddha "in a way that matched Victorian taste… His Buddha is part romantic hero, part self-reliant man, and part Christ without being Christ" (Fields 1992, p. 68). The deep-rooted psyche of Western superiority and Christian cultural habitus deterred the full embracement of Buddhism among Europeans and Americans (Sutin 2006).

The convening of the 1893 World's Parliament of Religions in Chicago was a catalyst for cultural diffusion and growth of Zen Buddhism in America. Influential Buddhists from Asia attended and spoke at the Parliament and it promoted interest among intellectuals other than Orientalists and faddists. Zen was the first Buddhist tradition to take roots in America, largely due to: the enthusiasm of Paul Carus, a theologian and managing editor of Open Court Publishing Company; influential lectures of a Japanese Rinzai master, Soyen Shaku, and the writings of Shaku's student D.T. Suzuki, who "introduced paradoxical Zen thought to many fascinated Western intellectuals" (Coleman 2002, p. 8). Suzuki studied with Carus and his prolific writing was published through the Open Court Publishing Company. Until the 1960s, most materials about Zen in the English-speaking world were written by Suzuki (Layman 1976).

Local and global political events contributed to a revival of Western enthusiasm in Buddhism in the 1960s and 1970s. Similar to the Western intellectualists who turned to Eastern religions as resistance against Christian puritanism and the dissident Orientalists who deployed Buddhism against the empire in the nineteenth century (Cox 2013; Turner 2013), many Americans and Europeans turned to Zen Buddhism to deal with loneliness, powerlessness, and meaninglessness in the modern industrialized society (Fromm 1959; Riesman et al. 1967).

> By the 1990s, Buddhism is no longer exotic. Bits and pieces lie around in American culture. Health professionals have secularized meditation, often using it simply as a kind of tranquilizer. Christian clergy borrow the same techniques, using them to attract modern Americans searching for an experiential ground for their ultimate beliefs… Writers like Thomas Merton tamed Zen, convincing some that it was not a distinct religion but pure mysticism (Tamney 1992, p. 102).

Accounts of the historical engagement with Buddhism in America and the West provide a useful backdrop for the understanding of the seldom-acknowledged Buddhist influence on the third-wave behavioral interventions such as ACT. It also invites us to be open-minded in order to fully appreciate Buddhism and not necessarily attempt to comprehend it from a Western lens, which tends to be analytic rather than holistic and intolerant of paradoxes (Cheng 1973; Varnum et al. 2010).

Philosophy Underlying ACT: Functional Contextualism

ACT is underpinned by a philosophy of science called *functional contextualism*, which has its roots in *pragmatism* and *contextualism* (Hayes et al. 1999). Pragmatism is concerned with the effective realization of beneficial goals based on human necessities and desirabilities within the context that we live in (Rescher 2012). Contextualism is a worldview that can be understood through examining its *root metaphor* of "an-act-in-context," that is, in any life event, actions cannot be understood separately from its context, including its current and past history and environment (Fox 2006). It is noteworthy that key figures of American pragmatism, including William James and John Dewey, were in fact heavily influenced by Buddhism as they developed their philosophy, including the functionalist orientation of Buddhism (Scott 1995, 2011).

Functional contextualism is not interested in any ontological claims about "truth." Instead, the truth criterion is "workability"—that is, the truth of any idea or concept depends pragmatically on its success in achieving a stated purposive goal (Hayes et al. 1999). The specific stated goal of *functional contextualism* is to be able to predict and influence the psychological events of interest (i.e., thoughts, feelings, behaviors) by deriving empirically based concepts and rules and manipulating contexts.

Theory of the Mind and Understanding of Suffering in RFT/ACT

Based on functional contextualism, relational frame theory (RFT) is a scientific theory to explain complex human behaviors, including language and cognition (Hayes et al. 2001). According to RFT, human language, the use of symbols externally in communication or internally in thought, developed from our unique capacity to relate events arbitrarily in a specific way. Properties of relational responding include: mutual entailment, combinatorial entailment, and transformation of stimulus functions. Mutual entailment describes the bidirectionality of stimulus relations [e.g., if A is greater than B, then B is less than A—in the class of "relational frame" of comparisons (of quantities)]. Combinatorial entailment describes the relationships among more than two stimuli, which themselves are in mutual entailment (e.g., if A is great than B and B is great than C, then A is great than C and C is less than A). Transformation of stimulus function is when function of one stimulus in the relational network is altered based on the functions of another stimulus in the network and the derived relation between the two (e.g., if A is greater than B and B becomes anxiety-provoking, then A also becomes anxiety-provoking and even more so than B.) There are many different types of arbitrary relationships that can be formed. A particular kind of relational frame, deictic relations, specify relations with respect to the perspective of a speaker—such as I versus you, here versus there, now versus then. This gives rise to a sense of self, which may be critical for perspective taking.

Based on RFT, the clinical implication for ACT practitioners is that language and cognition can be seen as the root of psychological suffering, and as such, it is intrinsic and inevitable to the "normal" human condition (Hayes et al. 1999). This suffering comes from our inherent capacity to form arbitrary connections between events; the inability to let go of and function outside of this constructed illusory world; and the engagement in avoidant behaviors or actions dictated by unworkable rules rather than pursuing a meaningful life. The ability to make arbitrary comparisons and relationships can give rise clinically to thoughts like "I am less worthy than her" or "death is less painful than living." In fact, the concept of suffering is a psychological verbal construct, hence the useful therapeutic distinction between pain and suffering. The ACT consistent adage "pain is inevitable, suffering is optional" by Japanese writer Murakami Haruki expresses this point. Our capacity to think is often the root of psychological suffering due to verbal processes (i.e., when we get entangled in our thoughts and feel stuck, disappointed, angered, jealous, etc.), and it is also this capacity that makes us become aware of and judge that we are "suffering."

Understanding of Suffering and Theory of the Mind in Zen Buddhism

Suffering is one of the core concepts in Buddhist psychology and is part of The Four Noble Truths, one of the most widely known Buddhist teachings. They are: (1) there is suffering (*dukkha*); (2) the roots and nature of suffering (*samudaya*) can be known, and they arise from ignorance, attachment/desire, and aversion; (3) cessation (*nirodha*) of creating suffering or emancipation from suffering is possible (by letting go of the desire and attachment); and (4) the path (*marga*) to enlightenment or the path to liberate us from doing things that lead to suffering is the Noble Eightfold Path (Bodhi 1994; Nhất Hạnh 1991, 1999; Santina 1984). The Noble Eightfold Path, which will be described in detail in a latter section, can be grouped into three clusters: (i) Wisdom (prajñā)—Right View (samyag-dṛṣṭi) and Right Intention (samyak-saṃkalpa); (ii) Ethical Conduct (śīla)—Right Speech (samyag-vāc), Right Action (samyak-karmānta), and Right Livelihood (samyag-ājīva); and (iii) Concentration of the Mind (samādhi)—Right Effort (samyag-vyāyāma), Right Mindfulness (samyak-smṛti), and Right Concentration (samyak-samādhi)).

The first noble truth of *dukkha* or suffering is often misunderstood to mean that living is nothing but pain and suffering. Actually, suffering in Buddhism refers to being caught in a cyclic existence of dissatisfaction (*samsara*) arising from wrong perceptions or an ignorance of the Three Dharma Seals (Dharma mudra), leading to attachment, craving and grasping that fuel the samara cycle. The Three Dharma Seals are as follows: impermanence (anitya)—all phenomena change, arising and disintegrating; nonself (anatman)—there is no separate independent self/entities; and true freedom (nirvana)—extinction of ignorance can lead to liberation from the cycle of samsara (Nhất Hạnh 1999). Our attachment and desire for things to be permanent when they are not can become a source of our suffering (e.g., in grief and loss). Our perception of things being discrete entities also causes us to suffer as we develop dualistic thinking. For example, the distinction of me versus not me and mine versus not mine gives rise to emotions such as desire, jealousy, greed, and hatred.

According to Zen, the correct perception includes seeing everything as interconnected, invoked in concepts such as *interbeing* (i.e., any one thing or self is actually made of nonself elements and thus is dependent on and inseparable from other things) and *interpenetration* (i.e., one thing contains all existing things, and all things contain that one thing), and hence the transcendence of dualistic thinking is central to Buddhist teachings. The Three Dharma Seals constitute a way of understanding suffering as well as the key to truly perceive reality. "To get to that reality, we have to let go of the images we create in our consciousness and our notions of self and other, inside and outside. Our practice is to correct this tendency to discriminate and think dualistically, so that reality will have a chance to reveal itself" (Nhất Hạnh 2006, p. 57). In fact, this is applicable to all dualistic concepts so that we can "go beyond ideas of being and nonbeing, coming and going, same and different, birth and death" (Nhất Hạnh 2006, p. 184).

It may be difficult to accept or understand this let alone truly achieve this unless we have reached the proposed state of enlightenment. However, Thích Nhất Hạnh encourages us to begin on this journey by perceiving the cloud and rain as being in the flower rather than as distinct entities. We can understand this rationally—the cloud gives rise to rain that becomes part of the flower when it is absorbed. The challenge is to be able to reach this through perception and contemplation rather than intellectualized understanding, and to be able to experience other things in this similar interconnected way, transcending notions of time, space, or boundaries. Experiencing this kind of interdependence will make the distinction and boundaries between dependence, independence, and interdependence fuzzy—the boundaries themselves may or may not exist.

In this vein, in Buddhist psychology, the mind and body are recognized as one. Based on the Manifestation-Only school, there are eight different consciousnesses: store consciousness, manas, mind consciousness, and the five sense consciousness (Nhất Hạnh 2006). Each of these consciousnesses can be understood as representing a different layer or function of consciousness, yet they are also considered one consciousness. For instance, our store consciousness, the deepest "root" layer of consciousness "inter-be with other consciousnesses. The one contains and is made of the all, and the all contains and is made of the one" (Nhất Hạnh 2006, p. 77).

The store consciousness is the ground and storage of all mental phenomena (in fact, including all phenomena, if the dualistic distinction between psychological and real world is completely let go of). Psychologically, information that we have received and phenomena that we have experienced or perceived are stored and preserved metaphorically as "seeds" in our consciousness. For example, names, words, and related images that are learned through our current life experience become seeds in the store consciousness. Our store consciousness is also thought to include seeds that may not have been learned by an individual in this lifetime (Nhất Hạnh 2006). Transcending the constraints of time, space, or any kind of duality/boundaries (e.g., objective vs. subjective worlds, individual vs. collective consciousness), seeds may reflect influences that occur even before an individual's lifetime, by the society at large, as well as by the physical environment. Just as the cloud and rain are in the flower, there may be latent seeds in an individual laid down by his/her ancestors or former lives (i.e., transcending time through karma), by society (e.g., shared seeds in the collective consciousness; the impact of systemic factors like racism), and even by the physical environment (i.e., transcending space or boundaries and connecting what apparently are unrelated things or events like the "butterfly effect" in chaos theory).

Under certain conditions and context, latent seeds will become manifestations and conceptually develop into and experienced as "mental formations." The exact number of mental formations varies according to the specific Buddhist schools. A system taught by Zen Master Thich Nhất Hạnh includes 51 mental formations (Nhất Hạnh 2006).[1] There are five "universal" mental formations (contact, attention, feeling, perception, and volition), which manifest in all layers of consciousness. Five particular mental formations (zeal, determination, mindfulness, concentration, and insight) are associated with manas, mind consciousness, and the five sense consciousness. There are 11 wholesome mental formations (e.g., faith; inner shame or remorse; outer shame or humility; absence of craving; equanimity; nondiscrimination; nonviolence, etc.), 26 unwholesome mental formations (e.g., greed; craving or attachment; hatred, etc.), and 4 indeterminate mental formations.

The wholesome or unwholesome "mental formations" arise from wholesome seeds (e.g., love, compassion, peace, understanding, joy, etc.) and unwholesome seeds (e.g., greed, hatred, ignorance, pride, jealousy, etc.), respectively. This teaching has the function of preventing complete moral relativism and serves as a guide toward increasing our compassion and well-being while lessening our suffering. These seeds and formations are not dualistic in the sense of being categorically different or diametrically opposites, like good and evil, god and devil. Rather, the metaphors help us understand the karmic consequences of cultivating and expressing different kinds of seeds. Indeed, the path toward ending suffering involves cultivating the wholesome seeds while transforming unwholesome seeds through mindfulness and other practices.

Manas is the second deepest layer of consciousness, evolving from the store consciousness (Nhất Hạnh 2006). Manas is thought to grasp on to the "perceiver" aspect within store consciousness, cling on to a mental representation of it, and defend it, thereby creating an illusory autonomous and independent psychological self. This corresponds to learning deictic frames in RFT, i.e., learning the distinction between "I" and "not-I." Manas is driven by craving and delusions arising from unwholesome seeds, and thus its perception is distorted.

The five sense consciousness arises when our five sense organs acting as "sense base" (i.e., eyes, ears, tongue, nose, or body) are in contact with their corresponding "objects of the senses" (i.e., form, sound, taste, smell, and tactile sensation) (Nhất Hạnh 2006). Similarly, our mind consciousness arises when manas as the "sense base" is in contact with the "objects of the mind." The information that manas passes on to the

[1]For more details on the 51 mental formations, refer to chart available at Plum Village website—http://plumvillage.org/transcriptions/51-mental-formation/.

mind consciousness from the store consciousness is usually distorted because of the nature of manas, and therefore, our mind consciousness is also vulnerable to perceiving things with distortion.

Our mind consciousness operates in five different states of mind (Nhất Hạnh 2006). It can operate with sense consciousness (e.g., when we are aware of seeing or hearing something) or independently of sense consciousness (e.g., dreaming). It can operate in a dispersed way (e.g., our usual way of thinking, getting caught up in the past or future) or in an unstable way (e.g., in a state of psychosis). Finally, it can also function in a focused way through the training of *mindfulness*. Through the energy of mindfulness, mind consciousness has the increased capacity to be in direct perception of "thing-as-it-is" in the store consciousness as opposed to distorted mental representations offered by manas and thus, the capacity to transform unwholesome seeds. Mind consciousness is the source of all our actions in thought, speech, and behavior. With the state of mindfulness and the correct perception of impermanence, nonself, and interbeing, mind consciousness as the "gardener" will help cultivate the wholesome seeds in our store consciousness, ultimately bearing the fruit of enlightenment and cessation of suffering.

At this point, it is useful to note that the overall formulation of suffering caused by attachment to language and cognition in RFT and ACT bears some correspondence to Buddhism. The constructed relational frames in RFT, and hence our thoughts and psychological way of making sense of the world, may be seen as a natural cause of our belief in the illusions of permanence and selfhood in our psychological representation of the world. From a Buddhist perspective, true perception of reality arises when all constructed relational frames are let go of. This is consistent with the emphasis on the benefits of mindfulness meditation where the practice is not to attain more logical understanding but to loosen our attachment to all our words, thoughts, concepts, and language. It is also of note that Buddhist psychology has a lot of elaborations such as seeds and mental formations that are completely absent in RFT/ACT, as is further discussed in the next section.

Acceptance and Commitment Therapy and Relationship to Zen

ACT is the clinical application of functional contextualism and RFT. In clinical practice, ACT seeks to promote six psychological processes: defusion, acceptance, contact with the present moment, self-as-context, values, and committed action (Hayes et al. 1999, 2012). These six processes are all interrelated and enhance an individual's psychological flexibility, which is "the ability to contact the present moment more fully as a conscious human being and to change or persist in behavior when doing so serves valued ends" (Hayes and Strosahl 2004).

Cognitive defusion is the ACT process of relating to thoughts as thoughts, no more and no less. We often do not notice our process of thinking and relate to our thoughts as if they are *fused* with reality and that the two are equivalent, especially if we believe our thoughts to be logical and true. While our thoughts are indispensably helpful most of the time, they are but a tool and a mere representation of the real world. Even the truest thought is in effect just a thought. An ACT metaphor illustrates this—no matter how detailed and precise you think of a chair, you cannot sit on the chair in your thought (Hayes et al. 1999). In therapy, cognitive defusion exercises aim to facilitate clients to experience and gradually gain the capacity to defuse from their thoughts, regardless of whether they believe their thought to be true or not. This can be applied equally to all types of thoughts, including thoughts that often engender a sense of rigidity and "stuckness," including judgments or evaluations ("*I am an utter failure*"); assumptions ("*I will never succeed or get better*"); or rules ("*I can never do something that makes me feel anxious").* This allows us to relate to our thoughts differently when they are not helpful to us. For example, a client may be asked to repeat a word out loud for a minute and notice that the word begins to lose its meaning, or guiding a client to label or thank their thoughts (e.g., "here it goes… a judgment… thank you, mind, for giving me this thought") rather than engaging with the thoughts' content. Thus, unlike other types of therapies, the emphasis is not on evaluating the thoughts; gaining understanding and insight; nor changing them into more positive, desirable, or rational thoughts. The therapeutic aim is on increasing the capacity to flexibly relate to these thoughts in a defused way when these thoughts are not helpful; rather than adhering to concepts and rules when they are not beneficial in a particular context, it increases our behavioral repertoire and responsiveness to real-world contingencies, thereby promoting "workability" in life.

Similarly, in Buddhist psychology, suffering occurs when perceptions generated from seeds in our store consciousness are reified and treated as aspects of the ultimate truth. In this process of reification, reality is objectified and the object is apprehended as "an alien thing that is independent of its producer" (Moore 1995, p. 701). The reified mental image and representations (e.g., dreams, imagination, or perceived reality) are fueled by our "habit energies" derived from all sources of past and present experiences and thoughts, including those from our ancestors, friends and family, and society; they prevent us from seeing things as they truly are (Nhất Hạnh 2006). Through mindfulness practice, Zen Buddhists seek to de-reify habitual patterns of thoughts and socialized perceptions of reality and to extinguish the notions of permanence and duality.

Acceptance in ACT describes the state of openness and willingness to experience what is present *internally*, including thoughts, feelings, emotions, and sensations. It is not, as it is often misunderstood to be, the passive acceptance of the conditions that lead to suffering. Acceptance is distinguished from experiential avoidance (Hayes et al. 1996), where one may attempt to control, suppress, or withdraw from these aversive internal experiences. Experiential avoidance is thought to be at the heart of many forms of apparent psychopathology as well as other common difficulties presenting in therapy. The act of avoidance itself can sometimes directly lead to worsening symptoms, such as pain or anxiety, contributing to "dirty" psychological pain which compounds the "clean" original pain (Hayes et al. 1996). Persistent avoidance may also reinforce rigid unworkable avoidant behaviors, which become a barrier to doing meaningful activities.

Metaphors are often helpful to enable clients to reflect on the nature of avoidance versus acceptance. An example is the reflection of what happens if one engages in a tug-of-war with a stronger opponent, such as an imagined overpowering "anxiety" monster (Hayes et al. 1999). One might be using all of one's strength if the stakes are high and the tug-of-war takes place over a bottomless abyss between one and the monster. In this case, a viable option is to "let go" of the rope, even if this means having to continue to face the monster on the other side of the abyss. In this metaphor, acceptance is the "letting go" of the struggle, even if it does not eliminate what is feared. This is distinct from "giving up" as it takes courage to let go of the struggle to face what is feared. Other similar physicalized metaphors, such as the Chair Sculpture of Suffering (Fung and Zurowski 2016), may also be used to engage clients in a group format to explore the stance of acceptance. In this exercise, the group facilitator invites participants to use their own chairs representing coping strategies to cover up the "chair of pain" in the center of the group circle, thereby creating a "chair sculpture of suffering." The participants can be invited to observe that their coping strategies do not eliminate pain and discomfort (the center chair) but can add to suffering (overall sculpture), regardless of what the coping strategy is. They can collectively reflect on how much effort they have exerted in this process, as they sacrifice their own chair to build the sculpture. Clients often find this to be a nonblaming approach. Through this exercise, their efforts to cope are acknowledged, while they also become aware that their diligence in finding a cure rather than accepting what they feel may have compounded their suffering, especially if they have devoted a lot of resources to fighting pain, anxiety, or other internal discomfort.

In Buddhism, acceptance is also promoted, but quite differently from ACT. Mindfulness can be used to foster an acceptance stance in order to transform unwholesome seeds and mental formations, including negative thoughts and feelings. "It is important to learn to embrace our anger, to recognize it and allow it to be. Then we can touch it with our mindfulness in order to transform it… every time a negative formation is recognized, it loses some of its strength" (Nhất Hạnh 2006, p. 80). The notion of *emptiness* in Zen Buddhism, essentially the concept of nonself, that describes the lack of independent durable essential nature of any entity also offers the wisdom that promotes acceptance. In the Heart Sutra, Bodhisattva Avalokita says, "Listen, Shariputra, form is emptiness, and emptiness is form. Form is not other than emptiness, emptiness is not other than form. The same is true with feelings, perceptions, mental formations, and consciousness…" (Nhất Hạnh 2012, p. 411). Thus, emptiness includes the emptiness of form (a permanent body), feelings, perceptions, mental formations, and consciousness. Finally, the concept of karma and past lives (collective histories and conditions) can foster radical acceptance of both internal and external conditions. The law of karma describes the nature of cause and effect, sowing seeds (individually and collectively) will eventually bear their corresponding fruits, wholesome or unwholesome (Nhất Hạnh 2006; Santina 1984). Therefore, it is not a pessimistic fatalistic retreat, but a fundamental way of promoting acceptance of our current contextual circumstances and responsibility for our actions that influence the future. The notion of transformation of unwholesome seeds and mental formations; the realization of emptiness; and the understanding of karma all draw on unique beliefs of Buddhism that is not within ACT and, therefore, promote acceptance in a way that ACT does not.

Contact with the Present Moment in ACT refers to the deliberate practice of attending to what is present in the here-and-now. While there is only one reality which is embedded in the on-going "now," our capacity for thought allows us to get stuck thinking about the past, which might have been filled with anger, hurt, trauma, or regrets or paralyzed in fearing for an imagined future. Increased contact with the present moment may support us to decrease our suffering associated with getting stuck in the past or worrying about the future. This also involves taking ourselves off "autopilot" and allowing ourselves to be in fuller contact with whatever actions that are being engaged in including eating, walking, and other complex behaviors. This may lead to renewed appreciation of positive and other rewarding experiences. It increases our capacity to react more flexibly and appropriately to the situational context rather than by reacting based on learned habits, unworkable rules, or reactive impulses. In an ACT session, the therapist may simply draw the client's attention to and observation of the "here-and-now," including immediate feelings and thoughts, to increase contact with the present moment. The therapist may also encourage the patient to work on this skill during and/or outside the therapy session by doing formal mindfulness practice of being in the present moment and being aware of the here-and-now; these practice activities are often taken or adapted from traditional Zen Buddhist meditative practices.

From a Buddhist perspective, mindfulness unites the body and mind and enables us to be aware of our physical body (feelings and sensations), our perceptions (thoughts, ideas, and views), and our disposition (habit energies that work with our store consciousness). Mindfulness practice enables us to look deeply (*vipashyana*) to gain the understanding that is needed to transform our own suffering and the suffering of the world (Nhất Hạnh 1999). Mindfulness meditative practice is an important step in practicing the Noble Eightfold Path—with Right Mindfulness, we are able to develop Right View and Right Thinking, which is integral to Right Speech, Right Action, Right Livelihood, and Right Diligence, and the cycle of practice goes on (see below). Thus, mindfulness in Buddhism is grounded in the ultimate purpose of achieving enlightenment, which is not the purpose of ACT. In mindfulness-based psychological interventions, mindfulness is often taken to be a skill to decrease psychological suffering, detached from its spiritual roots.

Self-as-context is also referred to as the *transcendent self* or *observer self*. This concept helps clients loosen up their attachment to the *conceptualized self* formed by identification of the self with any kind of psychological content, such as thoughts (e.g., "I am my thoughts"), feelings (e.g., "I am happy"), roles (e.g., "I am a father," "I am a psychologist," etc.), personality traits ("I am shy"), sociocultural identities ("I am Caucasian"), memories, self-narratives, and body image. While these concepts and phenomena help a person maintain a coherent view of the self and guide function in our daily lives, this fusion may also lead to rigidity when the person is unable to make changes in his action patterns. For example, a person who identifies himself or herself as "damaged" may refuse to engage in intimate relationships. Strong attachment to self-concepts may also lead to suffering from perceived losses of the self. For example, a person who strongly identifies with being a parent may be unable to recover when their child dies and they feel a part of the self has died.

In contrast, self-as-context refers to the experience of the self as the context in which psychological content occurs as opposed to the contents themselves. This is most directly experienced as being the "I" (and "not you") in the "here-and-now" across time and space, hence the transcendent sense of self. Metaphors can be used to facilitate contact with this observer self, such as the commonly used chess metaphor (Hayes et al. 1999). While clients may be entangled with which chess pieces best represent their true selves or their correct thoughts, the clients are guided to notice the difference between seeing themselves as the individual chess pieces versus being the board that holds all the pieces. The chessboard continues to be there regardless of the chess pieces' positions, which side is winning, or which side is "correct." Rather than struggling with having positive beliefs or true beliefs about the self, realizing that the self-as-context can continue on regardless of content can be an empowering experience in increasing one's resilience.

As discussed, the loosening of our attachment to self-concepts can be found in the Dharma Seal of nonself (*anatman*), a key Buddhist doctrine. The notions of nonself and impermanence are intricately connected. Since all things are constantly changing, they are devoid of absolute identity, and therefore, "A is not A, B is not B, and A can be B" (Nhất Hạnh 1995, p. 39). Furthermore, the practice of looking deeply into our self (through mindfulness practice) enables us to step outside of our subjective self to better appreciate the reality of nonself and the principle of *dependent arising*, that is, the conditions necessary to make up our objective world in relation to others (Kalupahana 1988). It allows us to see the reality of interbeing, that is, we do not exist independent of others; the self is made only of nonself elements, and humans are made up of nonhuman elements (Nhất Hạnh 1999). Things come into manifestation when the right conditions exist, as Thich Nhất Hạnh writes: "All that is created and destroyed, all that can be obtained and lost, is conditioned. A thing is lost when the conditions are no longer favorable" (Nhất Hạnh 1995, p. 83). The wisdom behind The Three Dharma Seals is for us to recognize concepts as concepts (e.g., Buddha is God) and not to confuse concepts with reality (e.g., Buddha nature in human).

The Buddhist doctrines of suffering, emptiness, and nonself are often misunderstood as a religion of pessimism, nihilism, or self-denial. However, Kalupahana (1988) suggests that Buddhist psychology of the mind, which recognizes the five mutually dependent aspects of the conscious human personality (the material body, feelings or sensation, perception, disposition, and consciousness), provides a solution to the Cartesian dualistic conceptualization of the separate body and mind. Zen Buddhism, based on the Mahayana tradition, emphasizes that enlightenment is achieved through one's awareness and insights, which cannot be transmitted by the Zen teacher (Suzuki 1994). Zen practices of mindfulness and koan[2] function as paths to enlightenment that enable us to let go of the wrong view of an independent enduring self and to recognize that our subjective self ("I") exists only in the context of the objective conditions surrounding us.

Nonself in Buddhism may seem contradictory to the apparent enduring nature of self-as-context. It may be helpful to understand that self-as-context in ACT is not an ontological claim of an enduring spiritual self but a useful concept for psychological functioning; in RFT, the sense of self arises from forming deictic frames discussed above, as we learn to distinguish "I" versus "you." In fact, it can also be pointed out that a dualistic understanding of self versus nonself is not accurate in Buddhism, as both are ideas that need to be transcended in the ultimate dimension. "The notion of self relies on the notion of nonself. Both ideas are products of our conceptual mind… nonself is a crucial teaching… But the teaching is not something to worship… When we are able to touch reality, both notions will be removed" (Nhất Hạnh 2006, p. 164).

In summary, both Buddhism and ACT acknowledge the pragmatic use of self for daily functioning. ACT loosens attachment to conceptualized self when it is not helpful, but reinforces self-as-context as it is still rooted in typical Western psychology. Buddhism goes one step further than ACT as it advocates for giving up the need to hang on to a sense of an autonomous independent self in spiritual development, and does not view it necessary for psychological health, especially as it embraces interdependence and nondualism, notions that will avoid nihilism but are missing in ACT.

Values refer to what an individual person holds as being most important to them in their lives. This is distinguished from goals that are achievable. The commonly used metaphor is that values serve as a guiding direction while goals are individual destinations along the way. If one's path is obstructed along a guided direction, one can find alternative paths to express the underlying values, enhancing one's flexibility. As values are not something that is ever attainable or able to be completed like a goal, this broad sense of life direction engenders less fusion with ideas like failure. In ACT, clients are encouraged to reflect on and clarify what their freely chosen values in various life domains are, including how they want to behave in their workplace; how they want to interact with their friends and family; how they want to parent; how they would like to be in touch with their spirituality; how they want to contribute to the community, etc.

There is an inherent clinical assumption in ACT that clients' chosen core values contain social and altruistic aspects that can lead to a meaningful and fulfilling life (Hayes et al. 2012). An ACT therapist's task is not to judge the clients' values or impose their own social values on the clients but to help them clarify their values. Sometimes, apparent selfish interests that are being pursued are really a "means" to an "ends," a "pseudo-value," rather than true values that need to be teased out (e.g., if a person said his value is to make a lot of money, behind this could be his value in providing for his family and loved ones) (Hayes et al. 2012).

Unlike ACT which emphasizes freely chosen values, Zen Buddhist values are grounded in the Noble Eightfold Paths (see below) and the five mindfulness training or precepts. These values do not constitute absolute laws to govern one's action. In Zen Buddhism, "good is what produces good consequences (attha) and such consequences are dependently arisen, that is, they depend upon various factors pertaining within each context" (Kalupahana 1988, pp. 301–302

In Zen Buddhism ethics, a person is considered inherently ethical. However, people often act in unethical ways because their Buddha nature has been distorted by conditioning that arises from ignorance and attachment (Brazier 1996). One can reconnect to one's Buddha nature—the capacity to wake up, to understand, and to love—

[2]Koan is a riddle or story that is not to be solved by reasoning, but to be contemplated on through concentration and mindfulness to advance the study and practice of Zen.

through mindfulness practice. Zen Buddhist principles of ethics and notions of wholesome and unwholesome seeds in the context of the Noble Eightfold Paths may be useful in supporting clients to identify and clarify their values. Perhaps one of the most important Zen Buddhist values that may enhance the effectiveness of ACT is the unconditional compassion for the interdependent self and sentient beings. In Buddhism, compassionate acceptance is thought to transform habit energies that fuel unwholesome seeds in our store consciousness.

Committed Action

Ultimately, one of the emphases in ACT is to enable clients to act in alignment with their values and thereby to fully live their life with vitality and meaning, with an assumption that this potential is within each client. Clients are encouraged to use the other ACT processes to overcome barriers, freeing themselves from reasoning as barriers and various forms of experiential avoidance, in the service of their values. The commitment can be seen as the deliberate and persistent engagement in an ever-larger pattern of action to express one's values. In therapy, many kinds of common behavioral interventions, from exposure to behavioral activation to various kinds of homework, may be framed as committed action when linked with specific chosen values.

In Buddhism, actions (karma) are of three types: mind action (thoughts), speech action, and bodily action (Nhất Hạnh 2006). Thus, similar to functional contextualism, thoughts are treated as an action/behavior. Our mind consciousness can initiate actions that result in cultivating wholesome or unwholesome seeds. By practicing the Noble Eightfold Path, we learn to nurture and sustain wholesome seeds and mental formations, while returning unwholesome seeds and mental formations to the store consciousness. Speech and bodily actions are also thought to result in seeds that can transcend life-and-death in the store consciousness, and be transmitted continuously through our interbeing.

Ultimately, liberation from suffering is possible through acting in accordance with the Noble Eightfold Path. In Zen Buddhism, something is "right" when it is connected to the path of liberation from suffering, including the understanding of the Three Dharma Seals. The interrelated Noble Eightfold Paths are summarized here (Bodhi 1994; Nhất Hạnh 1999; Santina 1984):

1. Right View is our ability to distinguish wholesome roots or seeds (kushala mula) from unwholesome roots in the depth of our stored consciousness, and to let go of our perceptions.
2. Right Thinking occurs when our thinking is aligned with Right View and when our body and mind are in unity through the practice of mindfulness.
3. Right Mindfulness is at the heart of Buddhist teaching. Mindfulness (smriti) is returning to the present moment; Right Mindfulness embraces everything without judging or reacting; it is a practice of finding ways to sustain appropriate attention throughout the day.
4. Right Speech is being aware of the suffering caused by unmindful speech and the commitment to cultivating deep listening and loving speech to bring joy and happiness to others.
5. Right Action is closely linked to four of the five Buddhist precepts or mindfulness trainings: reverence for life; generosity and commitment to social justice; ethical sexual responsibilities; and mindful consumption.
6. Right Diligence or Right Effort consists of practices that are based on Right View: preventing unwholesome seeds in our store consciousness from arising; helping unwholesome seeds that have arisen to return to our store consciousness; watering wholesome seeds in our store consciousness to promote blossoms; and nourishing wholesome seeds that have arisen so they stay strong in our mind consciousness.
7. Right Concentration is the practice of cultivating a one-pointed mind of evenness; there are two kinds of concentration—active and

selective. In active concentration, the mind dwells on the present moment; in selective concentration, we select one object to focus on this object to gain insight and liberation from suffering.

8. Right Livelihood refers to earning one's living without transgressing the five Buddhist precepts or mindfulness trainings. Based on the Zen Buddhist doctrine of interbeing and interdependent co-rising, Right Livelihood is viewed not as a personal matter but our collective karma.

Clinical Application of ACT

ACT is based on a transdiagnostic model of human suffering that is not specific to a particular type of psychopathology. As discussed, it has been widely applied to many different clinical populations, including depression, anxiety, and psychotic disorders (A-Tjak et al. 2015; Ruiz 2010). It has also been applied to many non-clinical populations, such as for preventing burnout and addressing issues related to stigma. There is great variability in how it is applied, from traditional individual therapy to group therapy; from single-session to short-term to long-term therapy; from clinical setting to educational/work setting to public setting. To remain consistent to the ACT model, it is more important that the techniques are flexibly applied and consistent with its principles rather than rigidly striving to conform to rigid standards or structure (Hayes et al. 2012). The therapist's capacity to adopt an acceptance stance toward the patient and guide experiential rather than intellectual learning is a key.

Clinical Case Example

The following is a disguised composite case example illustrating how ACT was applied to foster acceptance, enhance resilience, and increase committed action. In this case, the client had been followed by a psychiatrist over several years from a chance inpatient encounter to continued outpatient follow-up. The use of ACT was embedded in psychiatric follow-up appointments longitudinally over the years.

Ms. Chen is a 42-year-old married woman, who immigrated from China to Canada around 5 years ago. Her first experience with psychiatry was being involuntarily detained at a hospital two years ago when she was three months postpartum. She presented with severe depression with anxiety and psychotic symptoms. She was initially reluctant to disclose much about her experience to the treating team. Her husband and 10-year-old son visited her regularly at the hospital, and the whole family minimized her symptoms because of the stigma around mental illness and the fears about being detained in a hospital. When she was connected to a Chinese psychiatrist who facilitated her dialogue with the treatment team and subsequent discharge, she became hesitantly more trusting with treatment. The therapeutic relationship with the psychiatrist gradually increased over time after her condition became more stable and the psychiatrist helped her negotiated through another child protection services issue as an outpatient.

Ms. Chen and her husband are well off. Her husband works in China most of the time operating a very successful business. They moved to Canada because of the one child policy and for their son's education. While she became less depressed with medication treatment, she continued to have significant anxiety symptoms. An ACT approach was used by the psychiatrist to engage the patient and facilitate her recovery. Through therapy, she became aware that both she and the psychiatrist could observe rather than to judge her thoughts, emotions, and imageries in her mind, and she gradually opened up much more about her experiences.

She disclosed that she actually had vivid hallucinations of herself throwing her child out of the window when she was hospitalized. For some time, she had also been experiencing visual hallucinations of her husband's face on the wall yelling at her. When she got agitated, she screamed back or threw things at the wall. At times, she experienced symptoms of dissociation because of her distress, including sleepwalking at night. She further disclosed about an emotional abusive cycle from her husband where he becomes verbally abusive and apologizes afterward. She talked about how this reminded her of being yelled at by her mother, who favored her other siblings in the family. Her parents gave her a boy's name and were disappointed that she turned out to be the third girl in the family. Her younger brother, however, had been showered with affection. Her mother also was particularly harsh on her since her appearance resembled her mother's critical mother-in-law.

Defusion exercises helped her slowly face some of her internalized deprecating thoughts about herself. In one exercise, she wrote down some of these thoughts on paper, read them backward, and began to experience these thoughts in a different way. Mindfulness exercises were introduced to further help her become an observer of her own thoughts rather than getting attached to the meaning of her thoughts. Self-as-context work helped her become less attached to her negative labels about herself.

At one of the turning points in treatment, the patient was facing an acute crisis, as she had to return to China to attend her aunt's funeral. She had not seen her mother for years. She remained terrified of seeing her critical mother. She was bitter that her mother continued to favor all her other siblings, even though she was the only child in the family who had been financially supporting her mother over the years. From time to time, her mother would express care and concern about her siblings' finances and compelled her to help them financially as well.

Through an intense guided imagery exercise, she was able to deeply get in touch with her past traumatic memories of being verbally abused by her mother. Physicalizing her emotions in her mind, including both her anger and fear, she was able to make room for these emotions in her heart. She was able to regain her strength by remaining in contact with the present moment of her as an adult and be in touch with her observer self. The idea of the double-sided coin of suffering and values was introduced. She was able to connect with her painful yearning for her mother's approval, and through this, get in touch with her values as a daughter and love for her mother.

The use of ACT helped the patient to face and relate to her mother in a more mindful compassionate way. She became aware of how frail and old her mother was. She had become more accepting of her mother, while allowing herself to be aware of, and yet not controlled by, various kinds of negative thoughts and emotions about her mother. Forgiveness and acceptance from an ACT perspective and compassion and loving-kindness from the Zen perspective were discussed. At this point, her hallucinations of her mother and husband scolding at her dramatically decreased. She felt more empowered to relate to her husband. She took active steps to confront her husband about his behaviors. She chose to remain in the relationship and has been asserting her boundaries more decisively. Her sense of helplessness and suicidal ideation has resolved and has been dedicating her time to care for her children and resume some long-distance work in China.

Discussion

Despite a lack of explicit reference to the application of Zen Buddhist philosophy in ACT, we have shown that ACT is aligned with some of the principles and practices of Zen Buddhism. Namely, as in Zen Buddhist practice, ACT uses experiential exercises that support clients to gain insights about their attachment to concepts and stuckness in their habit energies. It emphasizes the importance of context in understanding one's suffering.

However, we have also discussed a number of important differences between Zen Buddhism and ACT. ACT does not have the goal of achieving nirvana or liberation from samsara. It does not teach any of the Three Dharma Seals specifically, including the concept of impermanence and nonself. Hence, interdependence and nondualism are not really discussed in ACT. ACT does not consist of sets of precepts or specific values, nor the idea of cultivating wholesome manifestations and seeds and transforming unwholesome ones.

These differences encourage ACT clients to develop psychological flexibility and achieve liberation based on their own set of values and religious beliefs. However, this may also potentially pose challenges and contradiction when one's values are not aligned with the emphasis of context in both ACT and Zen Buddhism. For example, beliefs in certain dogma as the absolute nonnegotiable truth may lead to certain stuckness (e.g., eyes-closed meditation invites the devil; homosexual practice is evil; substance abuse is a moral flaw, etc.)

While mindfulness meditative practices have been adopted in Western psychology, it is often adopted as a standalone technique or skill to be practiced independent of one's belief system or value. In Zen Buddhism, mindfulness practice is a focused practice, that is, being mindful of something (e.g., being mindful of the reality of nonself, or the seed of anger in store consciousness). In the absence of Buddhist understanding of interdependent arising, nonself, impermanence, and nonduality, it may be difficult for some ACT clients to sustain attainment of defusion or experiences of self-as-context.

Thus, if some of the core concepts of Zen Buddhism can be integrated into ACT and the clients are open to this, certain ACT processes may be more effectively grasped. Many of these concepts do not contradict RFT, but simply have not been articulated or elaborated in ACT. Illusions of permanence and independence can be introduced and become the explicit focus of defusion exercises and mindfulness practice. Contemplation of interdependence may also be embedded in a more extensive exploration of values. For example, a typical ACT values exercise may consist of contemplating one's funeral and what one would want our loved ones to say about ourselves. This can be restructured to allow deeper contemplation about our interconnected relationships, as is done in other Asian psychotherapies like Naikan therapy, where the client is rigorously invited to contemplate three questions: "(a) "What did this person give to me?" (b) "What did I return to this person?" and (c) "What trouble did I cause this person?" (Ozawa-de Silva 2015). Similarly, rather than only focusing on *self-as-context* as ACT currently does, RFT researchers suggest that it may be in theory possible to discuss *other-as-context* (Stewart and McHugh 2013). As they are both transcendental, situated in the here-and-now, they can be linked as *self-other-as-context*—effectively an interdependent state of being. Whether a clinical technique can be derived based on this RFT hypothesis remains to be seen. It may be that this is only effectively achieved through the correct practice of mindfulness and deep contemplation on interdependence such that we are truly able to perceive the other in ourselves, the cloud in the flower, and ultimately the cloud and flower in all of us.

The Zen emphasis on interconnectedness, interbeing, and nonduality has other implications as well. In understanding the symptoms of any one individual (e.g., issues with substance abuse), Zen Buddhism is likely to take a broader perspective than most therapists and will cast the problem as not only within the individual, but also reflective of all history (personal and collective), of all societies (including all realms), and of all environments. The Zen Buddhist concept of interconnectedness can offer complex insights into the increasing acknowledgment of the social and structural determinants of mental health in the West (Allen et al. 2014).

Further, as everyone and everything is ultimately connected, Zen Buddhism is critical of quietistic, individualistic practice of attaining tranquility and spiritual perfection. Zen Buddhist practice, based on Mahayana Buddhism, emphasizes total immersion in the flux of everyday life (this part is similar to ACT); it also emphasizes compassionate engagement with the world (Feleppa 2009). In Zen Buddhism, also known as engaged Buddhism, Zen practitioners possess "the willingness and capacity of being there, listening, responding to suffering and helping beings" (Nhất Hạnh 1999, p. 239). Indeed, the volitional action of Zen Buddhists does not stop until all beings are free from suffering. Finally, the Sangha, a community of Zen Buddhist practitioners, is much more explicitly emphasized in Buddhism.

In parallel, but to a more limited scale, ACT also takes a larger contextual perspective than many other psychotherapies; ACT has been used successfully to combat stigma and motivate social justice actions (Fung and Wong 2014); and there is a value-based effort in building a mutually supportive community of practice, as exemplified by the Association of Contextual Behavioral Science. It may be fruitful for ACT practitioners to dialogue and discuss strategies in supporting clients to build communities of ACT practices that promote their well-being.

Conclusion

In summary, ACT is a mindfulness-based intervention with core therapeutic processes that are congruent to some of the Zen Buddhist teachings. Its underlying philosophy, functional contextualism, and scientific theory, relational frame theory, bear some semblance to Buddhist philosophy and theory of the mind, although they are also substantially different when we appreciate distinct Buddhist concepts such as emptiness and the elaborate postulates of the mind in the Manifestation-Only school of Buddhist psychology. The aim of ACT in alleviating suffering is similar to that of Buddhism, but the scope is more mundane, modest, and limited (to psychological problems in this life) and it is much less morally prescriptive. Key concepts, like impermanence and nonself, though not incompatible, are not explicitly included, likely due to cultural reasons or the legacy of the eighteenth century Enlightenment period in the West, whereby religions were separated from medicine and healing (Koenig 2000). Thus, a successful treatment with ACT may not necessarily lead to spiritual enlightenment or a sense of collective interconnectedness. However, a deeper understanding and potential integration of some of the Buddhist principles and teachings may help ACT practitioners to become even more compassionate and effective. It is hopeful that exploration, comparison, and integration of the wisdom from Buddhist and other spiritual traditions may gradually inform the future refinement of ACT and other psychotherapies for the benefit of all. As Maex noted, "It was a stroke of genius to take mindfulness training out of the Buddhist context, but the risk might be that, instead of opening a door to the Dharma, it might also close a door leading to the vast richness of that context full of valuable insights and practices" (Maex 2011, p. 166). Rather than being stuck in scientism or looking to abstracting and Westernizing traditional practices out of their context, it may be wiser, more pragmatic, and more effective for a therapist to respectfully and meaningfully incorporate the deeper wisdom embedded in the spiritual traditions, while conducting therapy in a culturally competent, safe, and respectful manner cognizant of the client's own worldview and seeking opportunities to enhance cultural exchange and expansion of one's worldview (Lo and Fung 2003; Seiden and Lam 2010).

References

A-Tjak, J. G. L., Davis, M. L., Morina, N., Powers, M. B., Smits, J. A. J., & Emmelkamp, P. M. G. (2015). A meta-analysis of the efficacy of acceptance and commitment therapy for clinically relevant mental and physical health problems. *Psychotherapy and Psychosomatics*, *84*(1), 30–36. http://doi.org/10.1159/000365764

Allen, J., Balfour, R., Bell, R., & Marmot, M. (2014). Social determinants of mental health. *International Review of Psychiatry*, *26*(4), 392–407. doi:10.3109/09540261.2014.928270.

Bodhi, B. (1994). *The Noble eightfold path: The way to the end of suffering* (2nd ed.). Kandy: Buddhist Publication Society. Retrieved from http://www.accesstoinsight.org/lib/authors/bodhi/waytoend.html

Brazier, D. (1996). *Zen therapy: Transcending the sorrows of the human mind*. New York: Wiley.

Cheng, C.-Y. (1973). On Zen (Ch'an) language and Zen paradoxes. *Journal of Chinese Philosophy, 1*, 77–102.

Coleman, J. W. (2002). *The New Buddhism: The Western Transformation of an Ancient Tradition*. New York: Oxford University Press.

Cox, L. (2013). Rethinking early Western Buddhists: Beachcombers, "Going native" and dissident orientalism. *Contemporary Buddhism, 14*(1), 116–133. doi:10.1080/14639947.2013.785242.

Davids, C. R. (1914). *Buddhist psychology: An inquiry into the analysis and theory of mind in Pali literature*. London: G. Bell and Sons Ltd.

Emerson, R. W., & Myerson, J. E. (2015). The transcendentalist. In R. A. Bosco & J. Myerson (Eds.), *Ralph Waldo Emerson: The major prose*. Cambridge: The Belknap Press of Harvard University Press.

Feleppa, R. (2009). Zen, emotion, and social engagement. *Philosophy east and west, 59*(3), 263–293.

Fields, R. (1992). *How the Swans came to the lake: A narrative history of Buddhism in America*. Boston: Shambhala Publications.

Fox, E. J. (2006). Constructing a pragmatic science of learning and instruction with functional contextualism. *Educational Technology Research and Development, 54*(1), 5–36.

Franklin, J. J. (2008). *The lotus and the lion*. Ithaca: Cornell University Press.

Fromm, E. (1959). *Escape from freedom*. New York: Holt, Rinehart and Winston.

Fung, K. (2015). Acceptance and commitment therapy: Western adoption of Buddhist tenets? *Transcultural Psychiatry, 52*(4), 561–576. doi:10.1177/1363461514537544.

Fung, K. P., & Wong, J. (2014). *Using ACT to address HIV/AIDS stigma in ethnoracial communities*. Presented at the 12th Association for Contextual Behavioral Science (ACBS) World Conference, Minneapolis.

Fung, K. P., & Zurowski, M. (2016). Chair sculpture of suffering exercise. In A. Peterkin & P. Brett-McLean (Eds.), *Keeping reflection fresh: Top educators share their innovations in health professional education*. Kent: Kent State Press.

Hayes, S. C. (2002). Buddhism and acceptance and commitment therapy. *Cognitive and Behavioral Practice, 9*(1), 58–66.

Hayes, S. C., & Strosahl, K. D. (2004). A practical guide to acceptance and commitment therapy. Springer Science & Business Media.

Hayes, S. C., Barnes-Holmes, D., & Roche, B. (2001). *Relational frame theory: A post-Skinnerian account of human language and cognition*. New York: Kluwer Academic/Plenum Publishers.

Hayes, S. C., Follette, V. M., & Linehan, M. (2004). *Mindfulness and acceptance: Expanding the cognitive-behavioral tradition*. New York: Guilford Press.

Hayes, S. C., Strosahl, K., & Wilson, K. G. (1999). *Acceptance and commitment therapy: An experiential approach to behavior change*. New York: Guilford Press.

Hayes, S. C., Strosahl, K., & Wilson, K. G. (2012). *Acceptance and commitment therapy: The process and practice of mindful change*. New York: Guilford Press.

Hayes, S. C., Wilson, K. G., & Gifford, E. V. (1996). Experiential avoidance and behavioral disorders: A functional dimensional approach to diagnosis and treatment. *Journal of Consulting and Clinical Psychology, 64*(6), 1152–1168.

Kabat-Zinn, J. (2011). Some reflections on the origins of MBSR, skillful means, and the trouble with maps. *Contemporary Buddhism, 12*(1), 281–306. doi:10.1080/14639947.2011.564844.

Kalupahana, D. J. (1988). The buddhist conceptions of "subject" and "object" and their moral implications. *Philosophy East and West, 38*(3), 290–306.

Koenig, H. G. (2000). Religion and medicine I: Historical background and reasons for separation. *International Journal of Psychiatry in Medicine, 30*(4), 385–398.

Layman, E. M. (1976). *Buddhism in America*. Chicago: Nelson Hall.

Lo, H. T., & Fung, K. P. (2003). Culturally competent psychotherapy. *Canadian Journal of Psychiatry, 48*(3), 161–170.

Maex, E. (2011). The Buddhist roots of mindfulness training: a practitioners view. *Contemporary Buddhism, 12*(1), 165–175. doi:10.1080/14639947.2011.564835.

Moore, R. J. (1995). Dereification in Zen Buddhism. *The Sociological Quarterly, 36*(4), 699–723.

Nhất Hạnh, T. (1991). *Old path, white clouds: Walking in the footsteps of the Buddha*. Berkeley, CA: Parallax Press.

Nhất Hạnh, T. (1995). *Zen Keys*. New York: Doubleday.

Nhất Hạnh, T. (1999). *The heart of the Buddha's teaching: Transforming suffering into peace, joy & liberation*. New York: Broadway Books.

Nhất Hạnh, T. (2006). *Understanding our mind*. Berkeley, CA: Parallax Press.

Nhất Hạnh, T. (2012). *Awakening of the heart*. Berkeley: Parallax Press.

Ozawa-de Silva, C. (2015). Mindfulness of the kindness of others: The contemplative practice of Naikan in cultural context. *Transcultural Psychiatry, 52*(4), 524–542. doi:10.1177/1363461514562922.

Rescher, N. (2012). *Pragmatism: The restoration of its scientific roots*. New Brunswick: Transaction Publishers.

Riesman, D., Gitlin, T., Glazer, N., & Denney, R. (1967). *The lonely crowd: A study of the changing American character, abridged and revised edition*. New Haven: Yale University Press.

Ruiz, F. (2010). A review of acceptance and commitment therapy (ACT) empirical evidence: Correlational, experimental psychopathology, component and outcome studies. *International Journal of Psychology and Psychological Therapy, 10*(1), 125–162.

Santina, P. D. (1984). *Fundamentals of Buddhism* (pp. 1–134). Singapore: Srilankaramaya Buddhist Temple. Retrieved from http://www.buddhanet.net

Scott, D. (1995). Buddhist functionalism—Instrumentality reaffirmed. *Asian Philosophy, 5*(2), 127–149. doi:10.1080/09552369508575416.

Scott, D. (2011). William James and Buddhism: American pragmatism and the orient. *Religion, 30*(4), 333–352. doi:10.1006/reli.2000.0292.

Seiden, D. Y., & Lam, K. N. (2010). From Moses and Monotheism to Buddha and behaviorism: Cognitive behavior therapy's transpersonal crisis. *Journal of Transpersonal Psychology*.

Stewart, I., & McHugh, L. (2013). Perspective taking. In T. B. Kashdan & J. Ciarrochi (Eds.), *Mindfulness, acceptance, and positive psychology*. New Harbinger Publications.

Sutin, L. (2006). *All is change: The two-thousand-year journey of Buddhism to the west*. New York: Little, Brown and Co.

Suzuki, D. T. (1994). *Zen Koan as a means of attaining enlightenment*. Rutland: Charles E. Tuttle Co., Inc.

Tamney, J. B. (1992). *American society in the Buddhist mirror*. New York: Garland Publishing.

Turner, A. (2013). The bible, the bottle and the knife: Religion as a mode of resisting colonialism for U Dhammaloka. *Contemporary Buddhism, 14*(1), 66–77. doi:10.1080/14639947.2013.785248.

Varnum, M. E. W., Grossmann, I., Kitayama, S., & Nisbett, R. E. (2010). The origin of cultural differences in cognition: The social orientation hypothesis. *Current Directions in Psychological Science, 19*(1), 9–13. doi:10.1177/0963721409359301.

Young-Eisendrath, P., & Muramoto, S. (2002). *Awakening and insight: Zen Buddhism and psychotherapy*. Hove: Brunner-Routledge.

Zen, Pain, Suffering, and Death

Gordon M. Greene

Keywords
Zen · Suffering · Pain · Buddhism · Behavioral health · Death

That's a stark chapter title. Pain, suffering, and death evoke some of our deepest sorrows, our deepest fears. But let's start this chapter with some other emotions. I'm at my mother's bedside shortly after she had died from the progressing problems caused by chronic obstructive pulmonary disease. It was evening, just one table lamp turned on, and I was the only person with her. The moment came when she took her last breath and then as the minutes passed came the common progression of changes when someone dies: Her skin began looking waxy, a bit yellow, and her mouth was wide open, impossible to close, try as I might before my sister arrived.

Maybe an hour passed before she came into the room, but I wasn't feeling time. I had been sitting there beside my mother, empty of thoughts for the most part, just full of the muscle-dragging sadness that comes with loss. My sister and I are close, and she was certainly close to my mother. A hug when she came but no real need for talking as we sat there, not really convinced that all the worries of my mother's care over the past year were over. It had been a slow progression as her lungs slowly failed and as her dementia made it harder and harder to reach her. But one highlight to her week was the visit to the hair parlor in the nursing home where she would have her hair "done." It reflected her lifelong discipline of dressing well and looking her best without making a fuss about it.

My sister and I sat, quietly, slowly staring through the door that death presents us and looking out into a different world, one without our mother in it. And then she breaks the silence. "You know, that is not a good look for her," meaning the wide-open mouth among other things. And I laugh in the way that only someone who has sat beside a deathbed can laugh. How perfect! How true! How easily my mother would have said the same thing if she had been sitting in my sister's chair. How loving …

G.M. Greene (✉)
Spring Green Dojo, Spring Green, WI, USA
e-mail: gmgreene@wisc.edu

G.M. Greene
Department of Family Medicine, University of Wisconsin School of Medicine and Public Health, Madison, WI, USA

G.M. Greene
Meriter Hospital, Madison, WI, USA

G.M. Greene
6743 Sneed Creek Road, Spring Green, WI 53588, USA

A. Masuda and W.T. O'Donohue (eds.), *Handbook of Zen, Mindfulness, and Behavioral Health*, Mindfulness in Behavioral Health, DOI 10.1007/978-3-319-54595-0_22

I tell this story because once we step inside the world of pain, suffering, and death, there are no real rules. All feelings, all emotions can be appropriate—not just the dark ones—and they wash through that world in mysterious ways. And sometimes in wonderfully healing ways.

Another story, this one in a hospital room just after an elderly man died. I had been with this man, serving as the hospital chaplain on duty that night, sitting there with his wife, his sister, and one of his granddaughters. This granddaughter was a vibrant young woman, maybe in her early 20s, and she was the person most attentive to her grandfather as he was dying. She spoke to him without obvious sorrow, using a tone of voice perhaps no different from what she would have used telling him of her eager plans after graduation. During this last hour of his life, she talked about her friends; she talked about the way he would hold her hand when walking as a young girl visiting him. She spoke about the things that she saw happening to his body as his heart continued to fail. And then he died.

She kissed him. She hugged her grandmother and her aunt. And then she said, "You know, I need to eat the biggest cheeseburger I can find." Like my own sister, she spoke seemingly without thought, addressing the kind of hunger that can follow the difficult physical work she had been doing with her grandfather. As we all laughed, the faces of the patient's wife and sister shifted, coming out of the initial numbness into the life still present in the room.

As I said, there are no real rules. Though maybe there is one: Don't stand outside the experience of pain, suffering, and death, your own or others. Go inside. This "going inside" has a particular meaning in Zen training and that is the theme that connects the many parts of this chapter. But let me say up front—"going inside" is not a mental exercise. It is physical work. It is manual labor. It is only through this whole-body perspective that I can effectively talk about pain, suffering, and death. And I'll also say up front—this "going inside" doesn't always distinguish between going inside yourself or going inside another. That's one of the dualities that Zen training is meant to resolve. And that resolution is then meant to be put to service.

Despite the broad nature of the word "Zen" in this chapter title, this chapter presents a very narrow Zen perspective on that world of pain, suffering, and death. But it is a fairly detailed perspective so I want to show the specific ground I stand on. I speak as someone training in the Chozen-ji line of Rinzai Zen for more than thirty-five years. Ordained in 1988 and receiving *inka* from Tenshin Tanouye Roshi in 1996, I currently serve as the founder and head priest at Spring Green Dojo, a Chozen-ji *betsuin*, in rural Wisconsin.

There are a number of other chapter authors in this book who have been colleagues during those decades of training and they have written about the ways in which Chozen-ji training is highly physical—developing breath, posture, and samadhi—under the myriad conditions that training in the formal elements of Zen present. As well as in the martial arts and the fine arts. This is the three-part *Zen—Ken—Sho* curriculum (training in Zen, martial arts, and fine arts) established by the late Omori Sogen Roshi of Koho-in in Tokyo and the founder of Chozen-ji. In my case, the martial arts are Yoshinkai Aikido, Kendo, and the Hojo sword form that comes out of the school of Kashima Shinden Jikishinkage swordsmanship. The fine arts practiced are nonfiction writing and calligraphy in the Jubokudo School that came through Tesshu Yamaoka and Omori Roshi.

As you will read, this three-part training provides the foundation for the ways in which I approach all pain, suffering, and death—that of others as well as my own. But the broadest application of this training has come through work as a hospital chaplain in two community hospitals. The work began in 2008 in the role of a night chaplain, responding to the full spectrum of needs ranging from tragedies in the emergency room to comforting elderly patients unable to sleep. The principles of this chaplain work were easily understood when I began but there were also techniques for which I sought more formal training through Clinical Pastoral Education (CPE), the training system through which a chaplain ultimately becomes board-certified in the USA. My current knowledge of this training system is limited, however, since I was only able to take enough time away from other responsibilities to undergo the first three months of the year-long training that is required before applying for board certification.

During the short time spent in formal training as a chaplain, I worked to articulate a muscular form of chaplaincy, describing the ways in which chaplaincy is manual labor, labor based on the strength that comes through breath and posture and the sensitivity that comes from use of the senses. Following that first unit of training, I became a part-time chaplain in a Catholic hospital as well as an outpatient chaplain in a rural medical clinic that serves people without health insurance. The work became embodying this new form of chaplaincy.

That is the particular flavor of Zen Buddhism that I know, and the particular application through training and serving others in chaplaincy. Out of all these experiences, a number of principles and tools emerge that anchor this particular approach to pain, suffering, and death.

Before addressing these, however, I should also mention one other professional experience that has influenced my work as a chaplain, namely the fifteen years spent as a faculty member of the medical school at the University of Hawaii. I was hired both as a medical educator and as a Zen priest in order to find ways to improve teaching about the ways in which the relationship itself between a patient and a physician can be therapeutic. The work was both satisfying and frustrating. The satisfying aspect was finding an affinity with a number of physicians and medical educators—people such as Jodi Halpern (2001), Cassell (1991), Brody (1992), and Stein and Apprey (1990)—who sought to deeply understand and articulate the nature of relationships in the clinical care of patients. Rachel Naomi Remen has also worked hard to develop a widely adopted and respected course for medical students—the Healer's Art—that explicitly works to develop the "therapeutic self" of a physician, a phrase that will be discussed later in this chapter in the context of chaplaincy.

But there was frustration to this work as well: the inability of most people to understand what it means to resolve the question of life and death, the traditional phrasing used in Zen to describe the assault on duality that a Zen student must undertake. That is, there is an unshakeable assumption within medicine that the patient and the physician are two things. In Zen, we wouldn't say they are one thing but we would say they are not two.

I'm using this background as a way to describe why in this chapter I don't draw upon the medical literature that describes research on communication between patients and physicians or the much more scant chaplaincy literature on communication and relationship between patients and chaplains. The principles and tools that I describe here don't come out of a dualitic framework; they come out of Zen training. And that is the permission I have given myself in this chapter—to describe the work of a chaplain as best I can in a non-dualistic framework. Instead of having the significant checks and balances that evidence-based medicine provides in clinical settings, all I have is my experience.

Still, in the Zen world that are indeed checks and balances of another sort—namely the ability to detect the difference between two and not-two, and ability that takes years to develop and decades to hone. The closest phrase we might have in English to describe this ability is "the ring of truth," a phrase that includes both the physicality of resonance and a standard of certainty. How to bring this ability into the world of clinical research is a big question. For the moment at least, perhaps the closest approach might come through the studies of the neuroscientist Richard Davidson though his work is currently limited to the brain rather than a whole-body approach (see

Davidson and Begley 2012, for an overview of his work).

Principle #1: The Fundamental Human Illness Is Duality—The Separation of Self and Other, Mind and Body, Life and Death

We could also say that duality is the principle cause of human suffering—the canyon that lies between what I have and what I want. One example of this comes from a native Hawaiian woman who met with a class of medical students just beginning their training at the John A. Burns School of Medicine at the University of Hawaii. A physician colleague and I had arranged for this woman to describe her experience with a number of chronic medical conditions, including painful neuropathy caused by diabetes and shortness of breath because of her congestive heart failure. She spoke at length and answered questions about her many symptoms and her medical care. Clearly, there seemed to be a gulf between what she had and what she must want—to be pain free, to be symptom free.

Then, a young woman in the class asked her, "Out of all these difficult symptoms you have described, which is the worst one?" Long pause, and then an answer, "None of them." Another long pause. Then, "I fell in love many years ago with a man. We wanted to be together but my father disapproved of him. He forbade me to be with him. But we were young, and knew what we wanted, and so we married. From that day forward, my father has never spoken to me. Twenty years now. These other things we have been talking about, do you think those are painful? Those are nothing. Losing my father—that is the worst pain." That was not the suffering these students thought they were evaluating. The duality was not between chronic pain and no chronic pain. The duality was not wanting to lose what she lost.

Principle #2: For a Priest in the Chozen-Ji Lineage, the Traditional Instruction Is "Given a Choice Between Heaven and Hell, Choose Hell."

Zen training hurts. It can feel like an assault on all that seems necessary for comfort. Physical comfort, emotional comfort, spiritual comfort. The monastic rule of setting the needs of others before your own sounds good, sounds virtuous, but only until you recognize that the unspoken part of the rule is, "all the time." The rule must be relentless because the natural human ability to seek comfort is relentless. The problem with this very human need for comfort comes when those who need comfort seek to ease the suffering of those who are suffering. The point isn't to be uncomfortable. The point is to not be stuck on whether there is comfort or discomfort at any point. We train in order to be free to work from either position without being attached to it.

One night when I was on night chaplain duty, I was asked to visit with a man who had been admitted to the hospital following a suicide attempt. I introduced myself and was told, "I don't need a priest. I need to die." I didn't say anything and just stood there. Finally he said, "I'm just playing along here so that I'll be discharged. I know what they want me to say. I had the dose wrong (of the medications he had overdosed with) and I'll get it right." The answer that came without thought was, "So let's go there. Tell me about being dead." And he proceeded to tell me, talking with the certainty of someone whose decision has been clearly made.

The uncanny feeling was that of stepping into the world in which he had indeed already died. I knew this feeling from my Zen training but had never experienced it elsewhere. We sat there for an hour, talking about children, and songs, and the hellhole of depression he lived in. By many standards, including those of my colleagues also training as chaplains when they heard about this encounter, I was too passive. The situation called for doing something, encouraging him, coaching him in some fashion back toward life. But my deepest instinct was to be there dead with him. To not let there be any gap—me on the side of the river called life and him on the side called death. The patient was indeed discharged the next day and I don't know the outcome. I'm guessing, but that is all I can do, that he is still alive. For that brief hour, he had not been alone in Hell.

Principle #3: Compassion Is a Visceral Experience, Not a Virtue or an Act of Moral Behavior

Compassion is as natural to a human being as breathing. It is not something that comes from theology or from moral training, or from a professional code of ethics. It is an expression of being alive. Still, it is all too common to be alive and to not experience compassion. When you live with the conviction that duality is the natural state of things rather than an illness, you cannot know compassion. For a Zen priest, the instruction is to "to become one with," to continually resolve duality. That is not an ideal or an abstract virtue or a metaphor. "Becoming one with" is simply the best way to describe a visceral experience.

The more common way to discuss compassion in Buddhism is to describe the Boddhisattva of Compassion, namely Avalokiteshvara in Sanskrit (Kannon in Japanese).

In paintings or statues, this figure is most often viewed as a woman, with a gentle posture and a half-smile. To the degree that any of us associate compassion with our own mother—the loving embrace, the forgiving smile—this depiction brings a great deal of comfort to Buddhists and non-Buddhists alike. As you might expect, however, the Zen perspective on compassion is not so easily categorized.

The defining sutra for this bodhisattva is *The Sutra of the Lotus Flower of the Wonderful Law*. Chapter XXV is entitled "The All-Sidedness of the Bodhisattva Regarder of the Cries of the World" and it starts like this:

> At that time the Bodhisattva Infinite Thought rose up from his seat, and baring his right shoulder and folding his hands toward the Buddha, spoke thus: 'World-honored one! For what reason is the Bodhisattva Avalokiteshvara named Regarder of the Cries of the World?'
>
> The Buddha answered the Bodhisattva Infinite Thought: 'Good son! If there be countless hundred thousand myriad kotis of living beings suffering from pain and distress who hear of this Bodhisattva Regarder of the Cries of the World, and with all their mind call upon his name, the Bodhisattva Regarder of the Cries of the World will instantly regard their cries, and all of them will be delivered. (Kato et al. 1975)

In a Western context, this description sounds as if there is a deity that can be called upon for delivery from suffering. And that fits with a common view of compassion: It is something that I offer to you the way I might offer a cool drink of water. The bodhisattva and the living beings are separate, you and I are separate. Compassion is offered from one to the other. But the translation of the name Avalokiteshvara—"Regarder of the Cries of the World"—is a much more useful way to view the nature of compassion. For this kind of listening to become compassion, it is a very active form, a physical form, of listening. Not just sounds heard but sounds entered into—sounds that one has become one with.

In that becoming, duality is eased and because duality is eased, suffering is eased. In other words, compassion is a physical act—the sensory ability and physical strength to hear all the cries of the world—not something one person gives to another. In Zen training, this work of becoming one with comes out of many years of strenuous training in the use of breath and posture. As I wrote at the beginning of this chapter, alleviating suffering is manual labor.

I'm standing now in the intensive care unit with a mother, both of us at the side of her daughter, a young woman who had overdosed on heroin. This woman had been declared brain-dead shortly after arrival to the hospital, but who was being kept on "life" support so that she could be evaluated as a potential organ donor. In what way was there compassion in the room?

The honest answer is that I don't know. But I do know that something happened as we spent hours together, both talking and sitting silently. The physical work that I felt myself doing was twofold: filling this skinny, brittle mother with my strength and entering with both feet into her sadness. I say "physical" because the work was to keep adjusting my breath and posture so that as much strength as possible was being given and to keep adjusting breath and posture so that I could feel her sadness as much as possible. That is the work of regarding her cries.

All the time that I am deepening breath and posture, I am being challenged by the sadnesses she keeps expressing, some from long ago and some freshly delivered as we sat through the day. There was the sadness that a mother should feel that her daughter's death was inevitable, given her heroin addiction; that a mother should feel that her daughter's early heroin use may have contributed to the suicide of her own father; that a mother should know that her daughter's boyfriend is being charged with homicide because of his role in her death; that a mother should worry that her one remaining child, a son in high school, may not know how to handle the loss of his father and his sister in the same year.

One after the other, these are hard to take. Hard to take because they trigger my own experiences of sadness and loss. So I feel each of her sadnesses strike my body as I learn them. I feel each of my sadnesses in my body as they are triggered, and all the while I am supposed to be optimizing the use of my breath and posture so as to give her strength, to give her myself. This is what I call "facing suffering"—the physical act of letting someone's suffering flood through you, feeling it fully, but not letting it wash you away. Difficult work, imperfectly done.

Those have been principles that guide my work as a Zen priest and as a hospital chaplain. But it is also helpful to think of the tools that help someone act upon those principles.

Tool #1: Ignorance—The Ability to Not Know Something

Recognition of the therapeutic power of ignorance came early during my fifteen years as a faculty member at the medical school in Hawaii. Soon after arriving, I had been asked to help develop a seven-week family medicine seminar series that focused on the therapeutic aspects of the patient–physician relationship. This work was particularly meaningful to me because of the difficulties my wife and I experienced talking with physicians after our youngest son was born with a condition later diagnosed as a form of cerebral palsy. We had every reason to expect a healthy baby but that is not who arrived the day he was born.

In one of these seminars, students would pair up and role-play difficult conversations, including one in which the medical student, acting as a physician, was asked to visit the parent (the other medical student) of a child just born, healthy and normal in all ways other than missing his right forearm, an unusual anomaly in the prenatal development.

During one such seminar, we had an odd number of students so I took on the role of the baby's father, sitting in a chair a few hours after delivery of my son, healthy but without a forearm, waiting for the family physician to arrive at the hospital for a visit. My "physician" made the expected knock on the imaginary door but did so with an anguished look on her face. I waited for her to speak. She was struggling until she finally burst out, "Dr. Greene. I don't know what to say."

This was a profound moment for me. Suddenly I'm crying, really crying, and she is crying, role-play forgotten. In her mind, she had failed the exercise, saying to me in my role as professor that she didn't know what to do with this scenario. For me, however, finally here was the voice of a physician I had been longing to hear ever since my son, my real son, was born. What could anyone possibly say when the baby just born looked like a blue hunk of meat? When said sincerely, as this student had just done, "I don't know what to say" can be one of the most healing things for a parent to hear—acknowledging that there really are no adequate words for what just happened.

By most measures of a medical school curriculum, this student had failed the exercise. Communication skills are highly valued, and this student had just admitted that she had no idea of what to do. And yet, her admission of ignorance was healing. This was a turning point for me in my role as a medical educator. In a setting where knowledge is valued almost above all else, I cultivated the power of ignorance of "I don't know' and this continues in my work as a chaplain.

Tool #2: The Therapeutic Self. Once You Know That You Are Not Limited by the Boundary of Your Skin, You Are Free to Create Yourself as an Instrument of Healing, Free to Use All of Your Senses Including Intuition

A chaplain or a Zen priest doesn't have much of a toolkit available when facing someone who is suffering. We don't have medications to offer or broad knowledge of community resources and the means of accessing them. We just have our self. That sounds limited but in the development of a chaplain or a Zen priest, that can be profound. In chaplain training, the work is primarily through the emotions. In Zen training, that work is primarily through the senses. This intense work is meant to shatter one's sense of self such that something much greater and larger can emerge. This something can be called no-self but that is not the opposite of one's ordinary sense of self but something in which there is no attachment to self.

Use of my senses became a critical aspect of my work as a chaplain. I didn't really expect this to be possible until I wrote one of my first CPE assignments, an essay meant to articulate our concept of care. I wrote in the voice of a fictional chaplain, experiencing the magical realism of a new kind of hospital.

> There did come a Saturday when I was on 24-hour call at the hospital. It was a day of calm – my patients seemed to be at some level of ease and the two pages of the day had been for patients who needed help but were not in crisis. It was late afternoon when I headed for that staircase, descended, opened the gate I had thought was impassable and went down one more flight of stairs. The stairway door opened into a grove of white oaks. It looked to be a woodland pasture, with wide swaths of grasses between the trees but there were also small cabins scattered about the grove. And nurses, physicians, lab techs, walking about in their familiar garb but far from their familiar habitats.
>
> A nurse recognized my gait as that of a chaplain and motioned me into a cabin with her. Here was a patient, her face showing the wrinkled strains of someone ill and freshly arrived in her search for care. She was resting in a chair as the nurse bought out sample after sample of cloth: some of silk, others of linen, some coarser, some woven. And with each one, she would invite the patient to touch it as she closed her eyes, the nurse watching what passed through this patient as she felt the cloth. And then there was a shift in the atmosphere of the room. The nurse told me, "this is how we choose the bed linens for this woman while she is with us on this unit."
>
> I felt free to move on from this cabin, stopping at another one as I overheard a conversation about food. And not just any food. A nurse with a newly arrived patient was asking for childhood memories of favorite meals or foods. Maybe a kind of squash and sage soup that was served when the weather turned cool in the fall. Maybe a certain kind of cookie in the oven near Christmas time. Or a peach, the first mouthful on a hot July day, mid-day when the air has gone still and all there is to existence is the heat and the sweet juice coming down your chin. And this nurse told me, "this is how we know what smells should come in the window throughout the day."
>
> I moved on, this time to a cabin where the patient was seated in a porch swing and the nurse was slowly testing different frequencies of the swing's movement. Watching the patient's face intently, there came a moment when she saw a broad smile and a slight relaxing of her patient's body. "Now we know how to move this patient's bed at night, matching the way his mother swung him in her lap that evening in May as they watched the full moon rise, waiting for his father to come up the sidewalk."

And I could hear music in the distance as I left this cabin, a cello playing the theme from the "Silk Road" suite by Kitaro. Oh, how that drew me to find the source, but I should have known. There was this woman with hair like spun gold, a woman who had appeared at magical moments throughout my life, now playing her old companion, a cello made long ago in a workshop near Cremona. And the sounds, the notes…as she played, it slowly brought into reality a caravan of travelers crossing the Gobi Desert. There were proud horsemen and sultry women and fat traders in the party and ragged monks toward the back who were carrying litters with people lying on them. And I realized that I was one of these monks, and that the load we bore was that of the clinic patients from the grove of white oaks. And all of them were being carried with the majestic rhythm of that cello – the sound of each note carrying us forward to the night's oasis, still some distance ahead.

For all of us, patients and travelers alike, with each step we became a little more transparent, a little more of the sandstone and the sky showing through us. With each pulse of a step, with each pulse of a note we became more transparent. And our breathing became longer and deeper, and became closer and closer to becoming the wind that had begun to stir as the first hints of dusk came on. You couldn't tell perhaps when it happened, but at a certain moment, if you had looked away and now looked back, all of us, camels, horsemen, monks, dogs, had dissolved into sandstone and sky and air. Yet still you heard the cello, and all had been healed… (Greene 2011a)

This piece was written quickly and without much thought. What struck me as I read it later was how I had articulated a core conviction, one impossible to discuss in a medical school setting, but deeply felt out of my Zen training. The conviction? All can be healed but only when any sense of a healer has dissolved. Having lived with my Zen teacher for so many years, I could watch him heal duality all day long in all that he encountered. And somehow, with some instinct, I could always tell that he himself was not doing anything. There wasn't a healer and someone being healed. There was just healing.

In this context, "dissolved" doesn't mean gone. It means still present but in a different form. Not so different from the way in which the blades of a moving electric fan are both there and not there. This is the working of that no-self.

Tool #3: The Verbatim—A Particular Format for Reporting on a Patient Encounter That Can Show These Principles and Tools at Work

The last tool to be described is a verbatim, a technique used frequently within the training of hospital chaplains. This form of reporting on a patient encounter is centered on a capture of dialogue with the patient (hence "verbatim") but the main feature is the degree of analysis across many dimensions that is also reported. To be effective, a chaplain needs a high degree of self-awareness during any given encounter with a patient or family member, an expectation that would also be familiar to anyone training in Zen. The format acknowledges that there cannot be an objective description of a patient without also including descriptions of everyone interacting with this patient.

I'll provide an example of such a verbatim by showing excerpts from one based on a case seen during my chaplaincy training. It is relevant to this chapter because it shows how clearly my Zen training influences my work with patients.

Date/Time of Visitation: September __, 2011

Visit Number/Length of Visit: 2nd visit, 60 min

Patient Age: 40 **Sex**: Male

Marital Status/Number of Children: married for 9 years, some children but all placed for adoption several years ago

Religious Preference: none

Admitting Diagnosis: "abdominal pain"

Additional Factual Information

A chaplain resident on-call first encountered this family on the previous Saturday night when the patient's wife went to the ER to get drugs to control her anxiety. Apparently, this was the second night in a row that she went to the ER for this reason. When I first saw the patient the next day during my 24-h weekend call, the patient was awake and his wife was present. Their story of their life seemed to overwhelm the story of the patient's most immediate illness, as serious as it was. (The ER physician's preliminary diagnosis included acute renal failure, inflammation of the pancreas, and hypertension.) Both the patient and his wife had previously diagnosed psychiatric problems. No money for rent (though he works) and soon to be kicked out of their apartment. No money for heat, no friends, no insurance. The wife saw no hope for their future. The patient disagreed, "It always works out." But this triggered louder lamenting from his wife that he is a dreamer and can't see the truth.

After seeing the patient on this initial visit, I went out to talk with the patient's nurse, asking her what they do when a spouse stays with a patient, not out of concern for the patient, but because they don't have another place to go. I was worried that the wife might be interfering with the patient's care. The nurse seemed eager to vent, saying, "We are seeing more and more of this (homelessness). It wasn't like this before. It is so hard on all of us. She is way more demanding than he is and he is the one who is sick."

Plans

Before going in for this second visit, my plan was to give him strength for his return to his difficult life. Checking in with his nurse first, she said that they had been getting ready to discharge him today but that now his physicians were worried about some heart arrhythmia and so were going to run more tests. I asked whether his wife was still so agitated. The nurse said that she was not in the room, but most likely was down in the family lounge for a while. I thought, "Good. Finally I'll get some time just with J_____." I felt that he could not speak easily about his own fears or concerns with his wife present and I wanted to explore these with him.

Observations

This was not an easy room to step into, given my earlier encounters with the seeming helplessness of this patient's living condition. His wife was unexpectedly present, sitting on the couch amidst tangled sheets and clothes, wearing a hospital gown. The shades were drawn almost shut. The room smelled of human sweat, smelling all the stronger as I got closer to the wife. Unlike during my previous visit, the patient himself was not as antic. His smile was less forced—still friendly but less of a mask. Still, the angry wife was the strongest source of gravity in the room.

The Visit

C: Chaplain **P**: Patient **W**: Wife

C1: Hi there. It's been awhile since I stopped by. I heard you might be leaving today so I wanted to come by and see how you are doing. (I'm standing on the hall side of the patient's bed at this point)

P1: Nope. Not yet. More tests today. I passed out in the bathroom.

C2: Is that good news or bad news? (moving to the foot of the bed in order to stand closer to his wife.)

P2: Hey! (talking to his wife) Move that stuff off the chair so the chaplain can sit. (I help her bundle up some clothes, which she then moves beside her on the couch. The chair is right beside his wife, close to the corner of his bed. The movement of the clothes stirs the air and the smell of stale human sweat in the room gets much stronger. I sit down and lean back like I'm there for a relaxed conversation with friends.)

C3: So, what's happening?

W1: I'm going to kill somebody. (Said with her familiar anger. The patient grimaces as she says this.)

C4: That bad, hunh?

W2: Dude! The fucking computer doesn't work. (She must have been down in the family lounge in order to use the Internet…) And I'm still the invisible one. No one wants to see me, hear me. Nobody wants to smell me—they didn't want me to have this gown but I'm sorry, I can't keep stinking up clothes. All I've got is this sweatshirt and if I keep wearing it while I go up and down stairs (here at the hospital—but, why no elevator…?), it will stink. I've got nothing else to wear… (I'm looking at her at first, but then I glance over at J______ to see how he is taking this all in…He looks powerless.)

C5: Well, I can see you (talking to the patient's wife). I can hear you. I had to stay over in the hospital Sunday night and I didn't take a shower before working yesterday. I didn't like smelling myself either. This place is supposed to be so clean and tidy. No stink allowed…

W3: Yeah, no poor people allowed…but that's *their* problem. We still have no place to go.

C6: I hear you…so, J_____, what happened to you last night? (He looks eager to answer now that the attention has come back to him.)

P3: Whoa! I got so dizzy (said happily, like he's glad to have a real symptom). I got up to take a piss and I was filling the whole bottle. I mean I was filling that whole thing up—it was just pouring out of me. And maybe it was just too much because I suddenly got dizzy. And I'm looking for a place to set it before I go down…

C7: And then you fainted?

P4: Yeah, straight down.

C8: Wow! I'm glad you didn't hit your head.

W4: Dude! That would have been a mess if you had dropped it. God, the smell would have killed me.

C9: And then what?

P5: Well, the doctor heard about it this morning and he's wondering about my heart now so they want to run some tests before I can go.

C10: I wasn't kidding about the good news/bad news thing …what do you think? You've been on a roller coaster with this discharge/no discharge thing. Are you OK being here a bit longer?

W5: Why doesn't anybody ask me that question? He's getting all the drugs. He's getting all the tests. I can't get nothing. I'm the bad guy. Always I'm the bitch. People look right through me.

C11: But you (said to the wife) understand that most people here see your husband as their patient, right? I've never seen a double bed here where they can plop you both in the same bed—you guys would need the deluxe version where each half of the bed has its own mechanics—yours can go up, but his can go down. I can't see you guys agreeing on how to arrange the pillows

P6: (Laughs) You got that right! We can leave her right over there on the couch!

C11: Those drugs might help you, you know … (spoken to the wife, referring to the bi-polar medications she supposedly left in the place where they were staying before coming to the hospital) Can anybody give you a ride to get your meds?

W6: Dude! I already told you about that bus transfer place. You think I want more of that "Hey, Baby…How about it?" crap? And do you think we've got friends? He called his boss last night, asking about the money from that employee support fund. All that guy had to say was "When are you coming back to work?" No "How are you doing?" Nothing!

C12: (Talking to the patient) Maybe you should do some of that pissing in the bottle at work. You know, you might just get dizzy again and who knows if you could keep from dropping it on the floor a second time. Whoops—sorry.

P7: (Laughs) Yeah! That would be just about right for him (the boss) Several more minutes of talk about their life once they get out of the hospital… Then, in closing.

C13: So, what do you think? (talking to the patient) If you could become anybody, who would you be?

W7: Cassandra! I don't have to become her—I am her. The gods cursed me to always speak the truth but have no one believe me.

P8: Yeah, and I've thought about being Alexander the Great.

C14: Yes indeed, I look at that profile and you look like you belong on a coin. (His wife does a belly laugh.) You know, Halloween is coming up and I think I can see you both pulling this off—Cassandra and Alexander (more laughter) … I do need to get going to see more patients now, but I'm going to keep thinking of you both. You guys have got guts—don't give up!

W8: No way, Dude!

P9: I haven't seen anybody make her laugh like this. I'm going to keep thinking of you.

Analysis—The Patient

Theological Concerns

I've been asking myself how I best serve patients in my role as a chaplain. I've come through a phase of recognizing how valuable it can be for patients to feel seen, gotten, heard, accepted. From the perspective of the training of a Zen priest, that is indeed the primary work: "to become one with" is the phrase used. That is not a "become one with" in your imagination but in a deeply visceral sense. The reason we stop there in describing the work—I think—is that once there has been that joining, whatever happens next emerges from a different context than the one in which there is a concrete patient here and a concrete chaplain over there.

But over the course of the last few weeks, I haven't been satisfied that "becoming one with" and then allowing the "more" to just emerge is sufficient. The pump has to be primed in order for the "more" to flow. The challenge I feel is that it is not enough to simply see a patient through their own eyes. Instead, when I can see through those eyes, how can I (meaning we) alter the nature of the reality we are experiencing? In other words, if I perceive that a patient suffers from an inability to experience transcendence in their life, can I (we) work from within to facilitate movement toward that experience? It becomes an unconscious intention in other words and what I now realize is that such an intention may not work intentionally unless the seed already exists in me as a chaplain.

I also realize that those things we see as diagnostic may also become therapeutic. In other words, diagnosing an inability to experience the transcendent also suggests the work to be done: namely facilitating a patient's search for the transcendent. I say "suggests" very carefully because the facilitation I am describing can never effectively be done from outside the patient's own experience. I feel that it can only be done from within that sensation of "becoming one with."

Psychological Concerns

The psychological concern that most comes to mind for me is: Why this particular dynamic between the patient and his wife? It clearly is a well-honed coping mechanism: She is the angry bitch and he is the happy-go-lucky guy, friend to all of mankind. Given his wife's very harsh and bitter persona, this is not a couple likely to have very much success in navigating life in normal society. And this is a man not likely to be able to focus attention on his own needs. She will never generate in others a desire to help her unless there is someone ready to walk into her particular version of Hell. And he will never be able to seek the kind of medical help he so obviously needs until he takes control of his needs instead of allowing her to dictate them.

Several questions come to mind. How did they hit upon this particular coping mechanism? Did they ever have a chance for another one? How well does this particular one serve them? Are they stuck with this one? At first glance, my label for this couple is "train wreck!" or "dysfunctional family." But "dysfunctional" is a tricky term. My feeling is that until one explores the way in which their roles actually serve a useful purpose, there is no way that any shift could take place.

There is just about everything to "fix" for this patient and his wife but my feeling is that this is one of those existential situations where the best approach is to recognize that not only is there no way to "fix" things for them, but also to recognize first that there is nothing that needs "fixing." That may sound bizarre but I mean that until one first finds and accepts their current, not potential, humanity, nothing more can happen.

Ethical Concerns

I don't see any real ethical concerns for this patient and his wife. I felt comfortable joining into their lives but did not feel a need for any kind of aggressive advocacy role with regard to his care. The care he was given seemed to be no different than the care that is provided to any other patient.

One issue this raises, however, is one of my attending to the patient's wife perhaps more than the patient himself. There were at least three sets of problems in their room: the problems the patient has, the problems his wife has, and the problems that exist in the two of them together. I felt that the bulk of my work focused on the last problem set, but that didn't leave much attention for the patient himself and that doesn't feel right.

Analysis—The Chaplain

This is the hardest section of this verbatim to write because this patient hits close to home for me. Initially, I felt very much engaged with this patient because his life and his dilemma present such a clear cry for help. There are no easy answers to his medical problems; there are even fewer answers to his social, emotional, spiritual problems. This is a true example of a situation where the only possible approach lies in "being" and not "doing," at least from a chaplaincy perspective. And I often feel most engaged in these situations. So that was what brought me back to this patient for a second visit even though he wasn't on any of my assigned units and I had no formal responsibility for providing his spiritual care.

I have come to recognize in the course of developing this verbatim—especially as I was recreating the conversation in the room when we were together—that I have a lot of self-identification with this patient. Just like good theater can take human behavior and exaggerate it to a point beyond reality—but do that in a useful way—I find that the extreme coping mechanism this patient and his wife displayed points a finger straight to my own heart.

Someone close to me came through a long stretch of time in which she was often angry, with me, with others, in ways that felt out of proportion to the circumstances. In the face of this, my role was to be the peacemaker, the Zen guy above it all, the guy who could explain why she would erupt so and ask for understanding from those she hurt. This was the coping mechanism we were locked into and it took a long time for me to see how damaging it was—to her, to me, to all around us.

Part of the coping was that I so clearly thought of the anger as her problem; I was just another one of the victims but because of my Zen training, I could rise above it. This was the story. But it was only once I could feel my own anger that things could begin to shift. I had to do two things: abandon that coping mechanism and be willing to risk the chaos that ensued; and I had to recognize how intimately I was tied into her anger and bitterness. I wasn't separate from that. I was very much part of it.

What was true then is not true today. The original coping mechanism is gone. Overall, I feel embarrassed to admit such things but it illustrates one of the early stages of "becoming one with," namely "I've had a similar experience, making it easier for me to get inside the emotions you are describing."

Pastoral Opportunity

The opportunity is to not lie—to not pretend all is well—to say sometimes how painful this is—to not look for a new coping mechanism—to live with the rawness that I feel. I've been acknowledged for my strengths for so many years that I have swept far under the rug the many years of helplessness I experienced during my life. I thought I had earned the right to say that I have succeeded, that I have overcome so many emotional barriers, that I don't have to look back. But when I do look back, I see myself looking at myself today. There are indeed many strengths in my life now but there are also times of fresh helplessness. I need to know those for the sake of all my patients (Greene 2011b).

End of Verbatim

I'll close with one more story and one more principle. The story is about an encounter with an elderly woman one evening when I was again on duty as a chaplain. I stepped into her darkened room without any particular goal other than to make a visit with a patient who had not been seen by a chaplain since her admission. She was lying on bed, wide awake, as I came to the side of her bed. I asked how she was doing. She said, "I have lost so much in my life." There were no pleasantries, no warm-up, just straight to the core of her suffering. This kind of immediate self-revelation from a patient had never happened to me before but in the context of my day, it was not surprising. Suddenly, I felt that I understood the core nature of chaplaincy.

Earlier in the day, I had my weekly private meeting with my chaplaincy training supervisor. Coming after of a number of intense patient encounters during the previous few weeks, I could finally feel several losses I had experienced in life. Ever since my youngest son had been born—the one who was so present during the patient–physician role-play described earlier—I had resolved that I would never feel loss again. That resolution wasn't conscious. Although it was present for all the years since his birth, I couldn't feel it in my body. Until that particular day when I could.

Because that physical sensation of loss was so fresh in my body, it was if I walked into that elderly woman's room with a neon sign blinking on my chest, saying, "I have lost so much in my life." So how could she not so easily feel safe saying the same thing? This experience was much different from the far more common version of empathic communication, dependent on words. This was a human experience of non-duality. This is the compassion described earlier in this chapter as "the expression of being alive."

References

Greene, G. (2011a). *"Projective character study," essay submitted for clinical pastoral education training program*. Madison, Wisconsin: Department of Spiritual Care, Meriter Hospital.

Greene, G. (2011b). *"Cassandra and Alexander the Great—Verbatim #2," essay submitted for clinical pastoral education training program*. Madison, Wisconsin: Department of Spiritual Care, Meriter Hospital.

Kato, B., et al. (Trans.). (1975). *The threefold lotus sutra* (p. 319). New York and Tokyo: Weatherhill and Kosei.

Bibliography

Brody, H. (1992). *The healer's power*. New Haven: Yale University Press.

Cassell, E. (1991). *The nature of suffering*. New York: Oxford University Press.

Davidson, R., & Begley, S. (2012). *The emotional life of your brain*. New York: Hudson Street Press.

Halpern, J. (2001). *From detached concern to empathy*. New York: Oxford University Press.

Remen, R. (no date). *The healer's art course*. At http://www.ishiprograms.org/programs/medical-educators-students/

Stein, H., & Apprey, M. (1990). *Clinical stories and their translations*. Charlottesville: University Press of Virginia.

Application of Zen Practices and Principles for Professionals/Advocates Who Work for Survivors of Trauma and Violence

Norma Wong

Keywords
Zen · Buddhism · Behavioral health · Mindfulness · Trauma · PTSD

As a matter of survival, people can permanently adapt to ways of living that include radical separation of mind, body, and spirit. This happens with the victims of violence, and professionals and advocates can experience its effects by proxy. Zen practices and principles offer ways of thinking and exercises to move beyond this survival mode.

By Norma (Ryuko) Wong Roshi, faculty of the Institute of Zen Studies, the Move to End Violence, and the Transitions Initiative of the Movement Strategy Center; strategy consultant; and teacher. The Catalyst Initiative of the George Family Foundation collaborated with the creation of this chapter, particularly with respect to trauma and secondary traumatic stress references.

Beyond Survival

Survival is a good thing. It is what we, as humans, are wired for. It means that we will fight to breathe, and we will run when there is danger. But what happens if we live at the edge of survival for too long? Do the traits that we are wired for begin to play out in ways that become destructive to our humanity? Is it possible to return to our full humanity and develop a state of being beyond survival?

These are questions that I first considered in working with Move to End Violence, a 10-year project of the NoVo Foundation with leaders in the fields of domestic violence, sexual assault, child abuse, and gender-based violence. A significant number of people who work in these fields are survivors themselves or have close relations to survivors. They are passionately drawn by their experiences to support other survivors, as well as to advocate with individuals and communities to interrupt and eliminate violence. The survival story is a heroic one, and part of the therapeutic journey is to be able to tell and own our stories, including the traumatic components. Later, I began to notice that the mind-body-spirit conditions of survivors of these types of violence are also present for many social activists who come from and have absorbed the pain of their communities, including indigenous people who live in survival of historical genocide. These leaders, advocates, and indigenous

N. Wong (✉)
Institute of Zen Studies, Honululu, HI, USA
e-mail: ankoin@hawaii.rr.com

A. Masuda and W.T. O'Donohue (eds.), *Handbook of Zen, Mindfulness, and Behavioral Health*, Mindfulness in Behavioral Health, DOI 10.1007/978-3-319-54595-0_23

people also happen to be strong, inspiring, highly functioning people.

Professionals and advocates who work with survivors of trauma and violence can become physically and mentally exhausted as a result of overworking and chronically carrying a heavy emotional burden. They can experience difficulty in being able to "turn off," and they can develop an unhealthy relationship with the concept of self-care. Although teaching self-care to others is an important part of healing for clients, practitioners and advocates have a tendency to stretch themselves too thin, only practicing self-care under extreme circumstances. Even then, it is not uncommon to hear self-care behaviors described as indulgent and selfish choices that quickly engender guilt in those conducting them. In working with strategic thinking, a tendency to lean toward the short-term is prevalent, and they almost always choose breadth over depth. Whereas it is very inventive in stretching limited resources, they have difficulty unleashing creative thought. As extraordinarily courageous people, many nonetheless avoid risk-taking. They yearn for spaciousness, but they immediately fill it up.[1]

In time, I came to understand these conditions as the natural result of living as a survivor and identifying closely with survivors. Even when they are no longer in the crosshairs of immediate danger, survivors will continue to think and behave in ways that served them in the past. Busy-ness is a friend for a survivor—a marker for self-worth and agency. The combination of saying busy and providing support for survivors and victims increases the likelihood of overextension. Survivors express tiredness and fatigue but do not acknowledge and are rarely alarmed by the very real impacts of tiredness on their bodies, psyche, and actions. Some are frequently overwhelmed by emotions.[2] Their worldview that spaciousness is an indulgence serves to keep it from being therapeutic, let alone a disciplined reality. A forced vacation is a barely controlled crash. Unable to exercise regular spaciousness, makes it much more difficult for survivors to think creatively, as creativity almost always arises upon a blank canvas. Risk-taking becomes more difficult as safety is paramount for survival. The cycle, as viewed from the outside, is destructive. When viewed from the inside, however, it is paramount to survival, as if the mind, body, and spirit separate themselves intentionally in order to move forward.

It is possible to reach a point, in the midst of experience trauma or after distancing oneself a bit, when finding a different way to be in the world feels plausible or at least worth trying for. From the perspective of a Zen practitioner, this is good and fertile ground.

We are indeed making headway in terms of interrupting habits and engaging in practices to cultivate more sustainable and powerful ways. However, survivor habits are deeply imbedded and require both vigilance and living differently. It is work in progress.

In this sense, it is useful to define habits and practices, at least in the context of this work.

Habits, as I learned from my teacher Tanouye Tenshin Rotaishi, are "unconscious, repetitive acts" (a successor of Omori Sogen Rotaishi who founded Daihonzan Chozen-ji in Honolulu, Hawaii, in 1979, the first Rinzai headquarters temple established outside of Japan). Human activity is riddled with habits that are patterned such that they escape our attention entirely. Because they are unconscious, even so-called good habits are unable to serve us. For example, most of us brush our teeth habitually, usually twice a day. However, your dentist may point out that you are brushing your teeth improperly, despite brushing them consistently, and will likely give you the same lecture each time with respect to the portion of the mouth that is ignored or the portion that is brushed in the wrong direction. Even good habits take up space in our unconsciousness and crowd out awareness. Moreover, the repetitive nature of habits imbeds itself into our cellular memory, making it much more difficult to interrupt them. From a Zen perspective, habits cover and hide the true person or nature within us.

Practices, on the other hand, are conscious, repetitive acts. Here, we come close, but not

[1] Killian (2008), Pfifferling and Gilley (2000).

[2] Summarized in Salston and Figley (2003).

quite akin, to the concept of *shugyo*. When my teacher asked his teacher, Omori Sogen Rotaishi, to come from Japan to Hawaii to train with students, it was this concept of *shugyo* that Tanouye Rotaishi was intending to help disseminate in the West. The closest we might get to a Western understanding of this concept may be something like discipline and forged understanding through practice—something like that. There is a quality, a quantity, and a consciousness to *shugyo*. Here, and in the way that it has been used in my applied Zen work, practice is about the conscious and regular engagement of learned physical activities and "ways of acting" so that and until it can become "ways of being."

One of the most pernicious habits we have is the way in which we breathe. A moderate rate of breathing (e.g., 10 times per minute) will yield 14,400 unconscious, repetitive breaths per day! That breathing happens regularly is absolutely necessary. That it is unconscious for the most part means that our bodies, and therefore our minds and our spirits, are engaged in the same habit action for the entirety of our lives … a minimum of 368 million times in the life of a 70-year-olds.

Many of the survivors that I have worked with alternate breathing patterns between a relatively rapid rate, frequently more than 20 times per minute, virtually holding the breath or breathing in such a faint and shallow way that breath is imperceptible. Physiologically, the breath appears to be higher in the chest. Using chest muscles naturally constricts breathing. This habit serves to reinforce anxiety, which can become distracting background noise or show itself in more demonstrative ways such as being compelled to talk.

From a Zen practice point of view, whether anxiety causes rapid, shallow breathing or the other way around is immaterial. The physical experience itself is a potent portal to shifting the mind-body-spirit condition. Attempting to make a person less anxious by dissecting reasons or other means of changing the mind such as repeatedly saying "I am not anxious" is ineffectual from a Zen practice point of view. Therefore, we simply focus on the practice of breath first by demonstrating, then practicing, and finally self-monitoring.

Although it is somewhat obvious, it is worth stating that a person cannot demonstrate if he or she is already breathing in a manner that is worthy of emulation. This, too, is a practitioner's way. The process of a person seeing and then emulating, trying and feeling, and observing for sense-making after trying and feeling is particularly important in work with survivors. The process itself reinforces agency.

Showing and demonstrating begin with the understanding that a breath that is low and slow, one that comes from a lower part of the body and is slower in execution, especially in the exhale of the breath, will make a person physically feel stronger and more grounded. In practice, it is a matter of partners standing facing each other with one gently but firmly pushing the other aside while the other breathes very high in the chest and very rapidly, and then repeating the gentle and firm push aside while the other breathes lower in the body in the region below the diaphragm and slower especially on the exhale. A high and rapid breath will yield a body that is easier to push. A low and slow breath will yield a body that is much more solid, both to the experimenter and to the pusher. This difference is particularly dramatic for first-time experimenters.

There is a famous saying "look under feet." This seemingly obvious aphorism is only apparent if one is actually aware of one's feet. In my work, I have found it to be a common phenomenon for survivors and activists experiencing secondary traumatic stress to have very little physical sensation below the part of the waist line which is above the belly button. The waist line is a particularly hard-cased barrier for survivors of sexual assault. Bringing the breath down to that place which is low so that it can be slow is a reintroduction to the connection of the upper body to lower trunk and extremities. Without dwelling on what is in between, we move directly to the feet. The instruction is given to gently push the ball of the feet into the ground at the same pace as the exhale. Being grounded is not a state of mind; rather, it is a state of physical being, that is, being and feeling connected to the ground. Attention is given to having as clean a practice floor as possible, encouraging people to take their shoes off for certain exercises. It is important also to spend time considering proper footwear that will allow for a flexible connection to the ground, especially in times of anticipated duress. For example, as a young upstart in the governor's office, I was known for wearing red sneakers on days in which difficult encounters were expected, normalizing the power practice (rather than the therapeutic practice) of having conscious feet.

Simply demonstrating over and over again does not result in a practice. The need to practice breathing presents a dilemma. Sitting quietly, as one might in meditation, is an anxiety-ridden exercise for many beginning sitters, as well as survivors for whom sitting quietly would not be safe unless you are hiding. Some even begin to breathe faster and have difficulty exhaling, drawn by habit to the sympathetic inhale and avoiding the parasympathetic exhale. As all martial artists and most athletes know, it is the exhale that renders a sense of grounded-ness and physical strength. However, if you are conditioned to inhale as a matter of survival, then merely telling someone that it would be more powerful to exhale is counterproductive because it places a person in an exercise in which they need to overcome the habit condition in order to receive and cultivate benefit.

Breath with physical movement holds more promise as a practice. In movement, there is less opportunity for thoughts to override the simple practice of breathing in and exhaling out low and slow. Breath can be coordinated with movement to reinforce the opening up of the inhale and the more powerful execution of the exhale in which posture improves over time. With a more erect and natural posture, the gaze can be "up and out," allowing for more physical and relational awareness and a general lifting of the spirit. Physical movement in and of itself is liberating, and breath with movement is a simple embodiment of liberation.

The type of movement practiced can be important. Yoga is a readily available breath and movement practice that can be locally sourced. However, the entry to yoga may be problematic for certain body types, disabilities, and those with self-judgmental attitudes. Powerful and energy-producing practices include dance (provided that the instructor emphasizes breath as part of the practice), tai chi, and gi gong. In my own practice and with my students, we practice a 10-step tai chi form that Dogi Kow Roshi originally developed to increase the breath and core strength for meditation. We also use a series of breathing exercises in which there is rhythmic and circular body movement. We choose exercises and practices that have low standards of ability at entry but can also be practiced at refined and vigorous levels by seasoned practitioners.

The expression of one's own voice is an important part of a survivor's healing. This is frequently exercised in story form; that is, being able to say out loud and to others what has happened, declaring that the violence and the harm is not because of a personal defect or failure to prevent perpetration. The liberation of a victim is to become a survivor. And what does it look and feel like to be liberated from survivor-hood without negating or compartmentalizing? Continued expression of survivor-hood can be problematic without going deeper than surface level.

In Zen, there is a predilection to avoid exercises that promulgate thoughts. Within the same time interval in which other facilitators are guiding journaling, art response, or deep conversations, my work with survivors and activists practices voice in its purest form: sound and vibration and resonance with others. A single vowel, whichever may be the favorite one chosen at the moment, vocalized in a low tone with as much volume as may be possible, for as long as the breath will take, in a room of people all doing the same thing, can in of itself create a healing moment.

Work on the physiological and psychological benefits and impacts of sound and voice work has primarily utilized mantras and recorded music. Along with breath (including meditation) and movement work, sound and voice, experienced by or even created by participants, brings about what is known as the relaxation response. When the relaxation response is stimulated or cultivated, less oxygen needs to be consumed by the body, there is less psychological distress, and there are other measurable physiological and psychological changes.[3] Instead of mantras and externally produced music, I use single-toned, loud, and resonant vowels. A partnered exercise with two participants taking each of the vowels in turn, with one vowel for each breath, creates an entirely different kind of relational connection that requires no words of explanation. Pairing tonal sounds at full volume with movement is extremely powerful; it is also a very good workout in building breathing capacity and core strength. The Spanish pronunciation of vowels is preferred over the English, as it is closer in tone to several Asian languages, as well as many of the indigenous language pronunciations, and has no "I."

Over time, survivors and activists can build resilience through breath, movement, and sound practice. Work and experimentation in this area is being conducted most notably with military veterans returning with symptoms of post-traumatic stress.[4] Studies and evaluative research using biofeedback measurements, before and after evaluation of ability to carry out everyday functions, quality of life satisfaction surveys, and other work are showing that mind-body experiential practices can move the dial in the positive direction for people who have had or continue to have trauma as part of their lives.

One of the tests of resilience that I utilize is whether there is a psychological and physical discomfort with shouting. Single-syllable shouting is an infamous signature of Zen, intended to cut through thoughts and practice complete expression in a single moment. It is startling to the casual observer, and as you may imagine, it can produce fear in a survivor or politicized negation in an activist. Just being able to shout, without the tensing of muscles or the residue of anger, without fighting or fleeing, is a physical sign that resilience is becoming deeper and broader. For practice, we shout the accompanying numbers in Cantonese while executing each of the 10 moves in the tai chi form.

Other forms of vocalization such as singing or chanting are good forms of practice, especially if practiced in group. Singing can have hidden challenges, such as drawing people into performance, which can limit or complicate the internal work, and the music and/or lyrics may trigger or influence emotions in unintended ways. Chanting, which is my preferred vocalized practice form, can be construed as a religious exercise. With these cautions, the singing and chanting forms are strong, embodied group practices for lay people and have been beneficial for some survivors and activists that I have practiced with.

Breathing, physical movement, and vocalization (both individually practiced and in pairs or groups) are embodied practices that reknit the conscious mind-body-spirit connection.

Many people live less physical lives simply because they can. Modern living coupled with trauma or agitation can actively "separate" the mind and the body. People describe being unaware of or not paying attention to long-standing, abnormal physical conditions. They may chronically ignore hunger or thirst and build habits around not eating, or overeating, or being chronically dehydrated, or using the facilities only when significantly uncomfortable as if the mind might be able to indefinitely control one's bladder. Survivors breathing at a rate of 20 rotations a minute are unaware of the rapidness of their breath, or the impact of this habit on their ability to think and act. The ever-present use of multiple information technology gadgets serves only to further separate people from their physical existence within the immediate environment.

The embodied spiritual practices, including my own path of Rinzai Zen, are built on the

[3]"Genomic Counter-Stress Changes Induced by the Relaxation Response," Dusek, Otu, Wohlhueter et al., 2008; see the work of James S. Gordon, founder and director with the Center for Mind-Body Medicine in Washington, D.C., with military veterans and survivors of conflict countries.

[4]Rosenberg (2012); "Journal of Traumatic Stress, Vol. 17, No. 2, April 2004, pp. 13–147, Treatment of Posttraumatic Stress Disorder in Postwar Kosovo High School Students Using Mind-Body Skills Groups: A Pilot Study."

premise of the mind-body-spirit connection. Practices of the body will support the work of the mind and the cultivation of the spirit. It is this mind-body-spirit connection that I draw upon in the methodology for applied work. By the time I am introduced to activists, organizers, leaders, and survivors, they have invested many years in the mind's work including leadership development, political and social analyses, strategy, psychotherapy, individual, group, and peer counseling. Their minds are well-developed, but nonetheless agitated, racing, and too crowded for creative thought. Doing more mind and thought work becomes less and less fruitful. In its stead, elements such as breath, voice, art, and physical movement are introduced as the means by which a person can not only learn new concepts, but also to reconnect themselves with all parts of who it is they are and who they are in the environment.

Some people will be especially attracted to the physical and psychological benefits and begin to practice on their own, outside of the group or coached settings. These are the people who are more likely to ask about learning meditation. A positive experience with meditation, at least among the survivors and activists that I've worked with, is related to the amount of work the person does beforehand to prepare for spaciousness.

Whereas many people consider meditation to be a practice of the mind, it is an embodied practice that requires significant physical activity and discipline. Any long-time practitioner knows that the quality and longevity of the breath, especially the exhale, will make a significant difference as will the relaxed state of muscles and limbs in a sitting or standing postural stance that supports focus and breath. Without the active participation of these physical elements, the mind will simply wander. Stillness and quiet, or rather, the opening of one's senses to everything and therefore embracing stillness and quiet is a cultivated state of the body long before it can reside in the mind.

Instead of directing a survivor to instruction in the form of meditation, I counsel beginning with a practice of self-care comprised of 15 min of spaciousness each day. 15 min is enough.

This is a practice that would feel familiar to those who practice mindfulness. In Zen, a teacher will counsel students to remember to prepare for meditation. If you just pull into the parking lot after an overfilled day, a few minutes late, rush to change clothes, bow hastily, and sit unceremoniously upon the zabuton slightly askew, many minutes of the sit will be unproductive as you strain to quiet an overbeating heart. Moreover, the sit will be just another activity in a long list of activities, rather than a practice about a way to live one's life.

Most survivors, especially high-functioning survivors, chronically fill their days with innumerable and overlapping activities. Multitasking is a run-of-the-mill modern disease to begin with; for survivors, extreme busy-ness is an act of power, of agency, and as a barrier to ward off demons and emotions. Spending fifteen minutes a day in just one simple activity of spaciousness can be an astonishingly unorthodox and somewhat radical action. The instruction of "one simple activity" should be a physical element intended to bring low-key personal enjoyment. Taking a walk without an iPhone or iPod; paying attention to the surroundings; and opening up one's senses to the heat, or cold, wind, or not, the sound and feeling of feet on the dirt path or grass; and walking only as fast as the quality of one's breath would qualify as one simple activity. Making a proper cup of tea with loose leaves instead of dunking a pouch until the water is brown, starting with boiling water and listening for the moment of the boil, picking a special cup with care and waiting for a proper steep until the fragrance tells you that the tea is ready, and taking time to enjoy the sip would also qualify. Weeding a garden, picking flowers, listening to live music or playing an instrument, watching children play at the local park, or singing along—all of these would qualify. Examples such as these are given, as the instruction of "one simple activity" would not be descriptive enough for a mind whose habits have crowded out the possibility of "simply" and "one."

The goal here is fifteen minutes a day, every day. It need not be the same activity, though people frequently remain in the groove of just one for several days on end. Many fall off the wagon, unable to maintain discipline on a daily basis. Here, there is the reminder of the very helpful reset button: taking a breath, exhaling low and slow, feeling feet on the ground and the spine straightening until you are taller, and essentially letting go and forgiving the past for the opportunity of the current moment. In this regard, we counsel an unlimited number of resets. Surviving traumatic events always has consequences, including those that are real and immediate, perceived and exaggerated. Therefore, a reset expressed simply as that, not as a letting go or a forgiving, is an important practice as is the reminder that we have an unlimited number of resets.

Once the fifteen minutes of spaciousness a day becomes an everyday practice for 21 days or more, then there is more fertile ground in the body and mind for meditation. Many are able to begin with and comfortably sustain a 30-min sit, two or three times a week, from this platform. Often, the practice becomes fifteen minutes of spaciousness followed by 30 min of meditation, taking it into the 45-min timeframe that is considered an optimal window for seasoned Zen practitioners.
Those survivors and activists that take on this simple practice frequently exhibit the condition known as the Beginner's mind. They will delight in the wonder and intensity of found beauty, express astonishment over sounds of previously unheard nature, and approach their simple and spacious practice with tear-producing sincerity.

It is at this point that survivors and activists begin to actively and vocally notice things about their everyday lives that are unsustainable, as if awakening to the reality of their existence. More importantly, many begin to make more healthy choices, which for others may seem ridiculously simple or absurd. An example may be hydrating properly, for example, because it is no longer a win to go to the bathroom once in a working day.

Still, the cellular memory of each habit is tenacious. This is what my teacher, Tanouye Tenshin Rotaishi, referred to as "habit energy": the way in which an unconscious repetitive act will trigger and be triggered, over and over again, creating its own reinforcing energy path that draws other habits and us into its vortex. Decision paths, such as the choice to take on too many responsibilities without cutting anything even in the face of mind and body recognition of its toll, are paths that are regularly chosen.

While the unlimited reset button is an invaluable tool throughout life, it in and of itself will not propel a person from the state of being called "survivor" to a place beyond that which we astonishingly do not have a familiar descriptor. Once a person begins to feel and to determinedly think about the possibilities of becoming more than a survivor, more intensive work is called for. A good sign that this stage has been reached is unapologetic dedication to a defined set of practices in such a way that requires the person to choose to *not* do something else. If the desire for spacious practice and the feeling of energy from self and others is about adding on to an otherwise overpacked life, then the survivor is still in the consumption stage of spaciousness rather than a self-generative stage.

What does intensive practice work look like? In some ways, this is uncharted territory. A good amount of work has occurred in a category called trauma-informed or trauma-specific approaches, which span identities from victim to survivor. Trauma as an event or series of events impacts physical and mental health over the course of a person's life, well beyond the event time horizon, and unaddressed, can significantly increase the risk of chronic mental and physical diseases as well as substance use. Although explored for decades by public institutions and service systems, the work is only beginning to have trauma-informed and trauma-specific work move beyond the naming of trauma to promote wellness and true recovery.[5]

[5]See "Trauma and Resilience," Wilder Research, in partnership with Mental Wellness Campaign, October 2014 Snapshot; SAMHSA's Concept of Trauma and Guidance for a Trauma-Informed Approach, Prepared by SAMHSA's Trauma and Justice Strategic Initiative, Substance Abuse and Mental Health Service Administration, July 2014.

Various transformative practices including the ones described here as well as an entire field of applied somatics are being used and experimented with for and by survivors and activists. Intensive practice work, however, intended to propel a practitioner willingly and by her or his own work into a different way of being, thinking, and acting, is still in the very early stages of development. Among the practice groups that I work with, a recent residential practice gathering of 40 survivors, activists, and Zen practitioners was a promising start. Activists and organizers in Los Angeles and St. Paul/Minneapolis, about twenty-five in each area, are meeting on a semi-regular basis as practice communities. Activists engaged as a national peer learning group are beginning to straddle the practice area between the self and the spiritual. One of the learnings from these experiences is that there are more people who are ready and eager for this than might be imagined. The mixture of beginners and practitioners is useful and inspirational. Beginners have models for emulation, and practitioners are moved in good ways by the sincerity of effort and depth of struggle of beginners. Another learning is that life-changing realizations can occur in the midst of great laughter which is a welcome departure from the dramatic, heart-wrenching work that many survivors and activists have equated with introspection and healing.

Whether it is beginner's practice or the more intensive variety, having a practice community can make a significant difference. While it is true that inner work is ours alone to do, it need not be attempted alone. The Buddha, the Dharma, and the Sangha are three treasures taught by Shakyamuni Buddha more than 2500 years ago, and they have proven themselves over and over again to being crucial to both self-development and spiritual enlightenment. The Sangha is a spiritual community, usually referring to a particular group of students and teachers who practice together. It is an important modality for spiritual training in that it supports, encourages, emulates, and reflects in ways that are not possible or are more difficult in individual practice. In fact, it is in Sangha that resonance and reflection can accelerate change as people practice, struggle, and celebrate together. In Sangha, we practice for each other as much as for our own selves. Thus, a practice community is constructed for and intended to go much further than group therapy. There is no graduation from practice; rather, practice itself becomes part of the repaired fabric of life, upon which more challenges and triumphs are probable.

In this article, I describe some of the mind-body experiential work that I and others are practicing with survivors, activists, leaders, indigenous people, and others who have experienced trauma and secondary traumatic stress. I practice as a Zen teacher and practitioner, and as someone who has worked in and with communities. Though I am neither a professional nor a service provider, there are some learned experiences and pitfalls that can be shared. Fundamentally, mind-body experiential work is about the experience. Therefore, it is important to be practicing with, rather than to require people to perform into a description. Performance of any kind can abbreviate results. Repetition is necessary in order to interrupt habits and engender more fruitful practices. Single demonstrations are not as useful as repetitive practices, which may mean finding different ways to practice the same thing in order to minimize loss of interest. Unless there is willingness, readiness, and openness, mind-body work is difficult to sustain. While it sometimes helps people to know that some of these practices are derived from age-old, traditional, and even sacred work, it is important for them to also know that as an applied methodology, "this" is not spiritual practice per se. Nonetheless, just by breathing more deeply and being fully integrated in one's body and mind, some people will begin to have deeper questions. These deeper inquiries should be explored in ways and means appropriate to the situation and the person. Finally, mind-body work is best coached by, taught by, learned from, a person who is farther into the work of mind-body connection and integration than the person who is being coached, being taught, and is learning. Emulation is the modern-day equivalent of apprenticeship. To effectively teach, one continues to learn and practice.

Why practice? In a chaotic and violent world, it would be convenient and indeed practical to be satisfied with the liberation of victims to the state of survivor-hood. Yet, it is quite possible (and shameful, really) that we give up too early on people, believing that once damaged only so much repair is possible. Instead, the restoration to original goodness is just one breath away, and another breath, and another. The potential of cultivation from the transcendence of suffering and hardship is part of the foundational mechanism of Buddhist teaching. There are survivors who are hungry for and open to the work necessary to move beyond their own survival story. Our collective humanity may depend on it.

References

Killian, K. D. (2008). Helping till it hurts? A multimethod study of compassion fatigue, burnout, and self-care in clinicians working with trauma survivors. *Traumatology, 14*(2).

Pfifferling, J. H., & Gilley, K. (2000). Overcoming compassion fatigue. *Family Practice Management*.

Rosenberg, T. (2012). For veterans, a surge of new treatments for trauma. *The New York Times*. September 26, 2012.

Salston, M. D., & Figley, C. R. (2003). Secondary traumatic stress effects of working with survivors of criminal victimization. *Journal of Traumatic Stress, 16*(2).

Zen Incarcerated: A Personal Essay

Jeffrey Schneider

Keywords

Zen · Behavioral health · Buddhism · Incarcerated · Mindfulness

I'm in a single cell 24 h a day 7 days a week. Every few days they will take me outside for a 30 to 45 min stroll by myself. I will be confined to this cell by myself with no interactions with any other inmates for the next year. This would drive most people crazy. I want to take advantage of this isolation.

From a letter from Joseph S., dated April 29, 2015
Alabama State Prison at Bessemer

"I constantly have to remind myself and find refuge in my dharma while in this cell. It is so depressing. It's almost like a cell of horrors…This building isn't a regular block how they have on the yard. There's no window to outside whatsoever. The one window they do have is at the front of the cell door and the only vie you have is a white wall 6 feet away. You can't see nothing down the hallway. And the cell is so small you can lay on the bed and touch the toilet. It feels closed in like a tomb. And it's all concrete. You know what happens when you leave batteries sitting on concrete right? The concrete drains all the batteries' energy. Well, that's what this cell is doin' to me.

From a letter from Mario R., dated April 29, 2015
California State Prison, Sacramento

In this chapter, I've been invited to describe and reflect upon my efforts as a Zen priest involved in work with prisoners. I came to the San Francisco Zen Center in 1978 with the goal of pursuing a life of service and practice. I have lived here ever since. My time at Zen Center has involved traditional monastic training as well as living and practicing in a busy city temple, which offers a variety of services to a predominantly lay community: a community that is predominantly white, educated, and middle-class. Please note that this is not a value judgment, but a statement of fact. Traditionally, when Buddhism has entered a new culture, it has first attracted the educated classes who have the leisure for study and practice. For the past several years, I have been a Zen Center's outreach coordinator. As such, one of my functions has been to oversee the programs described below.

J. Schneider (✉)
San Francisco Zen Center, California, USA
e-mail: outreach@sfzc.org

A. Masuda and W.T. O'Donohue (eds.), *Handbook of Zen, Mindfulness, and Behavioral Health*, Mindfulness in Behavioral Health, DOI 10.1007/978-3-319-54595-0_24

For many years, before being offered my current position as outreach coordinator at Zen Center, I was a pen pal to men in prison. It began when a friend of mine asked whether I would be willing to write to the cellmate of a man with whom she was corresponding, and I said yes. Since then, I have been a prison correspondent. In addition to being part of my current job, it is something that has always given me great satisfaction. I don't know why I have been drawn to this particular form of service, but I am grateful for the opportunity to be in touch with the men who've shared their lives with me.

The first time I visited the men's jail in San Francisco, I had the unsettling sense of disconnect, cognitive and emotional, that might have occurred had I stepped into a 1940s *film noir*. The bars, the officers carrying key chains weighted with big, old-fashioned keys, the heavy doors that seemed constructed only to slam with maximum impact, the *cages* filled with bunk beds and men, the harsh lighting, and the overwhelming noise—all of these felt like scene sets from a past that I imagined was confined to some other, less enlightened time. But, of course, the past, to quote Faulkner, isn't even past.

To be fair, I have to say that in my experience the men and women who work in the jail seem to be doing their best to make the best of a sad situation. I have rarely been met with anything but courtesy and helpfulness. The world of jail is the confluence of innumerable causes and conditions and the ability of most of us to influence that world can seem relatively minor. And to enter that world for the first time is unsettling.

What I felt, in retrospect, was not fear, really. I wasn't afraid of the prisoners or that somehow I wouldn't be allowed out. It wasn't claustrophobia, though the place could certainly induce it in any one prone. It wasn't even a righteous anger that people should be forced to endure such conditions.

I think what I experienced, and what I have to continue to recognize and work with, is something more like a creeping despair: What I could bring to these men in the short time I had with them that could possibly make any difference? What tools, after all, do I come equipped with? I'm not a lawyer or a doctor or a therapist or a social worker. I can't argue their case for them or find them work or housing when they are released.

What do I bring? A little meditation bell and some half-sheet giveaways with simple meditation instructions. And my experience. What I also bring with me is my anger, my despair, my impatience. In the words of one of the ceremonies we offer here at Zen Center "all my ancient twisted karma." I think this is important because I am constantly reminded that I am not different from the men I meet in jail. I have just as many unpleasant personality traits, just as dark a shadow as these men. But I've been luckier. I've been luckier in my birth and my education. I've been lucky that I've never been caught breaking the law. I've been lucky that I have encountered the dharma. If I have one tool that is the most useful, it is the sense that I am the same as the men I meet. Just as our bodies are almost identical—eyes, ears, nose, mouth, internal organs, etc.—so are our minds. To believe that our differences are those of kind rather than degree is what makes any sort of real connection impossible. And, of course, I also have the great gift of many years of meditation practice to share.

What else I bring in is my sense of acute failure. The failure that I have felt in my own life, as a person and as a priest, reminds me that I am not superior to any of those I encounter. My experiences of loss, of grief, and of powerlessness are potent tools for connecting with these men. Even if I do not share the particulars, nor ask for them of the prisoners I meet, those experiences inform my presence.

And, of course, I have the teaching and the practice of Buddhism. I can offer those techniques that may help to calm and quiet the raging or sorrowing mind. I can remind the men that they do not need to be slaves to the thoughts and feelings of the moment, those impulses of the mind and heart that have strewn so much destruction in their lives.

Although each of us who goes into the jail has developed his or her own routine, mine is pretty representative. After the men who have accepted the invitation to be part of the group have gathered, I introduce myself and ask each person for his name. Then, I describe what we'll be doing: specifically, that we will be trying a number of different practices, that each will be fairly brief, and that not everything we do will be useful to everyone equally. I encourage the men to use what works and in general to treat meditation as an experiment. "If you have some idea of the perfect meditator, and that's who you are trying to be, you'll just be setting yourself up for failure. But in an experiment, everything can be useful, even if it just shows you what doesn't work." Then, we do some stretching and a few simple yoga poses that can be done standing or sitting. I follow that with some very brief suggestions about posture: "Keep both feet on the floor, with your knees slightly apart to open the hip joints. Try to keep your spine straight and your head up with the chin slightly tucked in. Find a resting place for your hands on your lap. If you are comfortable doing so, close your eyes. If not, just keep the gaze downward in a soft focus. Take a few deep breaths and then allow the breath to find its own pace." After a few moments of silence, I lead the men through a guided meditation designed to relax the body.

Generally, after calming the body and slowing the breath for a while, I offer a *metta* or loving-kindness meditation. We do it for ourselves ("May I be happy; May I be free from fear; May I have joy in my life..."), for someone we already love, for someone we know who is suffering in some way, and finally for someone we don't like. I suggest that they don't pick their worst enemy in the world, but rather someone toward whom they feel irritation or dislike rather than violent hatred. Usually, I tell them that practicing *metta* for someone we really hate is at least at the Ph.D. level and we can work our way up to that gradually.

Depending upon the group and the ability of the members to sit still, I offer a three or five minute silent period, suggesting that they use a simple phrase ("breathing in/breathing out") in time with the breath. This is a practice for times of anxiety, fear, or distress. The mind is given a neutral phrase to keep it engaged, and the breath and the pulse gradually slow.

Our final practice is gratitude. Even in jail, there are things to be grateful for: "I give thanks for my eyes and that I can see...That I can walk... For clean water to drink..." I have found this a wonderfully useful tool for dealing with depression and self-pity.

Whether we do calming practices with the breath, or loving-kindness meditations, we can be together for a while in a place that is safe and peaceful. And, of course, I can never know what I've left behind. These practices may be forgotten the moment I walk out the door. Or they may be taken up from time to time and perhaps save someone from bringing more trouble on himself.

Zen, as all other forms of Buddhism, has undergone a sea change in its move to the West. This is not a new phenomenon in the two and a half millennia history of the religion. Each country, culture, each language and century has poured the dharma into its own mold. As opposed to a falling away from an imagined original purity, this adaptation may perhaps be seen as an extrapolation of what the Buddha taught, when he approved of his disciples teaching in the language of whatever land to which they travelled. He also compared himself to a physician, offering an appropriate medicine for each specific disease. So too, the teaching, while holding to the basics of wisdom and compassion, has given what is needed to those who are sick in spirit and mind. These sick ones in need of medicine are all of us who have yet to awaken from the daily nightmare of greed, hatred, and delusion.

Some of the particular ways in which Buddhism has accommodated itself to the West, at least in its social expressions, are through feminism, democratic institutions, and community service. In the USA, there are many Zen temples in which women serve as both religious and administrative leaders. Most American Buddhist practitioners would be both surprised and offended at the insinuation that women are not able to fill the highest temple offices. Obviously, this has not always been the case in the long history of the sangha. And it is still not so in other cultures in which Buddhism has been the majority tradition for centuries.

The idea that informed and committed lay persons should have an equal share in decision making is also predominantly a Western notion, based on the cultural norm of democratic representation. Once again, this is a new phenomenon in Buddhist history. It may perhaps be traced to the tradition of independent congregations in many American Protestant and Jewish denominations as well as that of representational government.

Generally speaking, in Buddhism the ideal of transformation is centered on the individual. This is in keeping with the understanding that reality is to be found in the specific, the particular, rather than in some Platonic ideal. In this way, practice is informed by the metaphysic. As the individual draws closer to awakening, he or she is more available, more able to be of service to others. This dedication to the well-being of suffering men and women is illustrated when the Buddha himself chose to teach and when he sent out his disciples "for the weal of the world." The underlying assumption is that the individual is the primary agent of positive change.

From what we can read in the early suttas, the Buddha seems to have largely accepted the social structures of his day. He certainly did not urge democratic or social revolutions, call for the overthrow of kings, etc. In this perhaps he was not so different from Paul of Taurus who called for slaves to be obedient to their masters (Ephesians 6:5).

This apparent lack of concern for social change and amelioration has been a Western criticism of Buddhism for a long time. It ties in with condemnations of Buddhism being pessimistic and nihilistic, which are not entirely charges only made by ill-informed critics in the past. And while these accusations are neither entirely accurate nor historically valid, it still must be said that there has not been anything in Buddhism throughout most of its history like Christian or Jewish social activism in the West.

That too is changing. The growth of what is often called engaged Buddhism has come to be a powerful force in the translation of the dharma. The basic premise is that as practitioners who have received the bodhisattva vows, we are charged to carry them into the world in ways that touch not only the individual, but also society as a whole. Thus, we see a Buddhist presence in the environmental movement, in various forms of social work among prisoners, homeless men and women, in the hospice movement, etc. Western Buddhists seek to bring the teachings and practices of the tradition into play in the wider field of social change.

We at the San Francisco Zen Center offer two services to prisoners as part of our outreach programs. Each week we (i.e., I or one of our volunteers) lead meditation groups in the women's jail, the men's jail, and the psychiatric unit of the men's jail as I've described above. Since all of these groups are comprised of people in jail rather than in prison, the turnover tends to be high. Sometimes, we'll see someone for three or four weeks, and then, he or she will be either released or transferred. This, of course, makes it difficult to build ongoing relationships with the members of the groups, to learn their stories, or to follow their progress. We lose them to prison or to the street. I have given my card and invited people to visit us at Zen Center if they would like to continue their practice. To date, no one has taken me up on the offer. Essentially, we are tasked with recreating the event each time we go in, usually with new individuals.

The second part of our outreach to prisoners is the correspondence program. We receive letters from prisons and jails all over the USA. Sometimes, the letters are from people who have very little idea about what Buddhism is, what Zen is. They have simply heard that it might be a way to lessen the suffering they experience. Sometimes, the letters are from those who have been reading and practicing for a while, alone, or (if they are very lucky) with a prison group. Each letter is answered individually. In response to a first request, along with a personal letter, we generally send some articles about practicing in prison and meditation instructions, together with an invitation to write again if the person has questions or would like more literature. We are also able, through the generosity of our supporters, to send Buddhist books into jail or prison at no cost to the recipient. Another service we offer is our pen pal program. We connect incarcerated practitioners with volunteer correspondents in the free world. As many prisoners are without local support for their practice, having a "good spiritual friend" on the outside can be a real lifeline. This program has been running for many years. There is always a waiting list for pen pals, but the prisoner who has requested one is encouraged to continue writing to us in the meanwhile. I've been fortunate to have gained a few long-term correspondents myself in this way. The conversation has become so intimate and long-standing that the idea of asking them to begin again with a new person is not something I can do. The quotations that head this chapter are taken, with their permission, from letters written to me by men who are my personal correspondents.

The suffering that some of these letters contain can feel overwhelming. Many of those who write to us are almost completely cut off from the outside world. Either they have no families or their families have become completely estranged. Many of these men have been in and out of prison for most of their lives and know almost nothing else. A large percentage of them have ended up where they are due to drug or alcohol addiction. As someone who has trained in the area of addiction treatment, I know that the reason many people begin using addictive substances is because these are the only tools available to lessen the suffering of intolerable situations. The men who write to us are not the well-educated businessmen who got caught with greedy hands in the till. By and large, they are the throwaways, the uneducated, the poor.

There are days I have to put the letters aside for a while and do something else. But often the courage, the willingness to learn, the openness, and the faith expressed (a faith that is often naïve or childlike in the best possible meaning of those words) can be tremendously moving. The name of our temple here in San Francisco is *Hosshin-ji* or Beginners' Mind Temple. It is this quality of mind that often comes through in these letters. Shunryu Suzuki Roshi, our founder, said that "In the beginner's mind there are many possibilities, but in the expert's there are few (Suzuki 1970, p. 21)." Meeting these beginner's minds, I'm often abashed at my own practice, but encouraged by the hopefulness of those who are newly engaged. To give an idea of the scope of the program, between April 2015 and March 2016, we responded to 613 individual letters, forwarded 845 letters to pen pals, and sent 375 books to individual inmates as well as five boxes of Buddhist books to different prison or jail libraries.

> A special transmission outside the scriptures;
>
> No dependence on words and letters;
>
> Direct pointing to the mind of man;
>
> Seeing into one's nature and attaining Buddhahood.

These four statements, attributed to Bodhidharma, the putative first Zen ancestor in China, do not seem at first glance to have much to do with the situation of a man or woman imprisoned in modern America. Those with whom we interact, either personally or through the mail, are not likely to be overly dependent upon Buddhist scriptures. At most a few might have a slight familiarity with the Bible and many have not even a glancing relationship with any sacred text.

It is no secret or surprise that the population of our jails and prisons is largely comprised of the poor and poorly educated. A fair number of these men and women are only marginally literate and unlikely to depend upon words or letters, theories of spirituality. This leaves directly pointing to the mind and attaining Buddhahood. Somehow even these slogans seem far removed from the reality of a noisy, brutal, crowded, and dehumanizing environment such as prison or jail.

In responding to the question of how the teachings of Zen inspire and are embodied in our outreach to prisoners, I think that we have to reach beyond Zen itself as a specific teaching or school and return to the basics of Buddhism. First to be considered are the differing experiences of the imprisoned individual and the person providing a service, either a pen pal or someone who goes into the facility to offer meditation. My own impulse to write to inmates and to engage in person can perhaps be understood in terms of the bodhisattva vow. In its most irreducible version, this states that "I vow to live and be lived for the benefit of all beings." Personally, I prefer this to the statement "Beings are numberless; I vow to save them." (In fact, both are used here at Zen Center in the same ceremony.) On the one hand, this is a conscious statement of intention, a solemn promise or assertion, undertaken as part of a religious practice. It is something, this vow, that I create by taking and, having taken it, give myself to as something greater than my personality or daily whims. On the other hand, however, it is a simple recognition of the inescapable truth that there is no such thing as personal salvation. We may wish to believe otherwise, but in fact—in fact and not in some ethereal theory—we are so intimately joined that we cannot separate ourselves out, expecting a separate peace. This is the faith and, more importantly, the experience, of those who aspire to awakening. My experience then comes both from a spiritual perspective (service as a religious duty, if you will) and from a deep place of recognized connection.

The experience of the person who writes to us or who attends the meditation group must be different. Obviously, each person will have his or her own unique experience as conditioned by background, personality, etc. But in a general way, it is still the experience of being one who receives. To be on the receiving end, to always be in a position of asking for what you need, is not an easy thing. In our liturgy, we use the phrase "the emptiness of the three wheels: giver, receiver and gift." However, this must have a different meaning to the "free-worlder" who is in a position to be in reciprocal relationships. This is why it is so important when a prisoner shares something of him or herself—a drawing, a poem, an experience. To allow someone to give is in itself a great gift.

To be powerless over almost every aspect of one's existence is something prisoners, hospital patients, the infirm or elderly in care facilities, and young children have in common. To cultivate patience and the ability to exert some conscious control over those small aspects of life subject to it (which in many such cases will only be the internal experience) involves major effort. Buddhist teaching and practice begin with the reality of suffering and of our lack of control over sickness, old age and death. This is perhaps where the experience of the prisoner and the practitioner coincide.

More often than not in practicing meditation with prisoners, we use techniques specific to particular, painful mental states, as described above. Obviously this is not Dogen's *shikantaza*, not formless meditation and perhaps not even Zen as such. Does it matter? Most of the prisoners I've encountered in jail are not specifically interested in Buddhism. A few are, and it's a pleasure to be able to provide them with further resources. But most are simply reaching out for anything that might possibly relieve some of the burden, both inner and outer, under which they struggle.

The correspondence program brings a different group to us. Because they are writing specifically to the Zen Center, most of them know they are in touch with a Buddhist organization. Some of those who write are already very engaged in practice and study and have been for some time. Some few are even lucky enough to be in places where there is a sitting group or weekly Buddhist service. Letters from these men are really a wonderful gift. I should mention here that I use the word "men" intentionally. For whatever reason, we receive almost no letters from women. Over the years, I've been involved with this project, perhaps as few as 1% come from female inmates. Often the probing questions are ones that will require me to look more deeply into my own practice and to sometimes research areas of Buddhist study that I haven't before.

Some letters come from those for whom the word "Zen" simply means something like peace of mind, who have little or no idea of Buddhist teaching or practice. These are often the most heart-rending letters to read. When I respond, I offer some simple instructions for meditation, respond to whatever questions they ask, and include an invitation for them to continue writing to us. And sometimes they do. And sometimes they write back that the practice has helped them deal with their situation a bit more easily. And sometimes, they don't respond. And, of course, the prison system being what it is, there is no way of knowing why.

The most difficult letters come from prisoners we can't help. These come from the ends of the spectrum, so to speak. On the one hand, there are the men who have heard there is a pen pal program, but have no interest in Buddhism, know nothing about it, and sometimes aren't even aware that they are writing to a Buddhist organization. They are just lonely and want someone to take an interest. These letters usually offer a description of the writer and perhaps the sort of music or television shows he likes, perhaps a little bit about his background: "I have a couple of kids, but I haven't seen them since I've been here. Their mother and I broke up." If we had a long waiting list of volunteers eager to write to prisoners, it would make me happy to provide the connection. In fact, we have a waiting list of prisoners who are interested in Buddhism, some of whom are long-time practitioners. I have to write back, explain the situation, and hope they will find other ways to connect with the outside world.

The other letters come from men who have been practicing for some time and have no real support where they are. They ask us to help find Buddhist teachers or clergy to visit. Sometimes, they ask how they can receive the precepts. As a lot of the prisons they write from are either rural or in areas with little or no Buddhist presence, it is often impossible to help with this. Even when they are in places not far from a temple or center, frequently the simple logistics and expense of time make it unfeasible for a priest or teacher to visit. (I once sent on a request for a visit to a priest I know. She replied that she no longer made visits to that prison. It was a 2 h drive for her and each time she tried to visit an excuse was made by the prison officials as to why she couldn't get in. Whether this was a simple run of bad luck or due to the fact that she was in an area not known for its openness to minority religions can't be known. But her experiences convinced her that as the sole priest of a temple, her time could be better spent.)

I have not been successful either in finding a way for prison practitioners to receive the precepts long-distance. The teachers I have approached about this feel strongly that the ceremony involves the face-to-face transmission and are not willing to confer the precepts on men they have not met in person. The best I can offer in such circumstances is to remind the person requesting the lay ordination that the precepts are not really given by the preceptor. We give ourselves to them. The teacher or officiant is in some way a witness or a holder of the tradition. But the real event is the vow the individual makes. Sometimes, I send a copy of the ceremony and suggest that the person take these vows in front of his friends, if possible, or simply recite them daily to himself.

> Avalokiteshvara, when practicing deeply prajna paramita, perceived that all five skandhas are empty and thus relieved all suffering.

These are the opening words of the Heart Sutra, chanted daily in Zen temples. Avalokiteshvara, whose name in one translation is "the one who hears [the cries of the world]", is the bodhisattva of compassion who is worshipped and invoked in many forms, male and female, throughout the Buddhist world.

There is a story about Avalokiteshvara I heard once, though I can't remember where and have been unable to locate the source for it in my searches. Perhaps this is the best sort of story. As it goes, he (or she) was sent by Amida Buddha into the deepest hells to preach the dharma there to the suffering beings and bring them hope of liberation. But the suffering was so great, and Avalokiteshvara's empathy so profound that he was unable to bear it and his head literally exploded. Gathering the pieces together, he returned to Amida in failure. Amida miraculously restored his head (or, in another version, used the pieces to create a multi-headed bodhisattva) and taught him the perfection of wisdom, the *prajna paramita*, so that he could witness and attend to great suffering without being destroyed by it.

The perfection of wisdom is, in this context, the teaching of emptiness. This is the extrapolation of the ancient Buddhist doctrine of the three marks of conditioned existence: that all conditioned things are impermanent (*anicca*), ultimately unsatisfactory (*dukkha*), and without abiding self (*anatta*). All things therefore are in constant flux determined by cause and effect, created by conditions and without independent being. At first glance, such a teaching can seem either a dry excursion into ontology or a rather nihilistic and depressing view of things. And yet, in the Heart Sutra, it is this wisdom which is offered as that healing teaching and practice which relieves suffering.

Emptiness is not only the lack of inherent existence, of own-being. It is also the teaching of interdependence and interconnectedness. If each thing is the result of innumerable causes and conditions, then each thing is the sum of everything is it not. A dandelion ultimately blooms because of the Big Bang. And so this teaching of the lack of individual essence is the basis of wisdom and compassion—wisdom arising from the suffering that sees itself in all other beings.

I was once, many years ago, fortunate enough to hear His Holiness the Dalai Lama speak to a relatively small group of people at Zen Center's temple, Green Gulch Farm. Of all the things he said, I remember only one. And this was that wisdom grows from compassion. I remember it because I was surprised. A relatively new student at the time, I thought it was the other way around: I'd do lots of meditation, get enlightened and then I'd be able to have compassion on all of the poor folks who weren't as advanced as I'd become.

I believe that those of us concerned with the various hells of jail and prison may do well to attend to the *prajna paramita*. So often we are confronted with situations over which we can exert neither control nor influence. Injustice (even in the name of justice), inhuman conditions, systems which operate in preferential ways, or sometimes sheer bureaucratic intransigence are factors that can easily lead to despair and the desire to simply withdraw. And more immediately, there are the men and women—the human faces, human voices—for whom we can do so much less that we wish we could. Showing up for an hour to lead meditation, writing a letter, can seem so little compared to the bottomless need, an ineffective response to overwhelming suffering.

In this teaching of perfect wisdom ("form is emptiness, emptiness is form") are embedded two points of view, often called the absolute and relative. In the relative point of view, there are individuals who suffer in their many ways. But, *and I believe this to be a very important thing to remember*, who have, and are entitled to, the dignity of their own suffering. Each prisoner, and each prison volunteer, has a unique history and individuality which must be respected and honored. If we forget this, we too easily become simply do-gooders, people who out of the kindness of our hearts reach down to our inferiors in order to somehow better them.

I think we must connect through our own suffering, through our own greed, hatred, and delusion, to those we would seek to serve. Not as people who have somehow risen above such impulses, who have successfully tamed the beast of the brainstem, but rather as those in more spacious prisons. Many years ago when I was practicing in Zen Center's mountain monastery, I was seated in zazen when the thought came to mind, "I want…" Oddly, I couldn't complete the sentence. So I ran through the things that I might want: food, sleep, sex, warmth, and a number of other things or situations. None of them was it. Finally, I became aware of a small voice at the back of my mind whispering: "I want. I want. I want." Our essential identity is perhaps not only something like the Buddha nature, but also the mind of wanting, and the mind of rage that arises when that wanting is thwarted. And of course, the basic delusion that keeps the whole tragic comedy going. We share this with our prisoner friends. I sometimes say that the basic difference between me and my prison pen pals is that I just didn't get caught.

In the midst of all of this, in the center of the fire, I think what may sustain our effort is faith.

Not faith in the sense of some assertion of belief, or in some naïve sense that "everything will work out somehow" but rather faith as a posture of mind. In fact, and in contradiction to most meanings of the word, faith in not-knowing. This faith finds itself in a litany like this:

> I think I'm wasting my time.
> But I don't know.
> I think what I offer isn't enough.
> But I don't know.
> I think I'm not wise enough, dedicated enough, skilled enough.
> But I don't know.
> I think.
> But I don't know.

This not knowing may be what allows us to continue, not knowing if we have planted some seed that may sprout in some unimaginable way. If the bodhisattva vows to continue to work for the benefit of all beings as long as there are beings to be saved, this not knowing may be the only stance which allows us to continue working against the odds.

As the title says, this is a personal essay and makes no claims to be anything else. My experience and my thoughts issue only from my limited point of view. In closing then, I offer them with the dedication of merit I use at the end of each meditation session in the jail:

> We dedicate the merit of our practice to the benefit of all beings in the ten directions, especially those imprisoned in body or mind,
> And for those who are in physical or mental distress of any sort.
> May they find ease, comfort and healing.
> May they be happy.
> May we be happy.
> May all beings be happy.

Reference

Suzuki, S. (1970). *Zen mind, Beginner's mind: Informal talks on Zen meditation and practice.*

Index

A. Masuda and W.T. O'Donohue (eds.), *Handbook of Zen, Mindfulness, and Behavioral Health*, Mindfulness in Behavioral Health, DOI 10.1007/978-3-319-54595-0

9783319545936